T0139805

Computational Pulse Signal Analysis

David Zhang • Wangmeng Zuo • Peng Wang

Computational Pulse Signal Analysis

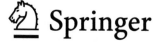 Springer

David Zhang
School of Science and Engineering
The Chinese University of Hong Kong
Shenzhen, Guangdong, China

Wangmeng Zuo
Harbin Institute of Technology
Harbin, China

Peng Wang
Northeast Agricultural University
Harbin, China

ISBN 978-981-13-3835-9   ISBN 978-981-10-4044-3   (eBook)
https://doi.org/10.1007/978-981-10-4044-3

This Springer imprint is published by the registered company Springer Nature Singapore Pte Ltd.
The registered company address is: 152 Beach Road, #21-01/04 Gateway East, Singapore 189721, Singapore

Preface

Traditional Chinese diagnostics is a fundamental component in traditional Chinese medicine (TCM). In general, there are four major diagnostic methods of TCM, i.e., looking, listening, asking, and feeling the pulse. Among them, pulse diagnosis (i.e., feeling the pulse) is operated by placing the three fingers of the practitioner at the wrist radial artery of the patient for analyzing the health condition. For thousands of years, pulse diagnosis has played an indispensable role in TCM and traditional Ayurvedic medicine (TAM). Due to its convenient, inexpensive, and noninvasive properties, even nowadays pulse diagnosis is still very competitive for disease diagnosis.

Recent studies have revealed that wrist pulse signal is a kind of bloodstream signal influenced by many physiological or pathological factors and can be applied for disease analyses. However, the practice of traditional Chinese pulse diagnosis (TCPD) extremely depends on the experience of the practitioners. The measurement and interpretation in TCPD generally require years of training of the practitioners. It is also difficult for different practitioners to share their feelings on the pulse signal. All these restrict its development and applications in contemporary clinical practice.

Fortunately, with the development on sensors, signal processing, and pattern recognition, considerable progresses have been achieved in computational pulse signal analysis. With the advances in sensor technologies, three types of sensors, e.g., pressure, photoelectric, and ultrasonic sensors, have been developed for pulse signal acquisition. To simulate the practitioners in analyzing the pulse signal, signal processing and pattern recognition methods have been developed. By far, pulse signals have been investigated for pulse waveform classification and the diagnosis of many diseases, such as cholecystitis, nephrotic syndrome, diabetes, etc.

In this book, we intend to provide an in-depth summary to the latest advances in pulse signal acquisition, processing, and applications in classification and diagnosis. The system design, model and algorithm implementation, experimental evaluation, and underlying rationales are also given in the book. Following the pipeline of computational pulse signal analysis, the book is organized into six parts. In the first part, Chap. 1 introduces the connection between wrist pulse signal and cardiac electrical activity, which lays a physiological foundation for pulse diagnosis. Subsequently, we provide an overview on the practice of TCPD and the pipeline of computational pulse analysis.

In the second part, pulse acquisition systems are introduced to capture pulse signals at representative positions, under various pressures, and from different types of sensors. In Chap. 2, we introduce a compound multiple-channel pressure signal acquisition system. By equipping with sensor array design and pressure adjustment, the system can capture multichannel pulse signals and is effective in measuring the width of the pulse. Chapter 3 integrates a pressure sensor with a photoelectric sensor to acquire more pulse information. The photoelectric sensor array is used to detect the pulse width and the center of radial artery, while the pressure sensor measures the pulsations with high resolution.

In the third part, several representative preprocessing methods are described for baseline wander correction and detection of low-quality pulse signal. In Chap. 4, we present an energy ratio-based criterion to evaluate the level of baseline drift and a wavelet-based cascaded adaptive filter to remove baseline drift. In Chap. 5, we consider two types of corruption, i.e., saturation and artifact. For the detection of saturation, we use two criteria based on its definition. For the artifact detection, we suggest a complex network-based scheme by measuring the network connectivity. Finally, Chap. 6 presents an optimal preprocessing framework by integrating frequency-dependent analysis, curve fitting, period segmentation, and normalization.

The fourth part introduces the feature extraction of wrist pulse signal. In Chap. 7, the Lempel-Ziv complexity analysis is adopted to detect arrhythmic pulses. In Chap. 8, the spatial features and spectrum feature are extracted from blood flow velocity signal. In Chap. 9, generalized 2-D matrix feature is extracted to characterize the periodic and nonperiodic information. In Chap. 10, complex network is introduced to transform the pulse signal from time domain to network domain, and multi-scale entropy is used to measure the inter- and intra-cycle variations of pulse signal.

The fifth part presents several representative classification methods for the recognition and diagnosis of pulse signal. In Chap. 11, the ERP-based KNN classifiers are developed for pulse waveform classification. In Chap. 12, a modified Gaussian model is used for modeling pulse signal and a fuzzy C-means (FCM) classifier is adopted for computational pulse diagnosis. In Chap. 13, the residual error of autoregressive (AR) model is utilized for disease diagnosis. In Chap. 14, we present a multiple kernel learning model for the integration of heterogeneous features for pulse classification and diagnosis.

Finally, in the sixth part, some discussions are provided to reveal the relationship between different types of pulse signals. In Chap. 15, we analyze the physical meanings and sensitivities of signals acquired by different types of pulse signal acquisition systems to guide the sensor selection for computational pulse diagnosis. In Chap. 16, a comparative study on pulse and ECG signals is conducted to reveal their complementarities. Finally, Chap. 17 provides a brief recapitulation on the main content of this book.

The book is based on our years of researches on computational pulse signal analysis. Since 2003, under the grant support from the National Natural Science Foundation of China (NSFC), we have published our first chapter on computational pulse signal analysis. Since then, more and more researches have been conducted in this ever-growing field, and we have systematically studied the acquisition, preprocessing, feature extraction, and classification of pulse signals. With several typical diseases such as gallbladder diseases and diabetes, we also show the feasibility of pulse signal for disease diagnosis. We would like to express our special thanks to Mr. Zhaotian Zhang, Mr. Ke Liu, and Ms. Xiaoyun Xiong from NSFC, who consistently supported our research work for decades.

We would like to express our gratitude to our colleagues and PhD students, i.e., Prof. Naimin Li, Prof. Kuanquan Wang, Prof. Jie Zhou, Prof. Lisheng Xu, Prof. Guangming Lu, Prof. Yong Xu, Prof. Jane You, Prof. Lei Zhang, Dr. Hongzhi Zhang, Dr. Yinghui Chen, Dr. Dongyu Zhang, Dr. Lei Liu, and Dr. Dimin Wang, for their contributions to the research achievements on this topic. It is our great honor to work with them in this inspiring topic in the previous years. The authors owe a debt of gratitude to Mr. Pengju Liu for his careful reading and for checking the draft of the manuscript. We are also hugely indebted to Ms. Celine L. Chang and Ms. Jane Li of Springer for their consistent help and encouragement. Finally, the work in this book was mainly sponsored by the NSFC Program under Grant Nos. 61332011, 61271093, and 61471146.

The Chinese University of Hong Kong   David Zhang
Shenzhen, Guangdong, China
July, 2017

Contents

Part I
Background

Chapter 1
Introduction: Computational Pulse Diagnosis

Pulse diagnosis is a traditional diagnosis technique by analyzing the tactile radial arterial palpation by trained fingertips; however it is a subjective skill which needs years of training and practice to master. Computational pulse diagnosis intends to employ some modern sensor and computer technology to make pulse diagnosis more objective. In this chapter, we will give an overview of computational pulse diagnosis. Firstly, the principle of pulse diagnosis and the traditional pulse diagnosis were introduced, and then the main concept of and the four stages of computational pulse diagnosis were introduced.

1.1 Principle of Pulse Signal

Pulse is a physiological phenomenon propagated throughout the arterial system and is usually viewed as a traveling pressure which is mainly produced by cardiac cycle [1]. The cardiac cycle refers to the sequence of mechanical and electrical events that repeats with every heartbeat; these electrical events can be found in ECG signal [2]. Figure 1.1 shows the changes of aorta pressure, ventricular pressure, and ECG in two cardiac cycles which would be helpful to illustrate the principle of pulse signal.

The ECG signal contains P wave, QRS complex, and T wave. The P wave is caused by spread of depolarization through the atria, and this is followed by atrial contraction; about 0.16 second after the onset of the P wave, the QRS waves appear because of electrical depolarization of the ventricles, which initiates contraction of the ventricles. When the left ventricle contracts, the ventricular pressure increases rapidly until the aortic valve opens. Then, after the valve opens, the pressure in the ventricle rises much less rapidly, because blood immediately flows out of the ventricle into the aorta and then into the systemic distribution arteries. The entry of blood into the arteries causes the walls of these arteries to stretch and the pressure to increase which produces the main peak of pulse signal. T wave represents the

© Springer Nature Singapore Pte Ltd. 2018
D. Zhang et al., *Computational Pulse Signal Analysis*,
https://doi.org/10.1007/978-981-10-4044-3_1

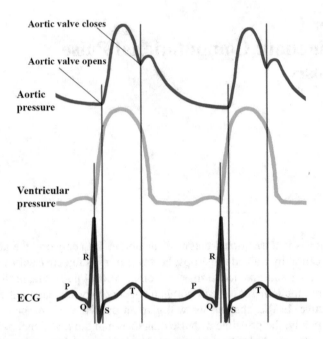

Fig. 1.1 The changes of aorta pressure, ventricular pressure, and ECG

stage of repolarization of the ventricles when the ventricular muscle fibers begin to relax. After the aortic valve has closed, the pressure in the aorta decreases slowly throughout diastole because the blood stored in the distended elastic arteries flows continually through the peripheral vessels back to the veins. From Fig. 1.1 one can see a secondary peak shows up in the aortic pressure curve when the aortic valve closes. This is caused by a short period of backward flow of blood immediately before closure of the valve, followed by sudden cessation of the backflow. [3] If an artery is close to the skin, one can feel the pressure change of the vessel by tactile arterial palpation; moreover, if a bone is under that artery, it would be easier to understand the fluctuations by pressing the artery against that bone, and this is the main principle of pulse. The neck (carotid artery), wrist (radial artery), and the ankle (posterior tibial artery) are the common places that can be used to measure the pulse signal; the wrist is the most popular positon among doctors and researchers. Moreover, as described in [4], "vascular properties in the upper limbs are less affected by ageing, arterial pressure, or various manoeuvers as compared to vessels in the trunk and lower limbs." In this book, we also refer pulse as the wrist pulse.

1.2   Traditional Pulse Diagnosis

Pulse diagnosis is to judge disease by means of fingertips palpating patient's pulse. It has played an important role in traditional Chinese medicine (TCM) and traditional Ayurvedic medicine (TAM) for thousands of years. [5–7] In addition, it is a

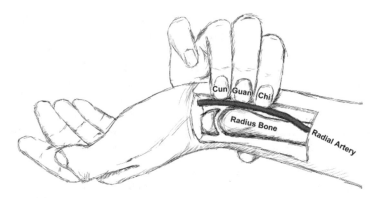

Fig. 1.2 Principle of pulse diagnosis

convenient, inexpensive, painless, bloodless, noninvasive, and non-side effect method promoted by UN [8]

The pulse originates from the heart, but the conditions of the skin, the thickness and elasticity of vessel walls, the composition of blood, and other parameters will also influence the fluctuations. Consequently, some of the healthy conditions that have connection with these parameters are able to manifest in pulse. In TCM and TAM, the practitioner puts three fingers on the three specific positions of the patient's wrist to adaptively feel the fluctuations in the radial artery and then analyze the health condition of the patient based on TCM theory and their experiences. Figure 1.2 shows the principle of traditional pulse diagnosis. From Fig. 1.2 we can see the relative positions between the three fingers, the radial artery and the radius bone during pulse diagnosis. In TCM, the three specific positions to put fingers are named as Cun, Guan, and Chi, respectively. The position Guan is at the end of radius bone, the position Cun is slightly before Guan, and Chi is slightly after Guan. In TAM, the same three positions are adopted, but their names are different with TCM. In these positions the radial artery is close to the skin, and the radius bone is just under the artery; thus they are optimal palpation positions. The practitioner presses the radial artery against the radius bone using different pressure to acquire more information about the vessel and flow in order to understand the health condition.

1.3   Computational Pulse Signal Analysis

Pulse diagnosis is an important noninvasive approach for health diagnosis in TCM; however the tactile arterial palpation actually is a subjective skill which needs years of training and long-term clinical experiences to master [9]. Moreover, for different practitioners, the diagnosis results may be inconsistent. To overcome these limitations, computational pulse signal analysis has recently been studied to make pulse diagnosis objective and quantitative.

Computational pulse signal analysis aims to employ some modern sensor technologies, signal processing technologies, feature extraction technologies, and machine learning technologies to objectify the process of pulse diagnosis.

The sensor technologies enable us to record and digitalize the pulse signal, signal processing and feature extraction technologies enable us to refine these signals and extract effective features for disease diagnosis, and machine learning technologies enable us to assist the diagnosis using computers. Thus, computational pulse signal analysis usually involves four stages, i.e., the acquisition stage, the preprocessing stage, the feature extraction stage, and the analysis (classification) stage.

Acquisition Pulse signal acquisition is not to acquire the pulse itself but to acquire the time series of some parameters which change with the pulsation. Some typical parameters are contact pressure, volume of radial artery, velocity of blood speed, etc. Let's use the contact pressure as an example: one can put a pressure sensor at the position Guan and press the sensor against the wrist lightly, the pressure sensor will measure the contact pressure in real time, and then one can get the pressure time series. That is a brief version of the principle, in fact one will need some more circuit to get the pressure signal, such as amplifier circuit, analog to digital circuit, and other control circuit to amplify and digitalize the pulse signal and transfer the signal into computer for pulse analysis.

Most of the time, different contact pressure will influence the sampled signal. Figure 1.3 shows a pressure series sampled in different hold-down pressure. When the pulse waveform amplitude is the highest among those pulse waveforms, it is named optimal pulse waveform, and usually the optimal pulse waveform was used for pulse analysis. In Part II of this book, we will further discuss some new method to acquire different type of pulse signal.

Preprocessing In most case, the sampled pulse signal is not good enough for pulse analysis; it usually contains some high-frequency noise and suffers from baseline

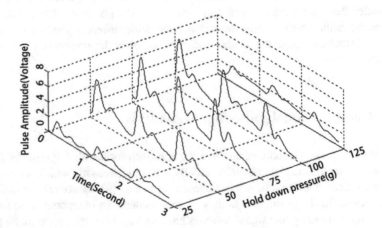

Fig. 1.3 Pressure pulse signal sampled in different pressure

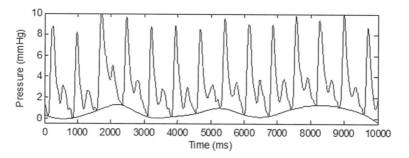

Fig. 1.4 Pulse signal coupled with baseline drift

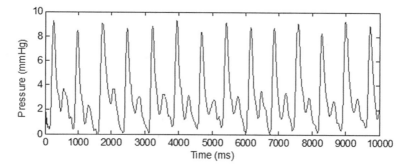

Fig. 1.5 Baseline drift removal based on high-pass filtering

drift (the start points of each cycle were not zero); moreover the signal may also contain saturation or artifact. The high-frequency noise is mostly attributed to power line interference, the baseline drift usually caused by breathing and body movement, saturation usually caused by large amplify parameters, and artifact usually caused by body movement such as arm twitching.

Preprocessing is to cancel these interferences and improve the quality of the sampled pulse signal. Let's use the baseline drift as an example. Figure 1.4 shows a pulse signal coupled with baseline drift. The baseline was also marked in the figure. From the shape of the baseline, one can see that the baseline in Fig. 1.4 was mostly caused by breathing. A simple idea of removing the noise and baseline drift is to use high-pass filter due to the frequency band of the baseline which was relative lower than the frequency band of the pulse signal. Figure 1.5 shows the result of baseline drift removal using high-pass filter. One can see that the drift is mostly removed, and the quality of the pulse signal is improved. However, the high-pass filter is not the best solution because the pulse signal may also contain some low-frequency information, and high-pass filter will result in information loss. Moreover, the result of the high-pass filter can only make the start point of each cycle roughly around zero but not exactly at zero. In Part III of this book, we will introduce some new technic to tackle the baseline drift, high-frequency noise, saturation, and artifact.

Feature Extraction Pulse feature extraction is to build an informative, non-redundant vector from the original pulse signal which is intended to be facilitating the subsequent pulse analysis. When performing computational pulse analysis, one of the major problems is the pulse signal which is a time series with thousands of points. Analysis with a large number of variables not only requires a large amount of memory and computation power but also it may cause a classification algorithm overfitting to training pulse signal and generalize poorly to new pulse signal. Thus, building a vector which contains as much diagnosis information as possible but removing the redundant information to make the vector very short to facilitating the pulse analysis is an important stage.

Fiducial point-based method is one of the simplest feature extraction method which has been widely applied in pulse diagnosis [10–14]. The idea is to use some special points in the signal such as peak of primary wave, dicrotic notch, and peak of secondary wave to represent the whole signal. By far, spatial features have been extracted based on the location and amplitude of the fiducial points and the shape between fiducial points. Figure 1.6 illustrates the fiducial points in the pulse signal, and their meanings are listed in Table 1.1, and the common fiducial features are listed in Table 1.2.

Except the fiducial point-based feature, sample entropy and PCA features are also commonly used in classification. In Part IV of this book, we will discuss the

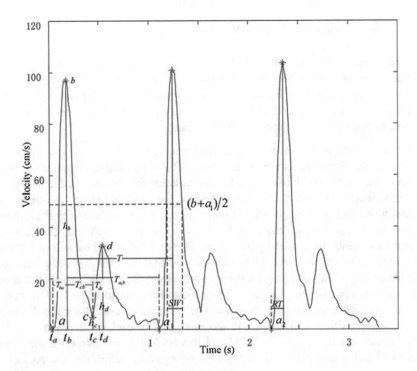

Fig. 1.6 Fiducial points and spatial features of pulse signal

Table 1.1 Meanings of the fiducial points

Points	Feature meaning
a	Onset of one period
b	Peak point of primary wave
c	Dicrotic notch
d	Peak point of secondary wave
a_1	Onset of the next period

Table 1.2 Common fiducial point-based features

Features	Meanings
SW	Time interval between half-peak points of the ascent and decent parts of primary wave
RT	Time interval between onset and peak of primary wave
T_{ba}/T	Ratio of time interval of ascent part of primary wave to the period
T_{cb}/T	Ratio of time interval of decent part of primary wave to the period
T_{dc}/T	Ratio of time interval of ascent part of secondary wave to the period
T_{a_1b}/T_{ba}	Ratio of time interval of ascent part to that of decent part
h_c/h_b	Ratio of amplitude of dicrotic notch to that of peak of primary wave
h_d/h_b	Ratio of amplitude of peak of secondary wave to that of peak of primary wave

fiducial point-based feature and some other features which are effective in pulse feature extraction.

Classification and Diagnosis Pulse analysis aims to provide some reasonable interpretation based on features extracted in the previous stage using machine learning technique. The basic idea of pulse analysis is using a lot of pulse features paired with certain health condition label to produce an inferred model, which can be used to classify new pulse signal with unknown health condition.

Support vector machine is one of the most popular machine learning techniques used in feature classification and is widely used in pulse analysis [15]. In Part V we will introduce some new classification methods which are effective in pulse diagnosis.

According to the four stages of computational pulse diagnosis, this book was divided into six parts: Part II to Part V correspond with the four stages, and Part I introduces the background of pulse diagnosis, Part VI discussed the connection and difference between different types of pulse signal and ECG. Part VI also summarized this book and pointed some future work.

1.4   Summary

In this chapter, we introduce the principle of pulse signal, the traditional pulse diagnosis and the main concept of computational pulse diagnosis. The four main stages for computational pulse diagnosis are presented, and we use some simple examples to illustrate the process of these stages.

References

1. S. Walsh, and E. King, *Pulse Diagnosis A Clinical Guide*, Sydney, Australia: Elsevier, 2008.
2. W. F. Boron, and E. L. Boulpaep, *Medical Physiology* United States: Elsevier 2016.
3. A. C. Guyton, and J. E. Hall, *Textbook of Medical Physiology*, Pennsylvania: Elsevier, 2011.
4. C. Chen, E. Nevo, B. Fetics, P. H. Pak, F. C. P. Yin, L. Maughan, and D. A. Kass, "Estimation of central aortic pressure waveform by mathematical transformation of radial tonometry pressure: validation of generalized transfer function," Circulation, vol. 95, no. 7, pp. 1827-1836, 1997.
5. S. Walsh, and E. King, *Pulse Diagnosis: A Clinical Guide*, Sydney Australia: Elsevier, 2008.
6. V. D. Lad, *Secrets of the Pulse*, Albuquerque, New Mexico: The Ayurvedic Press, 1996.
7. E. Hsu, *Pulse Diagnosis in Early Chinese Medicine*, New York, American: Cambridge University Press, 2010.
8. H. Wang and Y. Cheng, "A quantitative system for pulse diagnosis in traditional Chinese medicine," in Proc. IEEE Eng. Med. Biol. Soc. Conf., Shanghai, China, 2005, pp. 5676–5679.
9. R. Amber, and B. Brooke, Pulse Diagnosis Detailed Interpretations For Eastern & Western Holistic Treatments, Santa Fe, New Mexico: Aurora Press, 1993.
10. L. Liu, W. Zuo, D. Zhang, N. Li, and H. Zhang, "Combination of heterogeneous features for wrist pulse blood flow signal diagnosis via multiple kernel learning," IEEE Transactions on Information Technology in Biomedicine, vol. 16, pp. 599-607, Jul 2012.
11. D. Zhang, W. Zuo, D. Zhang, H. Zhang, and N. Li, "Wrist blood flow signal-based computerized pulse diagnosis using spatial and spectrum features," Journal of Biomedical Science and Engineering, vol. 3, pp. 361-366, 2010.
12. L. Xu, M. Q. H. Meng, R. Liu, and K. Wang, "Robust peak detection of pulse waveform using height ratio," in International Conference of the IEEE Engineering in Medicine and Biology Society, Vancouver, BC, Canada, 2008, pp. 3856-3859.
13. L. Xu, M. Q. H. Meng, K. Wang, W. Lu, and N. Li, "Pulse images recognition using fuzzy neural network," Expert systems with applications, vol. 36, pp. 3805-3811, 2009.
14. Y. Wang, X. Wu, B. Liu, Y. Yi, and W. Wang, "Definition and application of indices in Doppler ultrasound sonogram," Shanghai Journal of Biomedical Engineering, vol. 18, pp. 26-29, Aug 1997.
15. C. J. C. Burges, "A tutorial on support vector machines for pattern recognition," Data Mining and Knowledge Discovery, vol. 2, no. 2, pp. 121-167, Jun, 1998.

Part II
Pulse Signal Acquisition

Chapter 2
Compound Pressure Signal Acquisition

In traditional Chinese pulse diagnosis (TCPD), to analyze the health condition of a patient, a practitioner should put three fingers on the wrist of the patient to adaptively feel the fluctuations in the radial pulse at the styloid processes. Thus, for comprehensive pulse signal acquisition, we should efficiently and accurately capture pulse signals at different positions and under different pressures. However, most conventional pulse signal acquisition devices can only capture signal at one position and under a fixed pressure and thus only capture limited pulse diagnostic information. In this chapter, we present a solution to the problems of sensor positioning, sensor array design, pressure adjustment, and mechanical structure design, resulting in a compound system for multiple-channel pulse signal acquisition. Compared with the other systems, this system provides a systematic solution to sensor positioning, is effective in measuring the width of the pulse, and can capture multichannel pulse signals together with sub-signals under different hold-down pressures.

2.1 Introduction

Wrist pulse is mainly caused by the cardiac contraction and relaxation and thus can be regarded as a traveling pressure wave [1]. Besides, for pulse diagnosis, the movement of blood and the change of vessel diameter would also have influence on wrist pulse. For thousands of years, pulse diagnosis has played an important role in traditional Chinese medicine and traditional Ayurvedic medicine for disease analysis [2, 3].

Despite its success in history, pulse diagnosis actually is a subjective skill which needs years of training and practice to master [4]. Moreover, for different practitioners, the diagnosis results may be inconsistent. To overcome these limitations, computational pulse diagnosis has recently been studied to make pulse diagnosis objective and quantitative, and researchers have verified the connection of pulse signals with several certain diseases [5–16].

© Springer Nature Singapore Pte Ltd. 2018
D. Zhang et al., *Computational Pulse Signal Analysis*,
https://doi.org/10.1007/978-981-10-4044-3_2

In traditional Chinese pulse diagnosis (TCPD), to analyze the health condition of a patient, a practitioner should put three fingers on the three positions (i.e., Cun, Guan, and Chi) of the patient's wrist to adaptively feel the fluctuations in the radial artery at the styloid processes. Since it is generally believed that wrist pulse is a pressure signal, several pressure sensor-based devices have been developed for pulse signal acquisition [17–21].

For computational pulse diagnosis, it is crucial to comprehensively and faithfully measure pressure pulse signal. By far, a number of sensors and systems have been developed for acquiring pressure pulse signal. Hannu et al. reported a pressure pulse sensor based on electromechanical film [22]. Kaniusas et al. used magnetoelastic skin curvature sensor to design a mechanical electrocardiography system for the non-disturbing measurement of blood pressure signal [23]. For wrist pulse signal acquisition, Chen et al. presented a liquid sensor system to measure the pulse signal [24]. Tyan et al. developed a pressure pulse monitoring system [20]. Lu et al. presented a wrist pressure signal device with three channels of biosensors for telemedicine [19]. Wu et al. proposed an air pressure pulse signal measurement system [25].

However, most existing wrist pulse signal acquisition devices and systems suffer from several limitations. Conventional acquisition device requires the user to manually place the probe to the appropriate position based on the user's experience. Thus, the wrist pulse signals actually are the combination of acquisition device and manual probe positioning, and it would be difficult to guarantee the objectiveness of the acquired pulse signal. Except the device in [19, 21], the other pulse signal acquisition systems only use a single pressure sensor to capture pulse signal and thus cannot simultaneously acquire multiple-channel signals for comprehensive pulse signal analysis. Moreover, the vessel diameter described in [1] reflects the pulse width information in TCPD, but usually cannot be acquired by the existed acquisition device.

In this chapter, we develop a novel pulse signal acquisition system to overcome the limitations of the current devices. First, for each of the Cun, Guan, and Chi positions, we design a main sensor to acquire main signal and a sub-sensor array to obtain the pulse width information and thus can simultaneously capture multiple-channel pulse signals. Second, we provide a systemic solution to the sensor positioning problem based on the position of the radius bone and the mean responses of sub-signals and thus make the pulse signal acquisition more objective. Moreover, step motor is adopted for pressure adjustment so that the pressure can be precisely controlled and tuned.

The remainder of the chapter is organized as follows. Section 2.2 discusses the performance requirements of a practical pulse signal acquisition system. Section 2.3 presents the design scheme of the four major modules: mechanical structure, sensor, circuit, and software. Section 2.4 provides the experimental results to evaluate the proposed pulse signal acquisition system. Finally, Section 2.5 gives several concluding remarks.

2.2   Application Scenario and Requirement Analysis

In this section, we first introduce the diagnostic information carried by wrist pulse signal and present an analysis on the principles of pulse diagnosis in traditional Chinese medicine (TCM) and traditional Ayurvedic medicine (TAM). Then, following these principles, we discuss the requirements of a wrist pulse signal acquisition system.

Generally, the wrist pulse signal carries rich diagnostic information, which is effective for disease diagnosis. First, wrist pulse signal is mainly produced by cardiac contraction and relaxation, is closely related with central aortic pressure waveform, and is effective in revealing cardiovascular status [18]. Second, pulse signal also reflects the movement of blood and the change of vessel diameter [1], making it valuable in analyzing several non-cardiac diseases. Moreover, as described in [18], "vascular properties in the upper limbs are less affected by ageing, arterial pressure, or various manoeuvers as compared to vessels in the trunk and lower limbs."

In TCM and TAM, the practitioner puts three fingers on the three specific positions of the patient's wrist to adaptively feel the fluctuations in the radial artery and then analyze the health condition of the patient based on the wrist pulse signals. Figure 1.2 shows the relative positions between the three fingers, the radial artery, and the radius bone during pulse diagnosis. Following the principles of pulse diagnosis, we discuss the main requirements of a pulse signal acquisition system. First, most current devices require the user to locate the positions of Cun, Guan, and Chi based on their experience. For objective pulse signal acquisition, we should solve the positioning problem. In this chapter, based on positioning principle used in TCPD, we design a positioning system to make the acquisition more automatic and easy to use.

Second, we should design suitable sensors to acquire as much as the diagnostic information used in TCPD. Wrist pulse signal is a kind of pressure waveform mainly caused by heartbeat and blood movement, and thus we adopt the pressure sensor. Besides, pulse width conveys the information of the change of vessel diameter and is also very valuable in TCPD. To capture pulse width information, a sub-sensor array is adopted in our wrist pulse signal acquisition system.

Finally, we should consider the characteristics of TCPD to improve the acquisition efficiency and signal usability. In TCPD, the practitioner puts three fingers on the Cun, Guan, and Chi, respectively, and adaptively feels the fluctuations in the radial artery. To imitate TCPD, our system involves three probes to simultaneously capture the pulse signals from Cun, Guan, and Chi, respectively, and use the step motor for pressure adjustment.

2.3 System Architecture

In this section, we introduce the system architecture of the proposed wrist pulse signal acquisition system by providing our design scheme of mechanical structure, sensor, circuit, and software system. Before introducing the system architecture in detail, we first give the three-dimensional Cartesian coordinate system used in this section. As shown in Fig. 2.1, we use the position of Guan as the origin. The XOY plane is parallel to the palm. The X-axis is parallel to the middle finger, while the Y-axis is perpendicular to the X-axis. The Z-axis is toward the direction of the external normal of the inner palm. Besides, we use millimeter (mm) as the length unit.

2.3.1 Mechanical Structure

In this subsection, we design the mechanical structure to address the positioning and pressure adjustment problems, which allows the simultaneous acquisition of the pulse signals from the Cun, Guan, and Chi positions. Moreover, other factors, e.g., size, appearance, and usability, are also considered in the mechanical structure design.

Figure 2.2 shows the mechanical structure of the proposed wrist pulse signal acquisition system, where Fig. 2.2a is a schematic sketch and Fig. 2.2b is a photo of our device. From Fig. 2.2a, one can see that the main components of the mechanical structure are pedestal, slide rail, stopper bolt, probes, pressure adjustment units, and control levers. The pedestal is installed on the bottom of the device. Three pressure adjustment units are installed on the slide rail. A probe is installed under each of the pressure adjustment units. In the following, we provide the detail of the design scheme for these components.

To capture pulse signals from Cun, Guan, and Chi, we use three probes, i.e., probe of Cun, probe of Guan, and probe of Chi. Based on the anatomy of wrist and

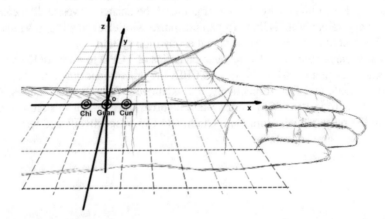

Fig. 2.1 The Cartesian coordinate system

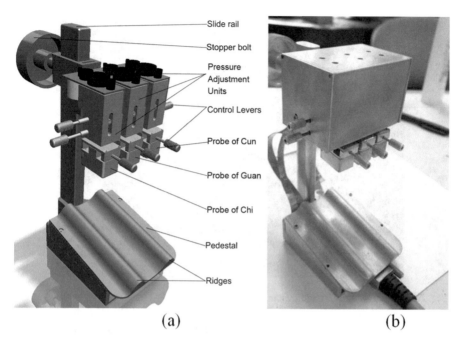

Fig. 2.2 The mechanical structure of our device: (**a**) schematic diagram and (**b**) photo

the TCPD principle, we design the pedestal and the three probes. Generally, the Guan position is adjacent to the styloid process of the radius. The Cun and Chi are in the front and the back of the Guan, respectively. In TCPD, when the middle finger is placed on the Guan position, the other two fingers, i.e., index finger and ring finger, fall naturally into their positions [1]. According to this principle the width of the probes is set to 10 mm, which is similar with the width of finger. To help the sensor positioning, we further design the pedestal installed on the bottom of the device by considering the wrist anatomy. As shown in Fig. 2.3, the styloid process is the end of radius bone and is a little larger than the other parts of the radius bone. This property can be utilized to locate the Guan position. Thus, we add two raised ridges on the pedestal to fix the styloid process of the radius bone. In this way, we can roughly locate the Guan position and then the Cun and Chi positions.

Given the pedestal and the probes, we design the sensor positioning and pressure adjustment components. As shown in Fig. 2.3, for sensor positioning, we add six control levers, where three of them (X-control levers) are used to adjust the positions of probes along X-axis, three (Y-control levers) to adjust the positions along Y-axis, and a stopper bolt to adjust the position along Z-axis. During pulse signal acquisition, we put the device among the wrist of the patient and use the two ridges to roughly locate the device along X-axis. Then, we use the control levers and stopper bolt to further adjust position of the probes along X-, Y-, and Z-axes.

Although the stopper bolt and slide rail can be used for pressure adjustment, it would add the same pressure on the three probes, and the adjustment is rough. In our

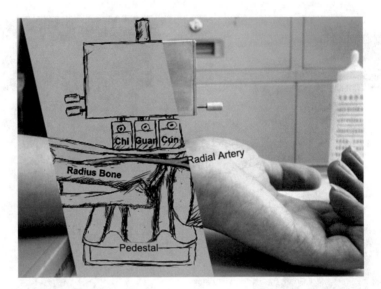

Fig. 2.3 The principle of locating Guan

device, we design three pressure adjustment units which allow the user to tune the pressure individually for each probe. The pressure adjustment unit is composed by power system and transmission system. The power system contains a reduction gear and a stepping motor, which is controlled by the software system to adjust the probe position and the hold-down pressure. The diameter of the step motor is restricted by the size of the probe and is set to be 10 mm. However, step motor with this size usually cannot provide sufficient torque. Fortunately, there is no strict requirement on the speed of the motor. So we use a set of reduction gear to exchange the speed for the torque. Another important component of the pressure adjustment unit is the transmission system, which includes the drive bolt, directional bolt, and other parts to transform the rotation of the motor to the movement of the probe along Z-axis.

Finally, we provide some numerical values on the evaluation of the sensor positioning and pressure adjustment performance. For sensor positioning along X-axis, the independent repetition test shows that the instrumental bias is 0.08 mm and the experimental standard deviation is 1.40 mm [26]. For sensor positioning along Y-axis, the discrimination threshold of the device is 1.0 mm. For pressure adjustment, the resolution is 0.005 N.

2.3.2 Sensor

In this section, we present the sensor design scheme, which includes a sub-sensor array to acquire pulse width information as well as sensor positioning along Y-axis and a main sensor for acquiring main signal.

Generally, we should choose the pressure sensor which is small in size and sensitive to pressure variation. By far, there are three types of pressure sensors available for pressure detection, metallic strain gauge (MSG), semiconductor strain gauge (SSG), and polyvinylidene fluoride (PVDF). The MSG is lack of sensitivity, the SSG and PVDF both meet the requirement, but the PVDF requires full shielding. So we choose SSG as the pressure sensor.

We use customized SSGs and elastic beams made of beryllium bronze to satisfy the size requirement of the pressure sensor. The SSGs are pasted on these elastic beams to measure the pressure. The change in pressure would make the strain gauges stretched or compressed and then cause the changes in resistance for signal acquisition.

The sub-sensor array of each probe was composed by 12 small elastic beams. The size of each beam is 0.8 mm × 8 mm. The gap between two beams is 0.2 mm. To obtain reliable pressure signal, the strain-voltage converter should be sensitive to extremely small changes in resistance. Usually, a Wheatstone bridge circuit [27] is used to convert the gauge's microstrain into a voltage change. When the resistances of all the four strain gauges in the bridge are absolutely equal, the bridge is perfectly balanced and the output of the Wheatstone bridge is zero. When any strain gauge is being compressed or stretched, the output departs from zero proportionally.

There are three types of Wheatstone bridges for strain-voltage conversion: full bridge, half bridge, and quarter bridge. Among these three types of bridges, the full bridge is the most sensitive. Moreover, the temperature error usually can be neglected because all four strain gauges are pasted close to each other and both the temperature and their temperature coefficient are nearly the same. However, the full bridge would occupy the larger spaces and need more wires, but the space for the sensor is quite limited. In order to control the sensitivity and accuracy, as shown in Fig. 2.5, we add another elastic beam above the sensor array as a main sensor. The main sensor has a larger elastic beam and has sufficient space to apply a full Wheatstone bridge. Meanwhile, the beam is much longer so that the sensitiveness would also increase. To achieve the largest output, four strain gauges are pasted on the elastic beam, two are in tension and the other two on the opposite side are in compression.

The structure of the main sensor is shown in Fig. 2.4. The length of the beam L is 16 mm. The height of the beam $h = 0.6$ mm is calculated by

$$h = \sqrt{\frac{6FL}{Ew\varepsilon}} \times 10^3 \qquad (2.1)$$

where $F = 20$ N denotes the maximum force that can be measured by the system, $E = 1.3 \times 10^{11}$ Pa denotes the elastic modulus of the beryllium bronze, $w = 6.4$ mm is the width of the beam, and $\varepsilon = 6 \times 10^{-3}$ is the limit strain of the strain gauges.

For each sub-sensor, the quarter bridge is adopted for strain-voltage conversion, where one strain gauge is pasted on each beam and three completion resistors on the printed circuit board, as shown in Fig. 2.5. Since the quarter bridge only uses one

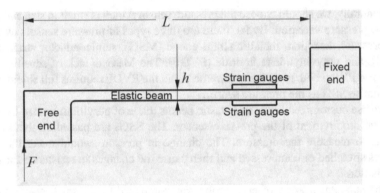

Fig. 2.4 The main sensor

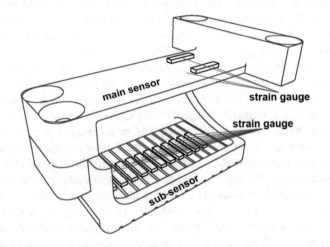

Fig. 2.5 The architecture of the sensor

strain gauge, the sensitivity is only a quarter of the full bridge. Fortunately, the sub-sensors are small in size and are densely arranged, and the relative difference between signals is reliable and consistent for pulse width analysis and Y-axis positioning. Based on the main sensor and the sub-sensor array, Fig. 2.6 shows a sketch figure and a photo of the probe adopted in our device.

2.3.3   Circuit

The circuit system is composed by the analog circuit and the digital circuit, which is used for pulse signal processing, transmission, and controlling of the pressure adjustment units. Figure 2.8 shows the schematic diagram of the circuit system.

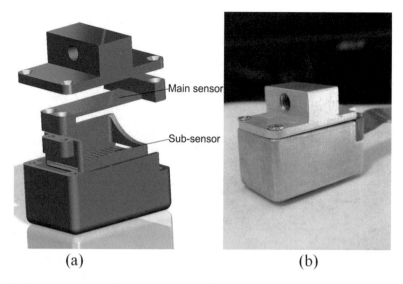

Fig. 2.6 Probe design: (**a**) schematic diagram and (**b**) photo

Analog Circuit The original pulse signal induced by the changes in resistance is weak. The non-ideal characteristics of Wheatstone bridge and the hold-down pressure would cause the analogical signal to contain both alternating current (AC) component and direct current (DC) components. So the analog circuit system is designed for the filtering and amplification of the signal, as shown in Fig. 2.7.

For each channel of pulse signal, two amplification units and two filtering units are adopted. First, both the AC and the DC components are amplified by using a preamplifier. We set the gain of the preamplifier to 10. Second, to remove the DC component, we use an AD8620 to construct a high-pass filter to remove the 0–0.05 Hz low-frequency components of the signal. Third, another amplifier composed by AD8620 is adopted to amplify the voltage signal to the interval of −5 V to +5 V. Finally, to remove the interference of alternating current, we use a 100 kΩ resistor and a 39 nF capacitor to construct a first-order low-pass filter which can remove the high-frequency interference. The transition band of the low-pass filter is 0–40 Hz, and the attenuation at 50 Hz is -4.1 dB. Because the diagnostic features generally are extracted from the 0.1 to 30 Hz frequency components of pulse signal, it is safe to use the high-pass and low-pass filters mentioned above for removing the DC component and the interference of alternating current.

Digital Circuit The digital circuit system is used to digitalize the amplified analogical pulse signals, transmit them to the computer, and control the motors. As shown in Fig. 2.8, the major components of the digital circuit system are the multiplexer (MUX), the analog to digital converter (ADC), the microprogrammed control unit (MCU), the motor controller, etc. In digital circuit design, the MUX unit is composed by eight eight-channel multiplexers make a sixty four channel multi-

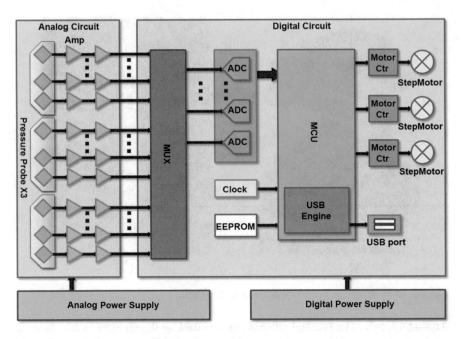

Fig. 2.7 Schematic diagram of the circuit system

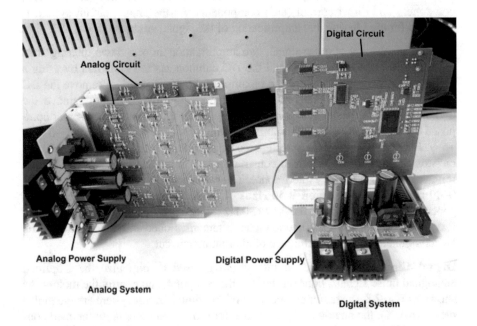

Fig. 2.8 Photograph of the circuit system

plexer (CD4051), the major component of the ADC unit is a high-speed 12-bit ADC MAX115, and we choose EZ-USB FX2 as the MCU.

Noise Suppression During signal acquisition and processing, noise would be inevitable. Thus the suppression of the noise would be a critical issue for the design of practical pulse acquisition system. In the following, we provide our strategy to suppress the noise from three aspects: design and choice of the preamplifier, power supply, and circuit layout.

First, the pulse signal before preamplification is weak, and we should be careful not to let the noise introduced by circuit destroy the signal. In our preamplification, the AD620 instrumentation operational amplifier is adopted to suppress common mode noise.

Second, we compare several candidate power supplies and choose the one with low noise and sufficient power. We consider three types of power supplies: chemical, switching, and liner power supplies. For chemical power supply, the power and voltage is low and cannot meet our requirements. For the switching power supply, the noise is severe. Thus, we choose the liner power since of its low noise level and sufficient power supply.

Third, in circuit layout design, the circuit for power and ground is wider than the circuit for signal, and we use two separated power supplies for digital circuit and analog circuit to reduce the high-frequency interference from digital circuit. Figure 2.8 shows the photograph of the circuit system.

Software Architecture The software system is designed for the control of the sampling process and for the browsing of the main signals and sub-signals. As shown in Fig. 2.9, the software graphical user interface (GUI) includes five main modules: control unit, database management unit, main signal display unit, sub-signal display unit, and pressure adjustment unit. During pulse signal acquisition, the control unit allows us to control the sampling procedure, and the database management unit allows us to edit the information of the volunteer and save the pulse signals. With the main signal and sub-signal display units, the user can browse the acquired signals in real time. Moreover, the pressure adjustment unit allows the user to adjust the hold-down pressure also in real time. For safety, we set the allowable interval of the hold-down pressure within 0 N to 5 N. Once the hold-down pressure reaches to 5 N, the system would restrict the step motors not to further increase the hold-down pressure.

2.3.4 Summary

In this subsection, we summarize the main advantages of our device for compound pulse signal acquisition and sensor positioning. First, compared with other pulse acquisition systems, our device can acquire more comprehensive pulse signals. The system consists of three probes to simultaneously capture three-channel pulse

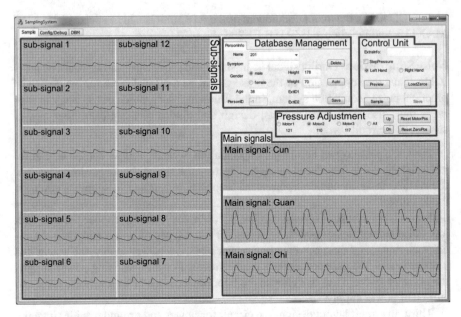

Fig. 2.9 The GUI of the acquisition system

signals from the Cun, Guan, and Chi positions. In each probe, we design a sub-sensor array to acquire 12 channels of sub-signals.

Second, our solution to the sensor positioning problem is systemic. Generally, the positioning accuracy of our device is sufficient, and the procedure of positioning could be finished within 1 min. For X-axis positioning, we could use the two ridges in the pedestal (Fig. 2.2) to quickly find the rough positions of Cun, Guan, and Chi. During pulse signal acquisition, we only required to tune the X-axis levers no more than 2 mm to accurately locate the sensor positions along X-axis. For Y-axis positioning, we can calculate the mean responses of the 12 sub-sensors in real time and tune the levers until the 6 or 7 channels of sub-signals are much stronger than the sub-signals from the other channels. For the positioning along the Y-axis, we provide two kinds of pressure adjustment modules: firstly, we can use the stopper bolt to adjust the position along Z-axis; moreover, we design the pressure adjustment unit composed by power system (including reduction gear and stepping motor) and transmission system, which allow to adjust the pressure along Z-axis individually for each probe in the software GUI.

2.4   System Evaluation

In this section, we first present several examples of the pulse signals, which indicate that our device can acquire rich wrist pulse signals. Then, we conduct a series of experiments to show that multichannel pulse signals can be used to improve the classification performance for disease diagnosis. Finally, we give a discussion by comparing our device with several other devices reported in recent literature.

2.4.1   Sampled Pulse Signals

As shown in Fig. 2.10, our device can acquire three channels of pulse signals from Cun, Guan, and Chi under different hold-down pressures. Moreover, for each channel, we can also acquire 12-channel pulse sub-signals by using the sub-sensor array.

Figure 2.11 shows all the signals acquired from one person's Guan position, which include 12 channels of sub-signals captured by the sub-sensor array and 1 channel of main signal acquired by the main sensor. Compared with the sub-signals, the main signal is more robust, which should be attributed to both the combination of the sub-sensors and the usage of the full Wheatstone bridge. So our device can acquire pulse signals from Cun, Guan, and Chi with satisfactory signal quality.

For each position, the 12 channels of sub-signals can be used for both the sensor positioning of the probe and the extraction of the pulse width feature. We use the mean responses of each of the 12 sub-sensors to locate the position of the blood vessel. The initial mean responses of these sub-sensors may be like Fig. 2.12a, where one can observe that sometimes the maximum mean pressure might not locate among the center of the 12 channels. In these cases, we could tune the position of the probe along the Y-axis until the 6 or 7 channels of sub-signals are much

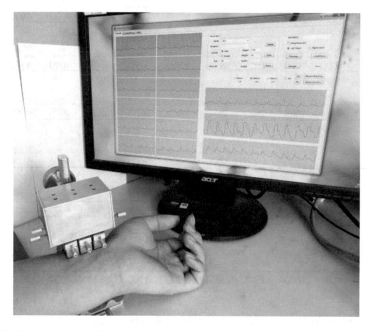

Fig. 2.10 Pulse signal sampling using our device

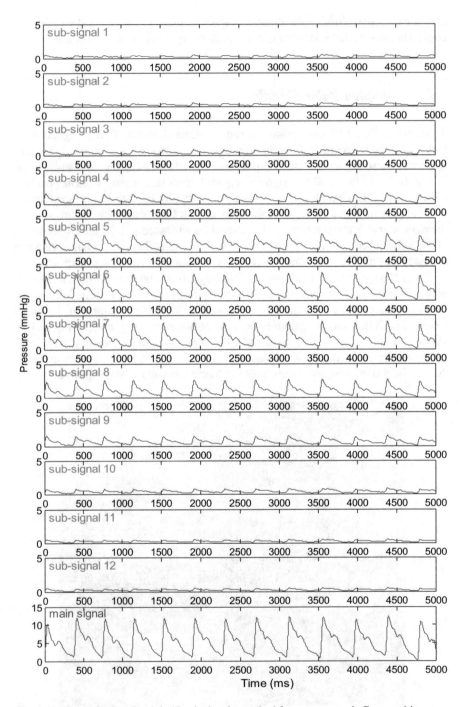

Fig. 2.11 The main signal and the 12 sub-signals acquired from one person's Guan position

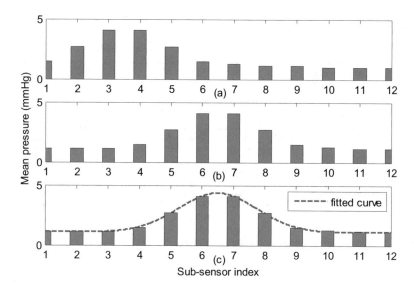

Fig. 2.12 The mean pressure responses of different sub-sensors: (**a**) before accurate positioning, (**b**) after accurate positioning, and (**c**) curve fitting

stronger than the sub-signals from the other channels, as shown in Fig. 2.12b. From Fig. 2.12b, we can further extract pulse width feature. As shown in Fig. 2.12c, we model the mean pressure of the 12 sub-sensor signals with a parametric Gaussian curve

$$f(i) = a \exp\left(-\frac{i^2}{2\sigma^2}\right) + C \tag{2.2}$$

where i denotes the index of the sub-sensor. After curve fitting, the value of σ can be used as the pulse width feature.

Figure 2.13 shows one person's pulse signals from Guan acquired under three different hold-down pressures. From Fig. 2.13, one can see that the difference is noticeable among pulse signals acquired under different hold-down pressures. So it would be interesting to investigate the connection between the pressure and the shape of the pulse signal. Moreover, by proper integration of features extracted from signal under different pressure, we might explore more valuable information for computational pulse diagnosis.

Finally, Fig. 2.14 shows the three main signals from Cun, Guan, and Chi acquired under the same hold-down pressure. One can see that not only the hold-down pressure but also the position would cause the difference in the pulse shape. In TCPD, the practitioner puts three fingers on Cun, Guan, and Chi, respectively, to feel the fluctuations in the radial artery for pulse diagnosis. So, the three-channel signals are also expected to provide richer diagnostic features for pulse analysis and diagnosis.

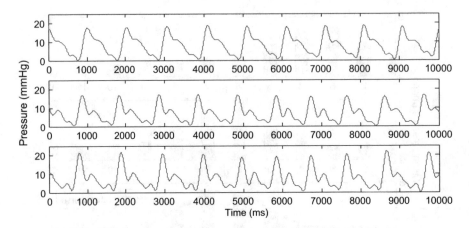

Fig. 2.13 Main signals from Guan acquired under three different hold-down pressure

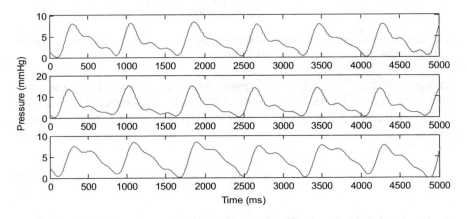

Fig. 2.14 Main signals from Cun, Guan, and Chi acquired under the same hold-down pressure

2.4.2 Computational Pulse Diagnosis

In this subsection, for experimental validation of the device, we first show that our device can acquire pulse signals with satisfactory quality for pulse diagnosis, and then conduct another experiment to validate the benefit of three-channel signals for computational pulse diagnosis.

In our experiments, we choose the classification problem of healthy persons with diabetic patients to evaluate the pulse signals acquired by our device. In TCPD, it is generally assumed that pulse signal would reflect the wrist blood velocity and viscosity. Recent studies have shown that the anomalies of blood viscosity are correlated with the condition of several diseases, e.g., malaria, AIDS, and diabetes [28]. In computational pulse analysis, researchers have also studied the problem of diabetes diagnosis based on pulse signal [14, 29, 30]. Thus, it is reasonable to use the diabetes diagnosis problem to conduct a preliminary evaluation on our device.

Table 2.1 Summary of dataset

	Age distribution				Gender distribution	
	1–40	40–50	50–60	> 60	Male	Female
Healthy	5	40	71	79	123	72
Diabetes	3	36	68	96	132	71

For experimental validation, we construct a dataset of three-channel pulse signals by collaborating with Hong Kong Yao Chung Kit Diabetes Assessment Centre. The dataset contains of 398 volunteers, including 195 healthy volunteers and 203 volunteers with diabetes. To avoid the potential influence of biological factors, we also ensure that the distributions of gender and age of volunteers with diabetes are similar with those of healthy volunteers. Table 2.1 lists a summary of the dataset.

For the preprocessing of the pulse signals, we adopt the denoising and baseline drift correction methods in [31]. For the feature extraction, we choose the multiscale sample entropy (SampEN) method [32]. Approximate entropy, sample entropy [33–36], and multiscale entropy [29, 30, 37–39] have been very successful in heart signal analysis and diabetes diagnosis. Besides, we also include the period of the pulse signal and the depth of the valley as the diagnostic feature. Figure 2.15 shows the distribution of four representative features, i.e., period, sample entropy under scale factor 10 (SampEn10), sample entropy under scale factor 50 (SampEn50), and sample entropy under scale factor 100 (SampEn100). One can see that the statistical distributions of features extracted from healthy volunteers are different from those features extracted from patients with diabetes. However, the difference between these two classes is complicated, and we cannot use some simple rules to classify healthy volunteers from patients with diabetes. Thus, based on these features, we use the support vector machine (SVM) for classification [40]. We adopt the tenfold cross-validation procedure and use the accuracy, sensitivity, and specificity [41] as the indicators of classification performance.

We first conduct an experiment to show that our device could acquire pulse signals with satisfactory quality for pulse diagnosis. Following the experimental setup adopted in previous computational pulse diagnosis studies, we only use the features extracted from main pulse signals from the Guan position for performance evaluation. Experimental results show that the sensitivity is 87.6%, the specificity is 83.1%, and the classification accuracy is 85.4%, as listed in Table 2.2. Compared with those reported in [7, 12], we can achieve similar classification accuracy, which implies that our device could acquire pulse signals with satisfactory quality for pulse diagnosis.

In the practice of TCPD, for comprehensive analysis, a practitioner should put three fingers on the wrist of the patient to feel the fluctuations in the radial pulse. Thus, in computational pulse diagnosis, the use of three-channel pulse signals is expected to benefit to classification performance. For classification based on three-channel pulse signals, we extract the same features as the single-channel experiment, then train one SVM classifier for each channel of pulse signal, and finally adopt the Bayes sum rule [42–44] to combine the output of the five individual

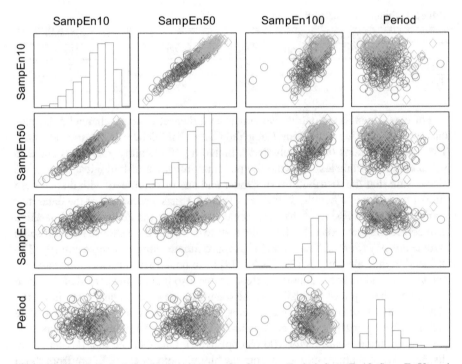

Fig. 2.15 The statistical distribution of four pulse features (Period, SampEn10, SampEn50, and SampEn100)

Table 2.2 Classification results

	Sensitivity (%)	Specificity (%)	Classification rate (%)
Single-channel	87.6	83.1	85.4
Three-channel	92.6	87.6	90.2

classifiers. Experimental results show that the sensitivity is 92.6%, the specificity is 87.6%, and the classification accuracy is 90.2%, as listed in Table 2.2. Compared with the accuracy obtained using the single-channel signals, the use of three-channel pulse signals would significantly improve the classification performance. We further adopt the McNemar test [45] to evaluate the statistical significance of the difference in classification rate obtained using single-channel and multiple-channel pulse signals. The result shows that the performance difference is statistically significant at $\alpha = 0.05$. If we adopt more proper feature- or decision-level fusion methods and make full use of both the main signals and the sub-signals from Cun, Guan, and Chi under different hold-down pressures, we expect that we could extract much richer diagnostic features and achieve much higher accuracy. Note that here we just use the diabetes diagnosis problem to conduct a preliminary evaluation on our device. For other disease diagnosis or TCM syndrome analysis problems, multi-channel signals may be more superior to single-channel signals.

Finally, we report the run time of the feature extraction and classification methods. All the experiments are conducted on a PC computer with i5-2400 CPU and 4G RAM. For each test sample, the average time of feature extraction is 0.467 s, and the average time of classification is 9.76×10^{-5} s.

2.4.3 Comparisons with Other Pulse Sampling Systems

We compare the proposed system with three pressure pulse acquisition devices and systems reported in the recent literature, as summarized in. We chose these three existing systems because these three pressure-based systems share several similar characteristics with the proposed system in sensor positioning, pressure adjustment, or compound pulse signal acquisition. From Table 2.3, our device is the only one that systematically addresses the X-, Y-, and Z-axes sensor positioning problems, while the other devices and systems either definitely require the user to put the sensor to proper position or just address the Y- and Z-axes sensor positioning. Besides, our device can simultaneously acquire three channels of main signals from the Cun, Guan, and Chi positions. For each position, we can also obtain 12 channels of sub-signals. Thus our device can acquire more comprehensive multiple-channel pulse signals than the other systems.

We further compare the classification performance of different devices and systems. Note that in each reference the authors constructed their own dataset to evalu-

Table 2.3 Classification results

System	Tyan et al. [20]	Lu et al. [19]	Hu et al. [21]	This chapter
Positioning system	Y-/Z-axes	Manual	Manual	X-/Y-/Z-axes
Number of sensors	One	Three	$3 \times 4 \times 3$ sub-sensors	Three main sensors, 12×3 sub-sensors
Pulse width measurement	Yes	No	Yes	Yes
Pressure adjustment module	Step motor	Belt	Three independent step motors	Three independent step motors
Dataset	Myocardial ischemia (20)/ health (40)	Hypertension/health; coronary/health; pregnancy/health; cirrhosis/health; subhealth/health (1456 in total)	Validation on repeatability during 10-min period (the size of the dataset is not mentioned in [21])	Diabetics (203) /nondiabetics (195)
Results	p = 0.0039 (hypothesis testing)	75%; 100%; 93.02%; 97.02%; 52.30% (classification rate)	p = 0.05 (repeatability)	90.2% (classification rate)

ate the device or system based on different classification tasks, and Tyan et al. [20] only reported the p value of the hypothesis testing, and Hu et al. [21] only reported their results on repeatability validation. Thus, it is not fair to compare the performance of different systems only based on the reported classification rates. From Table 2.3, one can see that we use a relative large dataset to evaluate our device, and the classification rate is also relatively higher.

2.5 Summary

In this chapter, we design a novel compound pulse signal acquisition system based on pressure sensor. Compared with other pulse signal acquisition, the device has the following notable advantages. First, our device can acquire comprehensive multiple-channel pulse signals, i.e., three channels of main signals together with the sub-signals, and thus more diagnostic features, e.g., pulse width, could be extracted. Second, we provide a systemic solution for the X-, Y-, and Z-axes sensor positioning. For X-axis sensor positioning, the instrumental bias is 0.08 mm, and the experimental standard deviation is 1.40 mm. The discrimination threshold along Y-axis is 1.0 mm, and the resolution of pressure adjustment is 0.005 N. Finally, the experimental results show that the three-channel pulse signals acquired by the device can achieve higher classification accuracy than the single-channel signals.

References

1. S. Walsh, and E. King, Pulse Diagnosis: A Clinical Guide, Sydney Australia: Elsevier, 2008.
2. V. D. Lad, Secrets of the Pulse, Albuquerque, New Mexico: The Ayurvedic Press, 1996.
3. E. Hsu, Pulse Diagnosis in Early Chinese Medicine, New York, American: Cambridge University Press, 2010.
4. R. Amber, and B. Brooke, Pulse Diagnosis Detailed Interpretations For Eastern & Western Holistic Treatments, Santa Fe, New Mexico: Aurora Press, 1993.
5. Y. Chen, L. Zhang, D. Zhang, and D. Zhang, "Computerized wrist pulse signal diagnosis using modified auto-regressive models," Journal of Medical Systems, vol. 35, no. 3, pp. 321-328, Jun, 2011.
6. Y. Chen, L. Zhang, and D. Zhang, "Wrist pulse signal diagnosis using modified Gaussian Models and Fuzzy C-Means classification," Medical Engineering & Physics, vol. 31, no. 10, pp. 1283-1289, Dec, 2009.
7. L. Liu, W. Zuo, D. Zhang, N. Li, and H. Zhang, "Combination of heterogeneous features for wrist pulse blood flow signal diagnosis via multiple kernel learning," IEEE Transactions on Information Technology in Biomedicine, vol. 16, no. 8, pp. 599-607, Jul, 2012.
8. L. Liu, W. Zuo, D. Zhang, N. Li, and H. Zhang, "Classification of wrist pulse blood flow signal using time warp edit distance," Medical Biometrics, vol. 6165, no. 1, pp. 137-144, 2010.
9. D. Zhang, L. Zhang, and Y. Zheng, "Wavelet based analysis of doppler ultrasonic wrist-pulse signals," in Proceedings of IEEE International Conference on Biomedical Engineering and Informatics, Hainan, China, 2008, pp. 539-543.

10. D. Y. Zhang, W. M. Zuo, D. Zhang, H. Z. Zhang, and N. M. Li, "Wrist blood flow signal-based computerized pulse diagnosis using spatial and spectrum features," Journal of Biomedical Science and Engineering, vol. 3, no. 4, pp. 361-366, 2010.
11. D. Zhang, W. Zuo, Y. Li, and N. Li, "Gaussian ERP kernel classifier for pulse waveforms classification," in Proceedings of IEEE International Conference on Pattern Recognition, Istanbul, Turkey 2010, pp. 2736-2739.
12. Q. L. Guo, K. Q. Wang, D. Y. Zhang, and N. M. Li, "A wavelet packet based pulse waveform analysis for cholecystitis and nephrotic syndrome diagnosis," in Proceedings of IEEE International Conference on Wavelet Analysis and Pattern Recognition, Hong Kong, China, 2008, pp. 513-517.
13. S. Charbonnier, S. Galichet, G. Mauris, and J. P. Siche, "Statistical and fuzzy models of ambulatory systolic blood pressure for hypertension diagnosis," IEEE Transactions on Instrumentation and Measurement, vol. 49, no. 5, pp. 998-1003, 2000.
14. H.-T. Wu, C.-H. Lee, C.-K. Sun, J.-T. Hsu, R.-M. Huang, and C.-J. Tang, "Arterial Waveforms Measured at the Wrist as Indicators of Diabetic Endothelial Dysfunction in the Elderly," IEEE Transactions on Instrumentation and Measurement, vol. 61, no. 1, pp. 162-169, 2012.
15. P. Dupuis, and C. Eugene, "Combined detection of respiratory and cardiac rhythm disorders by high-resolution differential cuff pressure measurement," IEEE Transactions on Instrumentation and Measurement, vol. 49, no. 3, pp. 498-502, 2000.
16. J. U. Kim, Y. J. Jeon, Y.-M. Kim, H. J. Lee, and J. Y. Kim, "Novel fiagnostic model for the deficient and excess pulse qualities," Evidence-Based Complementary and Alternative Medicine, vol. 2012, no. 563958, pp. 1-11, 2012.
17. P. Zhang, and H. Wang, "A framework for automatic time-domain characteristic Parameters extraction of human pulse signals," EURASIP Journal on Advances in Signal Processing, vol. 2008, no. 468390, pp. 1-9, 2008.
18. C. Chen, E. Nevo, B. Fetics, P. H. Pak, F. C. P. Yin, L. Maughan, and D. A. Kass, "Estimation of central aortic pressure waveform by mathematical transformation of radial tonometry pressure: validation of generalized transfer function," Circulation, vol. 95, no. 7, pp. 1827-1836, 1997.
19. S. Lu, R. Wang, L. Cui, Z. Zhao, Y. Yu, and Z. Shan, "Wireless networked Chinese telemedicine system: method and apparatus for remote pulse information retrieval and diagnosis," in Proceedings of IEEE International Conference on Pervasive Computing and Communications, Hong Kong, China, 2008, pp. 698-703.
20. C. C. Tyan, S. H. Liu, J. Y. Chen, J. J. Chen, and W. M. Liang, "A novel noninvasive measurement technique for analyzing the pressure pulse waveform of the radial artery," IEEE Transactions on Biomedical Engineering, vol. 55, no. 1, pp. 288-297, Jan, 2008.
21. C.-S. Hu, Y.-F. Chung, C.-C. Yeh, and C.-H. Luo, "Temporal and Spatial Properties of Arterial Pulsation Measurement Using Pressure Sensor Array," Evidence-Based Complementary and Alternative Medicine, vol. 2012, pp. 1-9, 2012.
22. H. Sorvoja, V. M. Kokko, R. Myllyla, and J. Miettinen, "Use of EMFi as a blood pressure pulse transducer," IEEE Transactions on Instrumentation and Measurement, vol. 54, no. 6, pp. 2505-2512, 2005.
23. E. Kaniusas, H. Pfutzner, L. Mehnen, J. Kosel, C. Tellez-Blanco, G. Varoneckas, A. Alonderis, T. Meydan, M. Vazquez, M. Rohn, A. M. Merlo, and B. Marquardt, "Method for continuous nondisturbing monitoring of blood pressure by magnetoelastic skin curvature sensor and ECG," IEEE Sensors Journal, vol. 6, no. 3, pp. 819-828, Jun, 2006.
24. L. Chen, H. Atsumi, M. Yagihashi, F. Mizuno, H. Narita, and H. Fujimoto, "A preliminary research on analysis of pulse diagnosis," in Proceedings of IEEE International Conference on Complex Medical Engineering, Beijing, China, 2007, pp. 1807-1812.
25. H.-T. Wu, C.-H. Lee, and A.-B. Liu, "Assessment of endothelial function using arterial pressure signals," Journal of Signal Processing Systems, vol. 64, no. 2, pp. 223-232, 2011.
26. ISO, IEC, OIML, and BIPM, Guide to the Expression of Uncertainty in Measurement, Geneva: ISO, 1995.

27. B. Dobkin, and J. Williams, Analog circuit design: a tutorial guide to applications and solutions, America: Newnes, 2011.
28. D. A. Fedosov, W. Pan, B. Caswell, G. Gompper, and G. E. Karniadakis, "Predicting human blood viscosity in silico," Proceedings of the National Academy of Sciences, vol. 108, no. 29, pp. 11772-11777, 2011.
29. I. Wakabayashi, and H. Masuda, "Association of pulse pressure with fibrinolysis in patients with type 2 diabetes," Thrombosis Research, vol. 121, no. 1, pp. 95-102, 2007.
30. N. Arunkumar, and K. M. M. Sirajudeen, "Approximate entropy based ayurvedic pulse diagnosis for diabetics - a case study," in Proceedings of IEEE International Conference on Trendz in Information Sciences and Computing, Chennai, India, 2011, pp. 133-135.
31. L. Xu, D. Zhang, and K. Wang, "Wavelet-based cascaded adaptive filter for removing baseline drift in pulse waveforms," IEEE Transactions on Biomedical Engineering, vol. 52, no. 11, pp. 1973-1975, Nov, 2005.
32. L. Liu, N. Li, W. Zuo, D. Zhang, and H. Zhang, "Multiscale sample entropy analysis of wrist pulse blood flow signal for disease diagnosis," in Proceedings of Sino-foreign-interchange Workshop on Intelligence Science and Intelligent Data Engineering, NanJing China, 2012.
33. D. E. Lake, J. S. Richman, M. P. Griffin, and J. R. Moorman, "Sample entropy analysis of neonatal heart rate variability," American Journal of Physiology-Regulatory, Integrative and Comparative Physiology, vol. 283, no. 3, pp. R789-R797, Sep, 2002.
34. J. S. Richman, and J. R. Moorman, "Physiological time-series analysis using approximate entropy and sample entropy," American Journal of Physiology-Heart and Circulatory Physiology, vol. 278, no. 6, pp. H2039-H2049, Jun, 2000.
35. L. Xu, M. Q. H. Meng, X. Qi, and K. Wang, "Morphology variability analysis of wrist pulse waveform for assessment of arteriosclerosis status," Journal of Medical Systems, vol. 34, no. 3, pp. 331-339, Jun, 2010.
36. S. M. Pincus, "Approximate entropy as a measure of system-complexity," Proceedings of the National Academy of Sciences, vol. 88, no. 6, pp. 2297-2301, Mar, 1991.
37. M. Costa, A. L. Goldberger, and C. K. Peng, "Multiscale entropy analysis of complex physiologic time series," Physical Review Letters, vol. 89, no. 068102, pp. 1-4, Aug 5, 2002.
38. M. Costa, A. Goldberger, and C. K. Peng, "Multiscale entropy to distinguish physiologic and synthetic RR time series," in Proceedings of Computers in Cardiology, Memphis, America, 2002, pp. 137-140.
39. M. Costa, A. L. Goldberger, and C. K. Peng, "Multiscale entropy analysis of biological signals," Physical Review E, vol. 71, no. 021906, pp. 1-18, Feb, 2005.
40. C. J. C. Burges, "A tutorial on support vector machines for pattern recognition," Data Mining and Knowledge Discovery, vol. 2, no. 2, pp. 121-167, Jun, 1998.
41. A. G. Lalkhen, and A. McCluskey, "Clinical tests: sensitivity and specificity," Continuing Education in Anaesthesia, Critical Care & Pain, vol. 8, no. 6, pp. 221-223, 2008.
42. J. Platt, "Probabilistic Outputs for Support Vector Machines and Comparison to Regularized Likelihood Methods," Proceedings of Advances in Large Margin Classifiers, pp. 61-74, 2000.
43. D. Jia, N. Li, S. Liu, and S. Li, "Decision level fusion for pulse signal classification using multiple features," in Proceedings of IEEE International Conference on Biomedical Engineering and Informatics, Yantai, China, 2010, pp. 843-847.
44. J. Kittler, M. Hatef, P. W. Duin, and J. Matas, "On Combining Classifiers," IEEE Transactions on Pattern Analysis and Machine Intelligence, vol. 20, pp. 226-239, 1998.
45. Q. McNemar, "Note on the sampling error of the difference between correlated proportions or percentages," Psychometrika, vol. 12, pp. 153-157, 1947.

Chapter 3
Pulse Signal Acquisition Using Multi-sensors

In this chapter, we integrate a pressure sensor with a photoelectric sensor to make a fusion sensor which can acquire the pulse from different approaches. We designed the multichannel sensor arrays structure and introduced the pulse analysis algorithm and classification methods. Experiments on disease classification are carried out to test the system performance with multichannel and different sensor arrays. The results show that the novel system is not only able to distinguish between healthy pulse samples and subjects suffering from diabetes but also good at obtaining more information than the conventional pulse system with single channel or simplex-type sensor.

3.1 Introduction

Pulse diagnosis is known as one of the four examination methods in traditional Chinese medicine (TCM) diagnosis which consists of observation, listening, smelling, and pulse feeling. In ancient times, Chinese medicine physicians diagnosed the pathological changes of organs by feeling the artery pulse [1, 2]. The pulse is transmitted by blood flow through arteries from the heart. Hence, it is affected not only by the conditions of the heart beatings but also by the conditions of nerves, organs, muscles, skin, arterial walls, blood parameters, etc. [3]. According to this principle, wrist pulse is usually regarded to give more body information than the electrocardiogram (ECG), which results in broader applications in health status analysis [4–11].

In TCM, a Chinese medicine practitioner took pulse by putting fingers on the patients' wrist at certain positions [1]. However, the pulse diagnosis skill requires several years experience to practice and master. Sometimes it may be not accordant among different practitioners because of the subjective judgment [12]. Compared with the finger-feeling diagnosis, a scientific way of pulse diagnosis is using the sensing elements to simulate the functions of fingers and transforming the physical

© Springer Nature Singapore Pte Ltd. 2018
D. Zhang et al., *Computational Pulse Signal Analysis*,
https://doi.org/10.1007/978-981-10-4044-3_3

signals into digital signals [13]. The quantification of the pulse diagnosis solves the problem of obtaining the objective pulse signals [14]. The pulse information which includes strengths, amplitudes, fluency, shapes, widths, variations of the rhythm, and so on are obtained from the digital pulse signals for further processing [3].

Recently, there are two kinds of pulse devices that have been reported. One is called pulse oximeter, applied with a probe attached to the patient's finger [15, 16]. It is a noninvasive method for measuring the oxygen saturation of arterial blood. Because the pulse rate always agreed with the heart rate on the basis of ECG, the oximeter has been widely used in cardiac monitoring [17]. A research group of the National Dong Hwa University in Taiwan [4] declared they successfully developed the artery health prediction system by detecting finger pulse. Humphreys et al. [9] presented a system capable of capturing two photoplethysmography signals at two different wavelengths simultaneously to give a quick indication of the cardiac rhythm. There is no doubt that the pulse oximeter is the big advance in acquiring the physiological blood signals. However, a falsely high or falsely low reading will occur in the pulse oximeter when hemoglobin binds to something other than oxygen [16]. Physiologists also demonstrated that the pulse waveform changes when the blood moves apart from the heart. Thus, the pulse waveform of the finger is different from that of the wrist [18]. As a result, the finger pulse feeling disagrees with the pulse diagnosis in TCM. It is insufficient to analyze the health status just through the artery oxygen saturation.

The other kind, operated with probe attached to the patient's wrist, is developed for objectifying TCM. Many sensor types such as polyvinylidene fluoride (PVDF) [19], optical sensor [15, 16], air pressure sensor [20], and ultrasonic Doppler sensor [5] have been introduced for the pulse acquisition. But these systems ignore the static contact pressure information. According to traditional Chinese pulse diagnosis (TCPD), Chinese medicine practitioners feel the pulsations by touching on the wrist vessel with three fingers and pressing with certain strength. The pressure levels are then divided into three patterns, Fu, Zhong, and Chen, corresponding to the levels of pulse depth under skin. It is an important symbol for judging the patient's physical conditions in TCPD [1]. Therefore, it is necessary to get the static contact pressure in pulse-collecting platforms.

Although the pulse system with pressure sensor is capable of obtaining the depth information [21, 22], it is short in acquiring the weak pulsations with high quality. The touch sensation is easily disturbed by the surrounding noise while feeling the weak physiological signals under skin. It is a fatal flaw of the pressure sensors, and the system performance needs to be robust under various conditions. Each sensor type is with its specific characteristics and complements to each other, whereas previous systems only apply single-type sensor. It is known that single-type sensor cannot replace the finger-feelings comprehensively and lose pulse information inevitably [23]. Therefore, we should keep the advantages of each sensor type and combine them together to obtain more arterial pulse information. Meanwhile, because most of the pulse systems are designed with a single-point transducer [24–32], it brings the problem about sampling location criterion. The three positions, defined as Cun, Guan, and Chi in TCM, have significant different meanings and provide a standard for pulse location [1]. The analysis of a wrist radial artery needs both temporal and spatial dimensions [22].

In this chapter, we propose a novel multichannel wrist pulse system with different sensor arrays to get rid of the problems of information loss. The pulse probe is composed of three independent channels, and each channel consists of an array of nine photoelectric sensors with one pressure sensor. The photoelectric sensor array is introduced to detect the pulse width information and to locate the center of the radial artery. The pressure sensor, regarded as the main sensing element, measures the pulsations with high resolution and the static contact pressure. Pulse waveforms are acquired from three channels corresponding to the position of Cun, Guan, and Chi. Step motors are used to adjust the static contact pressure applied on the radical artery, imitating the Fu, Zhong, and Chen of practitioners' feeling. Then, the pulse waveforms are processed using amplifier circuit followed by data acquisition circuit and finally displayed on liquid crystal display. The pulse signals collected by pressure sensors reflect the fluctuation of the vessel, and the signals collected by photoelectric sensors reflect the changes of blood volume. These two sensor types with different principles are combined to obtain more pulse information. We apply our system to the disease diagnosis and obtain satisfactory results. The experiment results prove that the proposed system has excellent performance in pulse acquisition and practical usage for auxiliary diagnosis.

3.2   Framework of the Proposed System

The proposed system consists of three main components: pulse sensors, sampling circuit, and user interface (UI) (Fig. 3.1). The sensor arrays first transform the physical pulse beatings into electric signals, and then the analog circuit follows to amplify the feeble physiology signals. Next, digital circuit is employed to implement the analog to digital (AD) conversion. Finally, the digital signals are transmitted to the UI at PC and stored in open database connectivity (ODBC) database through universal serial bus (USB).

The pulse from radial artery is usually taken as the TCM practitioners did for thousands of years. Feeling pulse is not as easy as it looks like, because pulse may be very weak in certain subjects such as the obesity group, or at certain parts. Generally, at Chi position one can hardly feel strong pulsations. Moreover, the

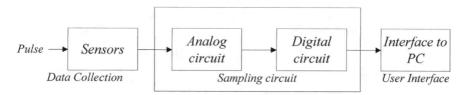

Fig. 3.1 Brief flow chart of the proposed pulse system

pressure applied on the wrist artery varies among subjects and also differs in the three positions [1]. Therefore, the pulse diagnosis needs the primary knowledge to ensure the approximate pulse position before the pulse-collecting stage. Otherwise, it will be time consuming and difficult to ensure the right positions of weak pulse signals.

3.2.1 Pulse Collecting

In TCM, practitioners took the pulse of patients by putting their fingers on a specific area of the wrist regarded as the position of pulsation, which is further subdivided into three adjacent domains named Cun, Guan, and Chi. As described in previous pulse research, each of the three parts corresponds to a specific inner body organ and brought different physical information [1]. Hence, the Chinese medicine practitioners used to press their index finger, middle finger, and ring finger upon the wrist of patients to feel the pulse at Cun, Guan, and Chi positions, respectively. Pulsations from the three body parts were considered for judging the health status [33].

Fig. 3.2 shows our wrist pulse system and the UI. We use the Velcro straps to fasten the pulse transducer instead of the traditional fixed support, because it is more convenient and flexible for clinical practice. The strap design also meets the further research trends of wearable devices. When acquiring subject's pulse, pulse beatings at the patient's wrist are first felt with our fingers, and the rough positions of Cun, Guan, and Chi are searched and ensured. Then, we just twine the Velcro straps around the wrist and easily adjust the positions and directions of the transducer to the right place by aligning each channel with the corresponding position. Because the pulse waveforms collected by the sensors are displayed on screen in real time as ECG, it is convenient and friendly for interaction. Further, the intervals between channels and the pulse center are subtly adjusted by the setting knobs to obtain stable pulse signals at higher amplitudes and less noise. If the optimal sampling position is ensured by watching the pulse performance in the interface, then the

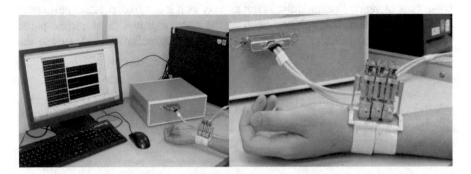

Fig. 3.2 Pulse acquisition system

Table 3.1 Fundamental working parameters of proposed system

System working parameters	Specifications
Working temperature	25±15 °C
Sampling frequency	500 Hz
Sampling time	60 s
Sensor force	1.00±1.00 N
Pressure pulse amplitude	0~3000 mV
Photoelectric pulse amplitude	0~2000 mV

pulse sensors are applied automatically with proper pressures by the step motors at the top of each channel. Therefore, pulse beatings at the wrist are felt by the sensors straight at the three body parts of Cun, Guan, and Chi. Then, we preview the collected pulse for a moment to check the signal stability. The pulse sampling phase starts following the preview stage.

During the pulse-collecting stage, subjects are required to hold a sitting position and to keep calm, which would reduce the noise caused by body movements and breathing actions. Meanwhile, the parameters and the positions of sensors are required to stay in a similar manner until the sampling procedure ends. In our experiments, pulse signals are taken from the left hand of patients uniformly. And the static contact pressures of sensors are controlled by the step motors instead of the manual operation, and thus more accurate pressure adjustment is realized. The whole collecting period lasts around 60 s for covering a complete and stable interval of multiperiod pulse. During this procedure, patients do not feel any discomfort as a result of the noninvasive approach. When collected pulse data meet the requirements of timing and quality, we stop the procedure, take down the straps, and store the database in a hard disk. The specification parameters of the proposed system are shown in Table 3.1 below. Our previous experiments have shown that this novel pulse system is robust through the repeatability and stability test.

3.2.2   Pulse Processing and Interaction Design

The sensing elements, which include 3 pressure sensors and 27 photoelectric sensors in total, constitute 3 independent sensor channels. Each channel which involves one pressure sensor and nine photoelectric sensors simulates a finger's function to feel pulse from one of the corresponding positions marked as Cun, Guan, and Chi. The sensor array in each channel response to pulse beatings and blood flowing transfers physical changes to quantitative electric signals. Pulse signals are then processed by signal amplification and filtering module, AD conversion module, and micro digital signal processing (DSP) module consequently. The digital pulse waveforms are finally sent to a computer through the USB interface for visualized operations and pulse database management.

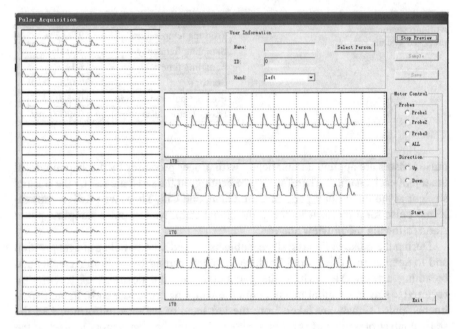

Fig. 3.3 UI of the pulse system

The software framework of pulse system involves interface-driven design, pulse control UI, and database operation. The proposed system shows digital pulse waveforms on computer screen (Fig. 3.3). Pulse signals sampled by the sensor arrays can be clearly watched in real time. The right part in the UI shows the pressure pulse signals of the three channels, and the left region of the interface gives a display of nine photoelectric signals from the channel selected. Through the operation on the graphical user interface, pulse data are then stored for further analysis in a database form, the content of which includes original pulse digital waveforms, subjects' information, channel information, sampling pressure, sampling time, and sampling rate. Meanwhile, it is also a standard template for recording quantized pulse information and related labels.

3.3   Design of the Different Sensor Arrays

The performance of the pulse system largely depends on the response of sensors. Thus, the sensor design plays an important part and makes our system distinctive compared with other previous pulse-taking platforms. Multichannel design and different sensor arrays are employed to obtain more information and standardize the sampling operations. The three independent channels correspond to the three body positions Cun, Guan, and Chi, and each channel is composed of a pressure sensor fusion with a photoelectric sensor array. The different sensor arrays complement each other to provide more features for pulse analysis.

3.3.1   Pressure Sensor

According to the previous researches, we choose traditional pressure sensor as the main sensing element in the proposed system, which is more similar in function to the physician's fingers when taking one's pulse. They sense the changes of pulse pressure at the wrist and obtain the pulsation information in the same way directly. Consequently, pressure sensor is closer to TCM in essence and easier to be understood and accepted both psychologically and in principle. The previous experiments about the pulse acquisition have shown that signals taken from these three positions do not carry identical information, because waveforms from each channel are obtained under different contact static pressure and they vary with each other in shapes and amplitudes.

Implementation of Pressure Sensor Array   Pressure sensor is a kind of widely accepted sensor to detect human pulse. It measures the changes of contact pressure upon the detector. Figure 3.4 shows the schematic representation of the pressure sensor structure. Cantilever beam is selected as the main measure elements, which presents elastic deformation when it is acted upon by a force at the free end. A contactor is placed at the bottom of this end, and an electric resistance strain gauge is laid on the top of cantilever beam. The electric resistance strain gauge changes its resistance value when deformation occurs. With this principle, we can transform the physical signals to electric signals through the interrelationship between pressure force and resistance value.

The whole operating procedure of taking pulse involves three stages: (1) The contactor is placed at the wrist upon radial artery to feel the pulse beatings with certain pressure. (2) The pulse beatings cause a periodic elastic deformation on cantilever beam as well as the strain gauge. (3) The deformation changes the resistance value of gauge and the electric lever of output signals.

In the proposed system, we select the TP2.6 series semiconductor gauge as the electric resistance strain gauge module, which has the advantage of high sensitivity and quick dynamic response. Its appearance and corresponding parameters are shown in Fig. 3.5a and Table. 3.2, respectively. It operates on the principle that the resistance of silicon-implanted piezo resistors will increase when the resistors flex

Fig. 3.4 Physic model of the pressure sensor. *1*: Fixed mount. *2*: Strain gauge. *3*: Cantilever beam. *4*: Contactor. *5*: Skin. *6*: Blood vessel

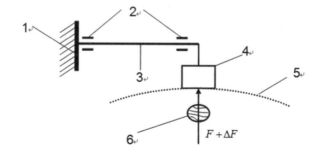

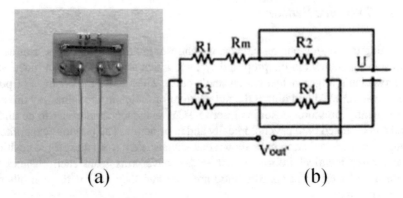

Fig. 3.5 (**a**) TP series semiconductor gauge. (**b**) Wheatstone bridge

Table 3.2 Parameters of semiconductor gauge

Gauge parameters	Specifications
Substrate size	5 mm × 3 mm
Silicon-strip size	2.5 mm × 0.2 mm × 0.04 mm
Resistance	1000 Ω
Sensitivity coefficient	150±5%K
Resistance-temperature coefficient	<0.40%per°C
Sensitivity-temperature coefficient	<0.30%per°C
Max operating temperature	80 °C
Operating current	5 mA
Ultimate strain	6000 $\mu\varepsilon$

under any applied force. The gauge is attached closely to the cantilever beam to sense its deformation and monitored with the Wheatstone bridge to transform this specific resistance change to the voltage change. In the bridge, three high-precision resistors (R2, R3, and R4) are fixed, and the strain gauge is inserted as the active resistor (R1). We add a series resistor (Rm) to compensate errors caused by temperature variations. Figure 3.5b shows the low power, unamplified, compensated Wheatstone bridge circuit design which provides inherently stable millivolt level outputs over the force range. Hence, the pulse beatings are converted into the electric signals accurately eventually.

Standardizations of Pressure Sensor Because the performance of the pulse system largely depends on the sensor specification and property, we propose several solutions to standardize the criterions of pressure sensors, including the pressure calibration and nonlinear response test. It provides information from two important aspects, the accuracy and dynamic region of the static pressure. The depth information of pulse, which is completely derived from the contact static pressure during the collecting phase, makes it necessary to develop the quantification technique accurately. For ensuring the dynamic region, we introduce a method to acquire the relationship between pressure and the signal output. Nevertheless, the contact pres-

Table 3.3 Pressure sensor standardization

Force (N)	Signal output(V)										Ave (V)
	1	2	3	4	5	6	7	8	9	10	
0.88	0.45	0.45	0.44	0.45	0.46	0.46	0.46	0.45	0.45	0.46	0.45
1.38	0.70	0.69	0.77	0.72	0.68	0.66	0.70	0.72	0.70	0.71	0.71
1.88	0.95	0.87	0.92	0.92	0.93	0.92	0.95	0.95	0.94	0.92	0.93
2.38	1.14	1.16	1.15	1.16	1.15	1.16	1.14	1.17	1.14	1.16	1.15
2.88	1.41	1.27	1.38	1.45	1.43	1.37	1.41	1.32	1.40	1.39	1.38
3.38	1.57	1.66	1.69	1.69	1.61	1.64	1.59	1.61	1.67	1.64	1.64
3.88	1.81	1.85	1.91	1.91	1.82	1.96	1.9	1.81	1.87	1.93	1.88
4.38	2.11	2.08	2.15	2.01	2.11	2.04	2.07	2.2	2.19	2.22	2.12
4.88	2.33	2.30	2.40	2.28	2.46	2.29	2.25	2.3	2.45	2.31	2.33
5.38	2.57	2.58	2.57	2.53	2.51	2.63	2.61	2.56	2.50	2.51	2.56
5.88	2.86	2.93	2.81	3.01	2.81	2.96	2.89	2.95	2.89	2.75	2.89

sure and the amplitude of pulse do not match a simple linear relationship. When the contact pressure exceeds a certain threshold, the amplitude will decrease. The related specific parameters of the proposed system and experiments results are given below.

The pressure calibration guarantees the accuracy of the pressure sensors in the proposed system. The baseline value of pulse waveform sampled by pressure sensor is influenced by the contact static pressure directly. Using the characteristic of the relationship between signal dc voltage and pressure value, we propose a standard pressure calibration procedure which is implemented in the following steps. First, we fix the sensor upside down on a platform, and then several weights are successively placed upon the sensor surface to acquire the dc voltage, and each stage is carried out for ten times to obtain the average dc level. Finally, the relationship between contact static pressures and the dc level are computed using the linear regression method.

Table 3.3 shows the outputs of a pressure sensor under different sampling pressures, and the fitting curves are obtained by fitting the pressure with dc voltage. Thus, the amplitudes of pulse baselines (dc level) are equivalently converted to the contact pressure through the one-to-one linear correspondence method.

For ensuring the dynamic linear region, we acquire the relationship between pressure and the pulse amplitude by adding contact force gradually for each channel, respectively. Results show that they do not match a simple linear relationship. When lighter contact pressure is applied, the amplitude of pulse waveform will increase when the pressure rises. If contact pressure exceeds certain value, then the amplitude will decrease. Therefore, the inflection pressure which corresponds to the pulse with highest amplitude is regarded as the upper limit of the dynamic linear region.

The proper pressure with the highest amplitude is not the same among the subjects. The experiments show that the pressure lies from 1.50 to 2.00 N when the pulse waveform reaches the max amplitude. Therefore, 2.00 N is selected as the max pressure when sampling the pulse. The amplitude and the pressure are almost

Table 3.4 Specifications of
the pressure sensor

Pressure sensor parameters	Specifications
Power	5~12 V DC
Contact force ranges	0~5.00 N
Sensitivity	24 m V/N
Ranges	60 mv~5VDC
Overload force	45 N
Linearity	± 0.1 N
Zero-drift error	± 0.5 mV
Sensitivity drift	± 1.2 m V/g

under the linear relationship when the pressure is below the extreme value. Table 3.4 gives the final specifications and parameters of the pressure sensors after the standardizations. It makes the pulse system more robust and normalized.

3.3.2   Photoelectric Sensor Array

Photoelectric sensor is selected as auxiliary sensor to detect changes of radial artery blood volume. It acquires the information of hemodynamic parameters and arterial stiffness, which makes it distinguished from the other sensor types. Consequently, photoelectric signals are regarded as a different way to obtain the information and a supplement to the pressure sensors. Because photoelectric elements are much smaller (such as charge-coupled device) in shape than the other types, it is easier to develop a high-density-integrated sensor array.

Principle of Photoelectric Sensor   Photoelectric sensor has the advantage of small size, high sensitivity, and less temperature influence. It has been widely used in the pulse oximetry system [34]. In the proposed system, a type of optical sensor known as near-infrared (NIR) light is selected as it can penetrate skin and reflect information below skin. According to the physiology foundation and our experiments, the penetration of NIR around 1000 nm is optimum for the pulse taking. Therefore, the model of 970 nm NIR sensor is chosen as the emitter. The inner structure of the photoelectric sensor is shown in Fig. 3.6. It is composed of a pair of optical emitter (NIR) and optical detector (phototransistor). The blood absorbs most of the NIR light, and the reflected light changes as the blood flow of the radial artery changes. Thus, we use this feature to transform the pulse flow into electric signals.

Motivation of Photoelectric Sensor Array   We designed a sensor array to enlarge the sensing area. Each array consists of nine photoelectric emitters and nine photoelectric detectors, which makes the number of sensing unit up to nine. As shown in Fig. 3.7, the sensor pairs are laid in two longitudinal rows with a light barrier in the middle. At the left side, we place nine photoelectric emitters with equidistant intervals of about 1 mm. The arrangement of emitters and detectors are set in a one-to-one relationship symmetrically.

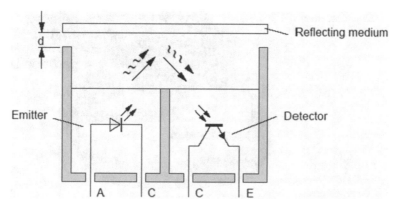

Fig. 3.6 Principle of the photoelectric sensor

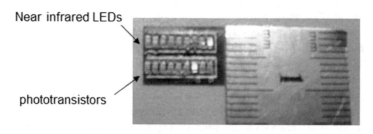

Fig. 3.7 Top view of photoelectric sensor array and the real object

At the pulse-collecting phase, each photoelectric sensor pair which involves one emitter and one detector works almost independently with the other sensors in the array. The motivation of this design belongs to the factor that radial artery varies in width among subjects and can be covered by nine sensor pairs in a lateral direction (Fig. 3.8). We define this feature as pulse width and add it into the feature space.

Moreover, the design of sensor array is also introduced for the requirement of ensuring pulse location. A wide coverage sensor array guarantees that the center of pulse is always under control and can be easily confirmed by comparing the amplitudes of pulse signals from the nine sensors of the array. Then, we adjust sensor probe in the horizontal direction to make sure that the center of pulse signal with highest amplitude is collected by the sensor in the middle of array.

3.3.3   Combination of Pressure and Photoelectric Sensor Arrays

Either of these two sensor types has its own characteristic. The pressure sensor which measures changes of throb force from the radial artery also acquires the information of pulse depth. The probe with three channels placed on the

Fig. 3.8 Simple schematic
diagram of array placement

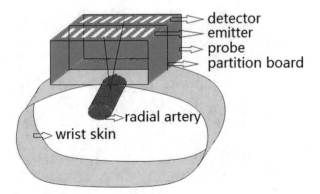

corresponding locations of wrist is applied with different external pressure which varies not only from individual to individual but also with the three positions to obtain an excellent pulse waveform. According to TCPD, the depth of pulse was always an important physiological manifestation and classified into three patterns named Fu, Zhong, and Chen. Each pattern represents a certain physical status in TCM. Naturally, this unique information that cannot be extracted from other non-pressure sensor types has been introduced into the proposed system to enrich the feature space. Our experiments have shown that it improves the final performance.

The photoelectric sensor which has the advantage of small size and high sensitivity is selected as subchannel in the proposed system. It provides another visualized way to feel the pulse in comparison with the pressure sensor as it detects the change of blood flow at the radial artery. To ensure the right position of pulse, we introduce the array design to cover the region. Besides, the information of pulse width, which reflects the degree of radial artery stenosis, is also obtained as it varies in amplitude with each sensor in the array. Considering these two sensor types with irreplaceable use value, fusion is adopted for this issue.

Different Sensor Arrays Fusion Principle Figure 3.9 shows the sensor fusion structure that is implemented in our system. The pressure and photoelectric sensors are integrated in a two-lever cantilever beam to combine their respective merits. There is a light-proof box containing a photoelectric sensor array at the bottom, and on the upside, a strain gauge is attached to acquire the contact pressure to the skin. These sensor elements are surrounded by metal shell.

The pulse-sampling principle is shown in Fig. 3.10. The photoelectric sensors which lie at the bottom receive reflected NIR light from the blood vessel directly. Meanwhile, the force sensor acquires the pressure variation of the radial artery under the skin transferred from the cantilever framework. Consequently, both of these two sensor types are compatible in the proposed system and collect pulse simultaneously.

Architectural Structure of Multichannel System Figure 3.11 shows the overall structure of the novel pulse probe with three channels. There are nine adjustable knobs in total, which are grouped into three directions. And every single channel is controlled by three of the knobs from each direction, respectively. We assume that

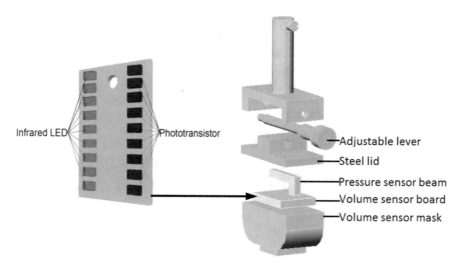

Fig. 3.9 Combination of pressure and photoelectric sensors

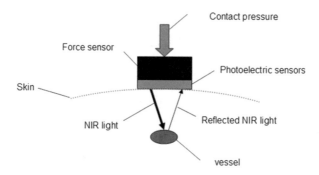

Fig. 3.10 Principle of the fusion sensors

there is a coordinate system. Step motors are applied in Z-axis direction to adjust the height of sensor arrays which reflects the contact pressure, while the distance among three channels is controlled by the Y-axis direction knobs to ensure the right positions of Cun, Guan, and Chi. The knobs in the X-axis direction guarantee that the center of pulse and the middle of photoelectric sensor array just coincide.

3.4   Multichannel Optimization

Pulse waveform acquired from multichannels brings more information than that from single-point transducer due to the complementarities. However, there is an inherent trade-off between channels and benefits. The increase is not satisfied just by adding more channels to the transducer, as uncorrelated or noised channels are

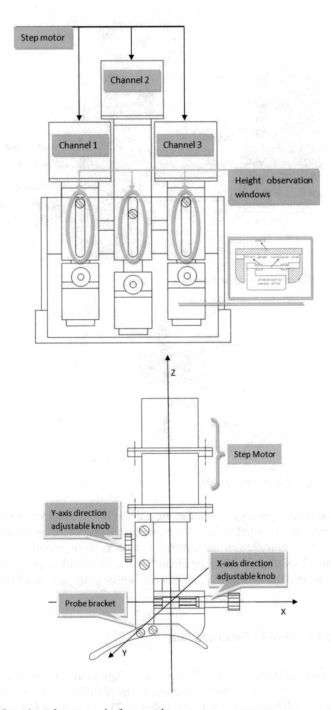

Fig. 3.11 Overview of sensor probe framework

bound to affect the performance. Therefore, the first proposed multichannel optimization, equal to the decision of pulse-taking positions, is developed through the experimental verification. It mainly consists of three steps, the Guan pulse with high SNR and stability is first selected as the reference. Then multiple linear regression is applied to compare the correlation relationship between the pulse of other channels and the Guan channel. Finally, the optimal selection of the channels is obtained based on the information measurement criterion.

3.4.1 Selection of Base Channel

Despite more than three positions at the wrist are available for pulse taking, standard Chinese pulse diagnosis is always limited to the Cun, Guan, and Chi, which are confirmed by experiences. In order to ensure the convincing pulse-taking positions at the wrist along the radial artery, we extend the three-point sensing into five-channel sensing. Figure 3.12 displays the candidate pulse-taking positions. Besides the traditional Cun, Guan, and Chi three points in TCM theory, we add another two positions alongside them which are named as 4th point and 5th point for convenience. The other positions at the wrist out of this area are not chosen, where one can hardly feel any pulsations as the radial artery goes deeper.

Figure 3.13 shows the coarse pulse signals without preprocessing, which are taken from the five candidate positions of one subject simultaneously. Waveforms from most of the channels are similar in shape except the channel-5, pulse signals of which are seriously corrupted by noises, baseline drift and outliers. Fig. 3.14 presents the partial enlarged view of an interval. The pulse signals are aligned and placed in one coordinate for comparison. It is obvious that pulse from channel-2 has the best performance with the highest amplitudes in contrast with the other four channels. And pulse from channel-5, which has the lowest amplitudes of all, almost

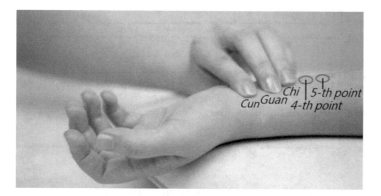

Fig. 3.12 The five candidate pulse-taking channels before optimization

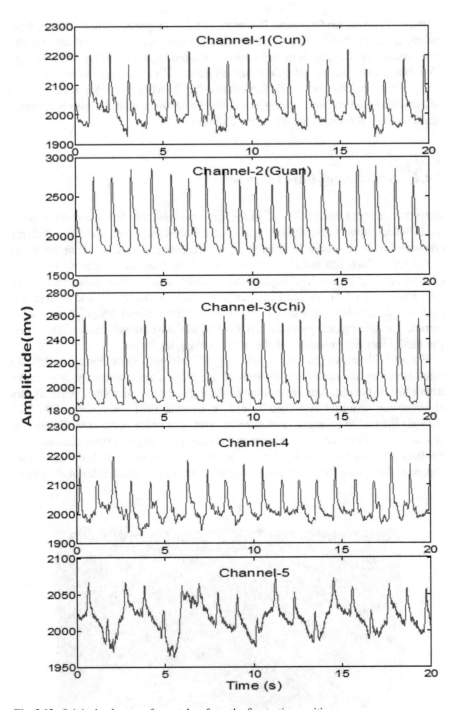

Fig. 3.13 Original pulse waveforms taken from the five testing positions

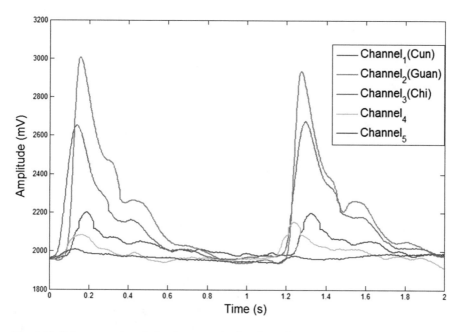

Fig. 3.14 Pulse comparison in details among the five channels

moves in a straight line. It is known that amplitude is the manifestation of energy, which determines the capacity to resist noises and remain stable.

Thus, the evaluation criterions, including signal-to-noise ratio (SNR) and pulse stability, are employed to measure the signal quality. Since the pulse information is concentrated in the low-frequency bands less than 10 Hz, signals are decomposed into signal and noise parts through a low-pass filter with 10 Hz cutoff frequency. SNR is defined as the ratio of the energy of pulse spectral graphs below 10 Hz to that above 10 Hz by the formula below.

$$\text{SNR}_{dB^4} = 10\log_{10}\left(\frac{P_{\text{signal}}}{P_{\text{noise}}}\right) \tag{3.1}$$

where P is the average power and the variance of the signal and noise are calculated as the signal energy and noise energy.

Pulse waveform is a typical periodic signal with similar shape in each cycle. Therefore, self-similarity is introduced to evaluate the pulse stability. Pulse from each channel is regarded as an independent class, and the segmented single-period pulse signals are for the elements of each class. In this chapter, the period segmentation is performed by using the adaptive sliding window method [35].

Suppose that we have segmented a set of N single-period signals, organized in a matrix $X_j = \left[\vec{x}_{1j},,,\vec{x}_{2j},,,\cdots,,,\vec{x}_{Nj}\right]$ for j_{th} channel. Figure 3.15 shows the normalized single-period pulse signals which are acquired from the five channels of a healthy subject within one sampling period. Each $\vec{x}_{ij}$ is normalized to the same length and

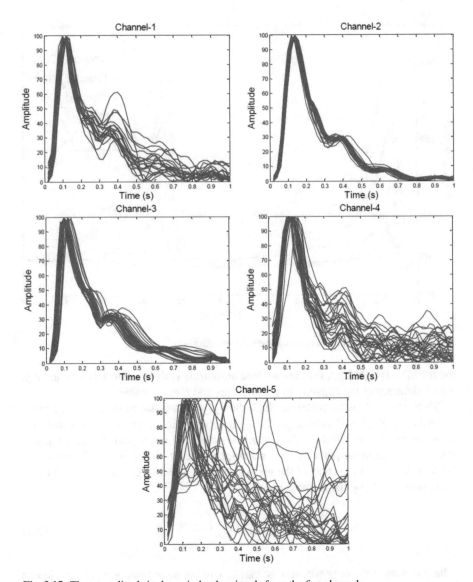

Fig. 3.15   The normalized single-period pulse signals from the five channels

amplitude. The self-similarity is then transformed into the form of inner-class divergence defined by the formulas below:

$$\vec{m}_j = \frac{1}{N} \sum_{i-1}^{N} \vec{x}_{ij}, j = 1, 2, \cdots, 5 \tag{3.2}$$

$$S_j = \frac{1}{N} \sum_{1-i}^{N} \left(\vec{x}_{ij} - \vec{m}_j \right) \left(\vec{x}_{ij} - \vec{x}_j \right)^T . \tag{3.3}$$

The subscript j is a mark of channel. The vector $\vec{x}_{ij}$ stands for the i-th single-period pulse of the j-th channel. And j m is the average single-period waveform of the j-th channel. The intra-class scatter matrix is defined by the matrix S_j, which measures the cluster degree. In general, single-period waveforms have high correlations with each other in the same channel. Inspired by the PCA method, we decompose the matrix S_j into the diagonal matrix.

$$S_j = P_j diag\left(\lambda_{j1},\lambda_{j2},\cdots\lambda_{jn},0,\cdots0\right)P_j^{-1},\qquad(3.4)$$

$$s_w^j = \prod_{i=1,2,\cdots,n} \lambda_{ji},\qquad(3.5)$$

where λ_{ji} is the nonzero eigenvalues of the matrix S_j. We define the dispersion measure s_w^j by multiplying λ_{ji} of each matrix S_j, repectively. As S_j is a positive definite matrix, there exists $\lambda_{ji}>0$. A more concentrated set will result in a smaller dispersion measure value.

We collect 465 pulse samples from 465 subjects in total with the proposed system. The average criterion results are shown in Table 3.5. Pulse signal with the highest SNR is obtained from channel-2 (Guan), and the intra-class distance is the smallest among the five channels. The signal energy and SNR gradually degrades in the other channels, since radial artery goes deeper apart from the Guan region. The signal energy of channel-5 is less than 1% of that of channel-2, resulting in the lowest SNR of all. Therefore, pulse waveform from channel-2 (Guan) is selected as the basic component. Figure 3.15 also illustrates that segmented single-period pulses from Guan stay in a more compact state. By contrast, pulses of channel-5 are easily disturbed by noise and stay in a chaotic state.

3.4.2   Multichannel Selection

The second stage is the multichannel selection. Pulse signals from multichannels are compared with the selected Guan pulse to select the channels with significant improvement. We intend to give an explanation about the reason why pulse should be taken at the Cun, Guan, and Chi three positions.

Single-period waveforms of Guan channel are selected and regarded as the reference. We randomly select half of them as base set, and the other part is regarded as

Table 3.5 Evaluation among the five channels

Channel	1	2	3	4	5
S_w	77.4	68.1	87.3	140.1	159.1
Signal energy	2.99e+07	7.17e+08	3.64e+08	1.78e+07	1.79e+06
Noise energy	1.04e+05	5.58e+05	7.99e+05	7.10e+04	1.34e+04
SNR(dB)	24.6	31.1	26.6	23.9	21.2

validation set. The base set is written as $X = [\vec{x}_1, \vec{x}_2, \cdots, \vec{x}_n]$. Each single-period waveform $\vec{x} = [\vec{x}_{i1}, \vec{x}_{i2}, \cdots, \vec{x}_{iL}]^T$ is normalized to the same length and amplitude. Then the multi-regression method is introduced to calculate the errors between fitting sets and the bases. For each fitting sample $\vec{y} = [\vec{y}_{i1}, \vec{y}_{i2}, \cdots, \vec{y}_{iL}]^T$, it is assumed to be generated by the following model:

$$\vec{y}_j = X\vec{\beta} + \vec{e}. \tag{3.6}$$

A generalized version of equation (6) is to find $\vec{\beta}$ such that the following objective function is minimized:

$$f(\vec{y}_j) = \min_{\vec{\beta}} \left\| \vec{y}_j - X\vec{\beta} \right\|_2. \tag{3.7}$$

Multi-regression approach is proposed for learning the optimal value for $\vec{\beta}$. The related algorithms are included in the toolbox of MATLAB.

Thus, the errors between fitting sets and bases are calculated. Through selecting proper error margins, we classify the single-period waveforms of the fitting sets into three patterns. The first pattern contains pulses represented by the reference (training samples from Guan channel) with little error. The second class is for pulses with additional information which are expected. The last pattern stands for the contaminated pulses.

The validation set is recognized as bringing no additional information as a result of the high correlations with base set. The maximum fitting errors of the validation set is defined as the lower limit of information threshold:

$$C_1 = \max_{\vec{y}_j \in \text{Channel}-2} f(\vec{y}_j). \tag{3.8}$$

If the fitting error of $\vec{y}_j$ is below C_1, it means that $\vec{y}_j$ belongs to the first pattern and brings no additional information.

The upper limit of the threshold is defined by the average fitting error among fitting sets:

$$C_2 = \frac{1}{M} \sum_{j=1}^{M} f(\vec{y}_j). \tag{3.9}$$

If the fitting error of $\vec{y}_j$ is bigger than C_2, it means that $\vec{y}_j$ belongs to the third class and brings no improvements to the pulse analysis. Fitting sets belonging to the second class are considered as bringing complementary information.

The fitting errors of fitting sets of a certain subject are shown in Fig. 3.16. The ratio of pulses belonging to the second class at each channel is defined as pulse information measure. It can be seen that fitting sets with errors between C_1 and C_2

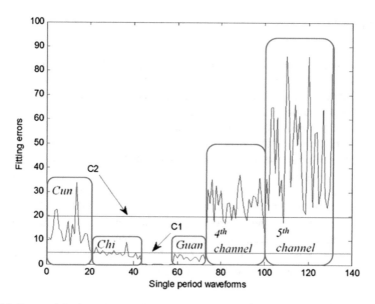

Fig. 3.16 Errors of single-period waveforms fitting to the basis

Table 3.6 Evaluation among the fitting sets

Channel	Cun	Chi	4	5
Information measure	79.0%	54.2%	24.1%	3.4%
Intra-class distance	59.1	54.5	64.0	103.1
Correlation coefficient	0.92	0.94	0.89	0.72

are mostly concentrated in Cun and Chi channel, which means that these two channels bring most of the pulse information. The fitting errors of the 4th channel and 5th channel exceed the threshold C_2, which demonstrate that pulse signals of these two channels are buried in the noises.

Table 3.6 presents the statistical results of pulse information measure, intra-class distance and correlation coefficient of the four channels compared with bases. The Cun and Chi channel are with information ratios up to 80% and 55%, respectively. The information ratio of Chi channel is lower than that of Cun channel as a result of the high correlation up to 0.94, which indicates that many fitting sets of Chi are classified into the first class with no additional information. The information ratios of channel-4 and channel-5 are less than 25%. Since the fitting sets from these two channels have low correlation and large intra-class distance, resulting in large fitting errors to the base set. Therefore, the Cun and Chi channel besides Guan are selected as the optimal channels for pulse taking based on the fitting evaluation. The result of multichannel optimization is also consistent with the significance of Cun, Guan, and Chi in TCM theory.

3.5   The Optimization of Different Sensors Fusion

The second improvement is the sensor fusion design. The motivation is to combine the advantages of pressure sensor and photoelectric sensor array. The pressure sensor, which detects the pressure changes at the wrist, obtains the pulsations directly. And the photoelectric sensor penetrates skin and reflects the blood information below skin. The fusion sensor acquires the pulse waveforms by different means. Therefore, not only the pulse rate, pulse width, and oxygen saturation are detected by the photoelectric sensor arrays, but also the shape and pulse depth are acquired by the pressure sensors.

The proposed system is composed of three independent channels corresponding to Cun, Guan, and Chi three positions. Nine sub-signals, photoelectric pulse, and one main signal, pressure pulse, are acquired simultaneously at each channel. It is necessary to reduce the data dimensions and to combine the features from different type of sensors. Since the pulse from Cun, Guan, and Chi bring supplementary information, the data dimension reduction is performed at each channel, respectively.

Since the pulse features from array signals are redundant due to the high correlations, we extract a representation of the array signals at each channel. The algorithm is described by the formulas as below:

$$\vec{x}_i \left[x_{i1}, x_{i2}, \cdots x_{iN} \right]^T, \vec{u} = \frac{1}{9} \sum_{i=1}^{9} \vec{x}_i, \tag{3.10}$$

$$S_w = \frac{1}{9} \sum_{i=1}^{9} \left(\vec{x}_i - \vec{u} \right) \left(\vec{x}_i - \vec{u} \right)^T. \tag{3.11}$$

The vector $\vec{x}_i$ denotes to the array signals with N sampling points. Matrix S_w denotes to the total scatter matrix of array signals.

$$\begin{aligned}
e_i &= \left\| \left(\vec{x}_i - \vec{u} \right) - \phi_1 \phi_1^T \left(\vec{x}_i - \vec{u} \right) \right\|_2 \\
&= \sqrt{ \left(\vec{x}_i - \vec{u} \right)^T \left(\vec{x}_i - \vec{u} \right) - \phi_1^T \left(\vec{x}_i - \vec{u} \right)^T \left(\vec{x}_i - \vec{u} \right) \phi_1 }. \\
&= \sqrt{ \left\| \vec{x}_i - \vec{u} \right\|_2^2 - \left\| \phi_1^T \left(\vec{x}_i - \vec{u} \right) \right\|_2^2 }
\end{aligned} \tag{3.12}$$

And ϕ_1 is the unit principal vector of S_w. The residual error vector $\left(\vec{x}_i - \vec{u} \right)$ is projected onto the principal vector ϕ_1, and e_i is defined as the projection error, which stands for the pulse energy deviating from the principal direction. Therefore, the most representative signal $\vec{y}$ of each array is determined by selecting the array signal $\vec{x}_i$ with the least value e_i:

$$\vec{y} = \underset{\vec{x}_1}{\arg \min} \sqrt{ \left\| \vec{x}_i - \vec{u}_2^2 \right\| - \left\| \phi_1^T \left(\vec{x}_i - \vec{u} \right) \right\|_2^2 }. \tag{3.13}$$

The simplified e_i consists of two parts. The vector $(\bar{x}_i - \bar{u})$ describes the similarity between array signal and the average, and $\phi_1^T (\bar{x}_i - \bar{u})$ denotes to the projection of the residual error on unit principal vector. In general, the pulse with the highest amplitudes is selected as it contributes the most to the principal vector. The array selection is performed to keep more pulse information and remove the redundant array signals.

Finally, pulse waveforms from 30 sensors are reduced to 6 signals. Each channel includes one pressure signal and one representative photoelectric signal. Pulse features extracted from the six signals are combined to form a feature vector in a serial strategy. The subscript pr_i and ph_i denotes to pressure and photoelectric pulse signal of i-th channel, respectively.

$$f = \begin{bmatrix} f_{pr1} f_{ph1} f_{pr2} f_{ph2} f_{pr3} f_{ph3} \end{bmatrix}$$
$$f_{pr/ph} = \begin{bmatrix} \vec{f}_{amp} \vec{f}_{fre} \vec{f}_{pca} \end{bmatrix}$$

$$(3.14)$$

The features of amplitudes, frequencies, and PCA components are extracted in our experiments. The pulse amplitudes reflect the energy information, and the frequencies describe the pulse period variance. We normalize the segmented single-period pulse waveforms of each subject to the same scale, calculate the eigenvectors and eigenvalues, and sort the eigenvectors by contribution degree. The first five eigenvectors and eigenvalues are selected as PCA features. The feature vector extracted from each signal contains 262 elements. And the fusion feature is 1572-dimension for one subject.

3.6 Experimental Results

Our goal is to compare the system performances before and after optimization. The experiments are performed on pulse database of healthy subjects and patients known to be afflicted with diabetes. Clinical medical studies demonstrated that the loss of arterial elasticity and endothelial function caused by certain disease such as diabetes results in decrease flexibility of vasculature and heightened stress to the circulatory system [36]. Many researches [12, 13, 35–39] have been published on this issue, which attracts increasing attentions.

In total, we collected 250 pulse samples from 125 healthy subjects and 125 diabetes patients, respectively. The database is built in Prince of Wales Hospital, Hong Kong. All patients were inpatient volunteers from the Hospital. The labels of the subjects are determined according to the recent health check. For each subject, the 3 pressure pulse and 27 photoelectric pulse from Cun, Guan, and Chi were acquired as one pulse sample. The distribution of the pulse database is ensured to avoid the influence caused by biological inter-patient variability. Table 3.7 lists the organization of the dataset. The age, BMI, and gender distribution are similar between healthy and diabetes patients.

Table 3.7 Data organization

	Age distribution			BMI distribution			Gender distribution	
	30~50	50~60	60~80	<20	20~50	>25	Female	Male
Healthy	30	47	48	4	83	38	51	74
Diabetes	57	91	102	6	161	83	103	147

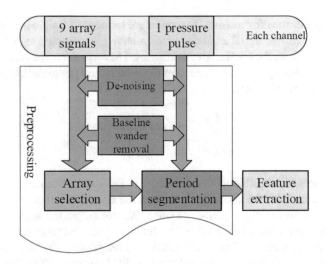

Fig. 3.17 The signal processing stage at each channel

Figure 3.17 shows the signal preprocessing stage before feature extraction. The original pressure pulse and array signals of each channel are preprocessed by the denoising, baseline drift removal, and period segmentation models sequentially. The array selection is used to obtain the most representative signal from the nine array signals. Then the fusion pulse features are extracted in the selected set. Next, the feature dimension is reduced by projecting the serial fusion features onto the PCA subspace. Last, SVM classifier is applied to predict the patterns of the testing samples. To reduce the influence caused by sample partitioning, the fivefold cross validation is employed in our experiments. We randomly divide the samples of each pattern into five equal folds. Each fold contains 25 different samples and each sample only belongs to one fold. In each cross validation, four folds are for training and the left for testing. The classification accuracy is obtained by averaging recognition rates of the fivefold cross experiments.

3.6.1   Experiment 1

In the first experiment, the performance between single-type sensors and fusion sensor is compared. The pulse at Cun, Guan, and Chi acquired by pressure sensor, photoelectric sensor, and fusion sensor are used to distinguish the healthy subjects

Table 3.8 Classification results of the sensors fusion

Channel	Before optimization		After optimization
	Pressure sensor (%)	Photoelectric sensors (%)	Fusion sensors (%)
Cun	77.2	58.4	77.6
Guan	85.2	63.6	85.6
Chi	72.8	56.4	76.8

from the diabetes patients, respectively. The classification results are shown in Table 3.8. It can be seen that pressure pulse is superior to photoelectric pulse in diabetes diagnosis, and pulse acquired from Guan channel achieves higher classification accuracy than that from the other two channels. That is why the former pulse acquisition platforms are generally designed by pressure sensor with single Guan channel. An accuracy of 85.2% is obtained in Guan position just by using pressure pulse features, and the recognition rate reaches 85.6% by extracting the fusion features of pressure and photoelectric pulse from Guan channel. Similarly, the performance of Cun channel increases to 77.6% by using the pulse from fusion sensors. The improvements of sensor fusion in Cun and Guan channels are not obvious as that in Chi channel. Because the photoelectric array design, which provides spatial information for pulse locations, guarantees the high quality of pressure pulse signals. However, the pressure pulse from Chi position are often unavailable due to the weak pulsations. Then the photoelectric signals provide significant supplements to the pressure pulses in Chi channel. Hence, the accuracy of fusion sensors at Chi channel is increased by 4%. The other reason is that, in the case of serial feature fusion at each channel, the dimension of feature vector is redoubled, and the accuracy estimation of principal vector is more difficult. Due to the dimensional increase and high correlation after feature fusion, estimation accuracy of PCA subspace is decreased and noise information is also increased. That is why the serial feature fusion strategy at Cun and Guan channel underperforms in this experiment. Conversely, the array pulses at Chi channel contains information which are not able to be detected by pressure sensors. This may be the key reason why sensor fusion at Chi channel outperforms the other channels in information fusion problems.

3.6.2 Experiment 2

In the second experiment, the performances of multichannel combination are compared. There are seven possible channel combinations: Cun, Guan, Chi, Cun plus Guan, Cun plus Chi, Guan plus Chi, and three channels. We do the experiment based on two sets of original pulse feature vectors: 262-dimensional pressure feature and 262-dimensional photoelectric feature. The fusion features of each candidate combination group are extracted.

Table 3.9 gives the classification results. The classification rate of single channel pulse reaches the best accuracy of 85.6% in the Guan channel. The performance is similar to the previous classification results of system with single channel [40, 21].

Table 3.9 Classification results of the multichannel

	Channel combination	Classification accuracy
Before optimization	Cun	77.6%
	Guan	85.6%
	Chi	7.8%
After optimization	Cun+Guan	90%
	Cun+Chi	84.8%
	Guan+Chi	88.4%
	Cun+Guan+Chi	91.6%

It demonstrates that the proposed system obtains quality pulse for diagnosis. The classification accuracy is significantly increased by using the pulses from two channels or three channels. The best accuracy of 91.6% is achieved by combining the pressure pulse features and array pulse features from all of the three channels. A ratio of 6% increase is obtained compared with the best performance of using single channel. The optimal design of multichannel is verified in this experiment, which implies that pulse from different channels bring complementary information. Based on the results of Experiments 1 and 2, we can draw the following conclusion:

- The classification accuracy is significantly increased after optimization.
- The performance of the proposed system is improved after channel combination, which demonstrate the "three regions and nine divisions" criterion in TCM clinical science.

3.7 Summary

This chapter proposes a novel wrist pulse system with multichannel design and different sensor arrays, which has broad applications in medicine diagnosis such as the healthy condition evaluation and the disease analysis. The framework of the system, pressure and photoelectric sensor design, novel array structure, and signal processing procedure are introduced. The optimization of the fusion strategy is discussed. Related experiments on diabetes diagnosis are developed to test the system ability and the accuracy is increased significantly after optimization. The experimental results demonstrate that the proposed system is better or at least not worse than the previous pulse acquisition platforms.

The novel design of our system mainly consists of two aspects, i.e., multichannel and sensor arrays. Each part is well analyzed and brings contributions to the whole system. The system is of practical applications in auxiliary diagnosis for patients who are suffering from diabetes. Compared with the traditional blood test, it has the advantages of no pain, no injection, and convenience, which is more acceptable in daily health monitoring.

References

1. B. Flaws, The Secret of Chinese Pulse Diagnosis. Boulder, CO, USA: Blue Poppy Enterprises, Inc., 1995.
2. M. Broffman and M. McCulloch, "Instrument-assisted pulse evaluation in the acupuncture practice," Amer. J. Acupuncture, vol. 14, no. 3, pp. 255–259, 1986.
3. C. T. Lee and L. Y. Wei, "Spectrum analysis of human pulse," IEEE Trans. Biomed. Eng., vol. BME-30, no. 6, pp. 348–352, Jun. 1983.
4. A.-B. Liu, P.-C. Hsu, Z.-L. Chen, and H.-T. Wu, "Measuring pulse wave velocity using ECG and photoplethysmography," J. Med. Syst., vol. 35, no. 5, pp. 771–777, Oct. 2011.
5. M. Saito, M. Matsukawa, T. Asada, and Y. Watanabe, "Noninvasive assessment of arterial stiffness by pulse wave analysis," IEEE Trans. Ultrason., Ferroelectr., Freq. Control, vol. 59, no. 11, pp. 2411–2419, Nov. 2012.
6. P. Dupuis and C. Eugène, "Combined detection of respiratory and cardiac rhythm disorders by high-resolution differential cuff pressure measurement," IEEE Trans. Instrum. Meas., vol. 49, no. 3, pp. 498–502, Jun. 2000.
7. J. M. Kang, T. Yoo, and H. C. Kim, "A wrist-worn integrated health monitoring instrument with a tele-reporting device for telemedicine and telecare," IEEE Trans. Instrum. Meas., vol. 55, no. 5, pp. 1655–1661, Oct. 2006.
8. H. M. Haqqani, J. B. Morton, and J. M. Kalman, "Using the 12-lead ECG to localize the origin of atrial and ventricular tachycardias: Part 2—Ventricular tachycardia," J. Cardiovascular Electrophysiol., vol. 20, no. 7, pp. 825–832, 2009.
9. K. Humphreys, T. Ward, and C. Markham, "Noncontact simultaneous dual wavelength photoplethysmography: A further step toward noncontact pulse oximetry," Rev. Sci. Instrum., vol. 78, no. 4, pp. 044304-1–044304-6, 2007.
10. C.-C. Tyan, S.-H. Liu, J.-Y. Chen, J.-J. Chen, and W.-M. Liang, "A novel noninvasive measurement technique for analyzing the pressure pulse waveform of the radial artery," IEEE Trans. Biomed. Eng., vol. 55, no. 1, pp. 288–297, Jan. 2008.
11. L. Xu, D. Zhang, K. Wang, and L. Wang, "Arrhythmic pulses detection using Lempel–Ziv complexity analysis," EURASIP J. Adv. Signal Process., vol. 2006, p. 018268, Mar. 2006.
12. W. C. Tang and H. J. Sun, "The detected method of multipath of pulse conditions and research of transducer," Chin. J. Traditional Med. Sci. Technol., vol. 7, no. 5, pp. 319–320, 2000.
13. L. Xu, K. Wang, and D. Zhang, "Modern research on traditional Chinese pulse diagnosis," Eur. J. Oriental Med., vol. 4, no. 6, pp. 46–54, 2004.
14. K. Amano, H. Kasahara, H. Ishiyama, and K. Kodama, "Diagnostic apparatus for analyzing arterial pulse waves," U.S. Patent US6 767 329 B2, Jul. 27, 2002.
15. J. P. Jaeb, D. W. Gilstad, and R. L. Branstetter, "Optical sensor for pulse oximeter," U.S. Patent US4 880 304 A, Nov. 14, 1989.
16. L. S. Lovinsky, "Urgent problems of metrological assurance of optical pulse oximetry," IEEE Trans. Instrum. Meas., vol. 55, no. 3, pp. 869–875, Jun. 2006.
17. T. Kageyama, M. Kabuto, T. Kaneko, and N. Nishikido, "Accuracy of pulse rate variability parameters obtained from finger plethysmogram: A comparison with heart rate variability parameters obtained from ECG," J. Occupat. Health, vol. 39, no. 2, pp. 154–155, 1997.
18. M. R. Neuman, "Measurement of blood pressure [tutorial]," IEEE Pulse, vol. 2, no. 2, pp. 39–44, Mar./Apr. 2011.
19. M. Toda and M. L. Thompson, "Contact-type vibration sensors using curved clamped PVDF film," IEEE Sensors J., vol. 6, no. 5, pp. 1170–1177, Oct. 2006.
20. T. T. Selvan and M. S. Begum, "Nadi aridhal: A pulse based automated diagnostic system," in Proc. 3rd Int. Conf. Electron. Comput. Technol. (ICECT), Apr. 2011, pp. 305–308.
21. P. Wang, W. Zuo, and D. Zhang, "A compound pressure signal acquisition system for multichannel wrist pulse signal analysis," IEEE Trans. Instrum. Meas., vol. 63, no. 6, pp. 1556–1565, Jun. 2012.

22. C.-S. Hu, Y.-F. Chung, C.-C. Yeh, and C.-H. Luo, "Temporal and spatial properties of arterial pulsation measurement using pressure sensor array," Evidence-Based Complementary Alternative Med., vol. 2012, pp. 1–9, May 2011, Art. ID 745127.
23. E. Kaniusas et al., "Method for continuous nondisturbing monitoring of blood pressure by magnetoelastic skin curvature sensor and ECG," IEEE Sensors J., vol. 6, no. 3, pp. 819–828, Jun. 2006.
24. M. R. Ram, K. V. Madhav, E. H. Krishna, N. R. Komalla, and K. A. Reddy, "A novel approach for motion artifact reduction in PPG signals based on AS-LMS adaptive filter," IEEE Trans. Instrum. Meas., vol. 61, no. 5, pp. 1445–1457, May 2012.
25. K. Q. Wang, L. S. Xu, L. Wang, Z. G. Li, and Y. Z. Li, "Pulse baseline wander removal using wavelet approximation," in Proc. Comput. Cardiol., Sep. 2003, pp. 605–608.
26. L. Xu, D. Zhang, and K. Wang, "Wavelet-based cascaded adaptive filter for removing baseline drift in pulse waveforms," IEEE Trans. Biomed. Eng., vol. 52, no. 11, pp. 1973–1975, Nov. 2005.
27. L. Xu, K. Wang, and D. Zhang, "Modern researches on pulse waveform of TCPD," in Proc. IEEE Int. Conf. Commun., Circuits, Syst. West Sino Expo., Jun./Jul. 2002, pp. 1073–1077.
28. L. S. Xu, K. Q. Wang, and L. Wang, "Pulse waveforms classification based on wavelet network," in Proc. IEEE-EMBS 27th Annu. Int. Conf. Eng. Med. Biol. Soc., Jan. 2006, pp. 4596–4599.
29. L. Wang, K.-Q. Wang, and L.-S. Xu, "Recognizing wrist pulse waveforms with improved dynamic time warping algorithm," in Proc. Int. Conf. Mach. Learn. Cybern., Aug. 2004, pp. 3644–3649.
30. M. F. O'Rourke, A. Pauca, and X.-J. Jiang, "Pulse wave analysis," Brit. J. Clin. Pharmacol., vol. 51, no. 6, pp. 507–522, 2001.
31. L. Wang, K. Q. Wang, and L. S. Xu, "Lempel–Ziv decomposition based arrhythmic pulses recognition," in Proc. 27th Int. Conf. IEEE Eng. Med. Biol. Soc., Shanghai, China, Sep. 2005, pp. 4606–4609.
32. L. Wang, K. Q. Wang, and L. S. Xu, "Lempel–Ziv decomposition based arrhythmic pulses recognition," in Proc. IEEE-EMBS 27th Annu. Int. Conf. Eng. Med. Biol. Soc., Jan. 2006, pp. 4606–4609.
33. S. Lukman, Y. He, and S.-C. Hui, "Computational methods for traditional Chinese medicine: A survey," Comput. Methods Programs Biomed., vol. 88, no. 3, pp. 283–294, Dec. 2007.
34. M. Nitzan and H. Taitelbaum, "The measurement of oxygen saturation in arterial and venous blood," IEEE Instrum. Meas. Mag., vol. 11, no. 3, pp. 9–15, Jun. 2008.
35. M. Nitzan, "Automatic noninvasive measurement of arterial blood pressure," IEEE Instrum. Meas. Mag., vol. 14, no. 1, pp. 32–37, Feb. 2011.
36. L. Xu, K. Wang, D. Zhang, Y. Li, Z. Wan, and J. Wang, "Objectifying researches on traditional Chinese pulse diagnosis," Inform. Med. Slovenica, vol. 8, no. 1, pp. 56–63, 2003.
37. X. Lisheng, W. Kuanquan, D. Zhang, and S. Cheng, "Adaptive baseline wander removal in the pulse waveform," in Proc. 15th IEEE Symp. Comput.-Based Med. Syst. (CBMS), Jun. 2002, pp. 143–148.
38. A. J. Joshi, S. Chandran, V. K. Jayaraman, and B. D. Kulkarni, "Multifractality in arterial pulse," in Proc. 19th Int. Conf. Pattern Recognit. (ICPR), Dec. 2008, pp. 1–4.
39. K.-Q. Wang, L.-S. Xu, D. Zhang, and C. Shi, "TCPD based pulse monitoring and analyzing," in Proc. Int. Conf. Mach. Learn. Cybern., 2002, pp. 1366–1370.
40. Y. Chen, L. Zhang, D. Zhang, and D. Zhang, "Wrist pulse signal diagnosis using modified Gaussian models and fuzzy C-means classification," Med. Eng. Phys., vol. 31, no. 10, pp. 1283–1289, 2009.

Part III
Pulse Signal Preprocessing

Chapter 4
Baseline Wander Correction in Pulse Waveforms Using Wavelet-Based Cascaded Adaptive Filter

Abstract Quantifying pulse diagnosis is to acquire and record pulse waveforms by a set of sensor firstly and then analyze these pulse waveforms. However, respiration and artifact motion during pulse waveform acquisition can introduce baseline drift. It is necessary, therefore, to remove the pulse waveform's baseline drift in order to perform accurate pulse waveform analysis. This chapter presents a wavelet-based cascaded adaptive filter (CAF) to remove the baseline drift of pulse waveform. To evaluate the level of baseline drift, we introduce a criterion: energy ratio (ER) of pulse waveform to its baseline drift. If the ER is more than a given threshold, the baseline drift can be removed only by cubic spline estimation; otherwise it must be filtered by, in sequence, discrete Meyer wavelet filter and the cubic spline estimation. Compared with traditional methods such as cubic spline estimation, morphology filter, and linear-phase finite impulse response (FIR) least-squares-error digital filter, the experimental results on 50 simulated and 500 real pulse signals demonstrate the power of CAF filter both in removing baseline drift and in preserving the diagnostic information of pulse waveforms. This CAF also can be used to remove the baseline drift of other physiological signals, such as ECG and so on.

4.1 Introduction

4.1.1 Pulse Waveform Analysis

Various civilizations have used arterial pulse as a guide to diagnose diseases [1, 2]. Traditional Chinese pulse diagnosis (TCPD) has been validated for more than 2000 years. Pulse diagnosis is convenient, inexpensive, painless, and noninvasive. These qualities make pulse diagnosis a valuable diagnostic tool, so it is not surprising to find an increasing interest in pulse research among medical researchers internationally. However, all pulse diagnoses methods require that practitioners have considerable training and experience. Fortunately, pulse waveform analysis not only can overcome this obstacle, but also makes pulse diagnosis more accurate [3–9]. Pulse waveform analysis employs a set of sensors to acquire and record pulse

© Springer Nature Singapore Pte Ltd. 2018
D. Zhang et al., *Computational Pulse Signal Analysis*,
https://doi.org/10.1007/978-981-10-4044-3_4

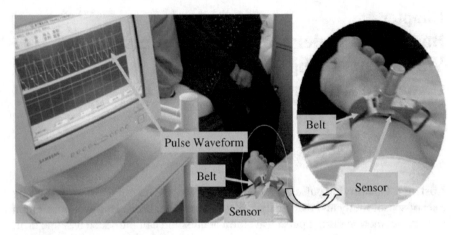

Fig. 4.1 The pulse wave acquisition system

waveforms and then analyze this series of pulse waveforms in accordance with medical theories.

Figure 4.1 illustrates our pulse acquisition device, which is comprised of a set of pulse sensors, an amplifier, and a computer. The sensor, named HMX-4, was made by Shanghai Medical Instrument Company. It is a strain cantilever beam transducer, which is different from the sensors used for studying western medicine. A belt-mounted sensor is used with the additional feature that the pressure could be gradually altered by means of a mechanical screw. This device can acquire a series of pulse pressure waveforms at different contact pressures. This series of pulse waveforms were regarded as pulse image of TCPD. From pulse image, we can measure TCPD information such as position, trend, width, shape, strength, rhythm, and so on. From the position, we can judge whether the pulse image is floating or sinking; from the trend, we can judge whether the pulse image is feeble or forceful and so on [10].

In the further pulse waveform analysis, we not only measure the features of pulse image, but also classify different pulse patterns. Li Shizhen (1518–1593 AD), a highly influential figure in Chinese medicine, has identified 27 different pulse patterns, distinctive in many aspects such as their positions, shapes, widths, strengths, trends, intensities, and rhythms [11]. These 27 pulse patterns relate to the syndromes in TCM. We take taut pulse and smooth pulse, two pulse patterns among the 27 pulse patterns, as examples. Taut pulse indicates the increase of the blood vessel's resistance of a body, while smooth pulse is strongly supportive of a diagnosis of phlegm-damp accumulation in the body.

Both the feature extraction and classification of pulse images require the raw pulse waveforms to have less distortion. Our pulse acquisition device has the bandwidth between 0.05 and 200 Hz with an almost linear response and thus will not distort pulse waveform; however, distortion can be arisen from subject's movement

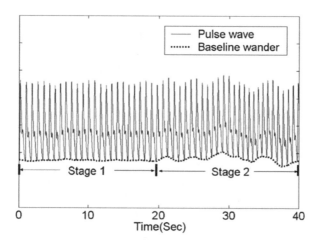

Fig. 4.2 Pulse wave and its baseline drift

and respiration. Fig. 4.2 shows a period of pulse waveform of a volunteer. At the first stage, the volunteer held his breath, illustrating that his pulse waveform is stable. While at the second stage, the volunteer took breath normally, which distorted the baseline of his pulse waveform, and the result is illustrated in the figure as the superposition of a quasiperiodic pulse and a relatively slow varying baseline drift. However, holding breath is unpractical for the long-term monitoring of pulse waveform and also can influence the original pulse waveform.

It is necessary to remove these subject-derived distortions of pulse waveform for further analysis. As far as pulse feature extraction and classification of pulse patterns are concerned, we want that all the onsets in every pulse period are exactly located at zero. Figure 4.3a illustrates some features extracted from a noise-free pulse waveform. As illustrated in Fig. 4.3b, an onset is the lowest point in each pulse period and is regarded as the starting point in every period of pulse wave. The pulse baseline is defined as the curve that connects these onsets. In Fig. 4.3b, the upper, middle, and lower panels are, respectively, the smooth pulse, normal pulse, and taut pulses. The h3 of the smooth pulse is lower than that of the normal pulse, and the h2 of taut pulse is higher than that of the normal pulse. The normal pulse, which is even and forceful, neither quick nor slow, has a medium frequency of 4–5 pulse beats per breath and a regular rhythm. In Fig. 4.3b, all the onsets are at zero level, and their baselines are the straight line across zero. If the pulses in Fig. 4.3b have been distorted by baseline drift, that is to say, these onsets of pulse drift to nonzero positions; the parameters such as h1, h2, h3, and so on will be influenced greatly. Hence correcting pulse baseline drift accurately is a key problem in pulse waveform analysis such as automatic processing of pulse waveforms, pulse visual diagnosis, and pulse pattern recognition. Recently, baseline drift removal is also mentioned for more accurate analysis of variability of pulse waveform and its parameters [12, 13].

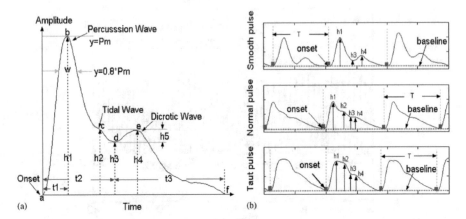

Fig. 4.3 (**a**) Scheme of some pulse's features. Pulse waveform is usually composed of percussion wave, tidal wave, and dicrotic wave. According to these waves, we extract some parameters for pulse pattern recognition, where h1, h2, h3, h4, h5, w, t1, t2, and t3 are the parameters and a, b, c, d, e, and f are the character points of pulse. Point "a" is the onset of pulse. (**b**) The smooth pulse, normal pulse, taut pulse and some of their parameters. The X-axis is the sampling point, and the y-axis is the relative pressure. The smooth pulse, whose tidal wave disappeared, has two peaks. Tidal wave of taut pulse is high and sometimes fuses with the percussion wave

4.1.2   Related Works on Baseline Drift Removal

A variety of techniques has been used to correct baseline drift in physiological signals. These techniques include ensemble averaging, polynomial interpolation, and filters such as time-invariant digital filters, morphology filters, time-variant digital filters, adaptive filters, and wavelet filters. Each of these techniques has distinct disadvantages if it is used to remove the baseline drift of pulse. The following will discuss their performances one by one.

The primary disadvantages of ensemble averaging are time-consuming and inadequate to remove baseline drift.

The performance of polynomial interpolation is unreliable because it depends on the accuracy of knot determination and may degrade when the knots become more separated. The linear interpolation may introduce more distortion, compared with cubic spline estimation [14].

Among time-invariant filters, finite impulse response (FIR) and infinite impulse response (IIR) filters have often been used to suppress baseline drift; only the filters with linear phase can be used. We tested a symmetric FIR digital filter and found that it did very little in reducing baseline drift.

Mathematical morphology is a nonlinear filtering technique based on local shape features of the signal. However, the choice of a structuring element sequence depends on the pulse rate and the pulse waveform shape [15].

Some time-variant filters are also presented because both physiological signal and its baseline drift are time varying. Sörnmo et al. used the time-variant filter to remove the baseline drift of ECGs [16], but their algorithm is complex, level dependent, or rhythm dependent. Zhu et al. used an adaptive filter to remove the baseline drift of ECGs [17–19]. However, this algorithm is time-consuming and suffers from converging problem. Moreover, obtaining a suitable reference signal is difficult for adaptive filter. Chiu et al. reduced the respiratory baseline drift in pulse by Wiener filter, and the result was unsatisfactory for lacking prior knowledge of the signal and noise [20]. The subject's pulse rate may vary, and the baseline drift of his pulses may vary too. Without little prior knowledge of a pulse and its baseline drift, time-variant methods cannot quickly trace the variability of a pulse and cannot accurately and satisfyingly remove the baseline drift.

Pulse waveform can be distorted greatly or slightly. Sometimes, they are distorted by respiration; sometimes they are distorted by motion artifact and sometimes by both respiration and motion artifact. The proposed wavelet-based cascaded adaptive filter (CAF) responds to these issues in that it does not require any reference input and in that the level of baseline drift can be evaluated simply by referring to the energy ratio (ER) of pulse waveform to its baseline drift.

This chapter is organized as follows. The CAF is described in Sect. 4.2. Section 4.3 discusses the effectiveness of the CAF and compares its performance with that of other filters using simulated pulse waveforms. In Sect. 4.4, the performance of the CAF in filtering the real typical pulse waveforms is studied. Some conclusions are offered in Sect. 4.5.

4.2 The Proposed CAF

This section describes the proposed CAF. At first, the basic idea of the CAF is outlined. After that, we explain the details of this CAF from three parts: the detection of baseline drift level, the discrete Meyer wavelet filter, and cubic spline estimation.

4.2.1 The Design of CAF

The proposed CAF is depicted in Fig. 4.4. The primary input signal is the pulse contaminated by baseline drift, and this filter does not need any reference input as the LMS adaptive filter does. Firstly, we decompose the pulse signal and compute its ER to detect pulse's baseline drift level. If the ER exceeds or is equal to the threshold, the pulse waveform just needs to be filtered by cubic spline estimation. Otherwise, the pulse will be filtered in two stages. The first stage is a discrete Meyer wavelet filter, and the second stage is cubic spline estimation. Pulse1, the output of the discrete Meyer wavelet filter, still contains a little baseline contamination and needs to be corrected to the zero level in order to meet the requirement of pulse waveform's analysis. As a result, the cubic spline estimation was applied to remove the remaining drift of Pulse1 and output the final result, Pulse2, at the second stage.

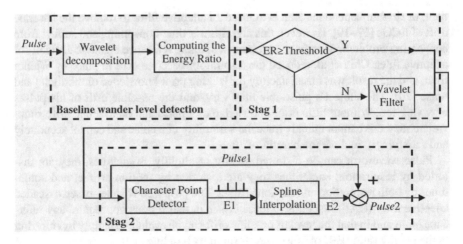

Fig. 4.4 The cascaded adaptive filter. It is composed of three parts: baseline drift level detection, Stag1, and Stag2. Level detection includes wavelet decomposition and ER calculation. In Stag1, if the ER of pulse wave is less than the threshold, the signal will be filtered using wavelet filter. Stag2 is composed of pulse onsets detector and cubic spline estimation

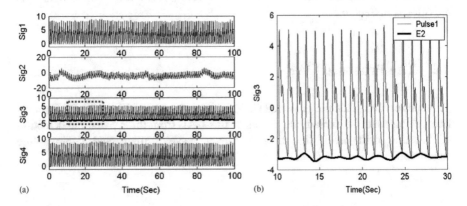

Fig. 4.5 Pulse waveform and some results produced by the cascaded filter, where (**b**) is the local enlargement of the third panel of (**a**)

Here, we take the onsets of Pulse1 as the knots for the later spline estimation. These knots can be easily obtained from Pulse1 with high precision using an algorithm based on pulse waveform's amplitude and derivatives.

To explain this CAF, we give an example in Fig. 4.5. In Fig. 4.5, Sig1 is the "clean" pulse waveform whose baseline does not drift. Sig2 is the contaminated signal that is simulated by adding baseline drift to the "clean" pulse Sig1. Sig2s ER of pulse signal to baseline drift is 2.1 dB. It should be filtered by the Meyer wavelet firstly. Sig3 are the semi-finished products processed by the CAF as illustrated in Fig. 4.4. Figure 4.5b is the local enlargement of Sig3, which is the third panel in Fig. 4.5a. Pulse1 is the wavelet's filtered result, and its ER increases to 56 dB. E2 in

Fig. 4.5b is the remaining baseline drift extracted by the cubic spline estimation. Sig4 is the final result filtered by CAF. The correlation coefficient of Sig1 and Sig4 is 0.99, showing that the majority information of Sig1 is preserved by Sig4.

The CAF algorithm is executed as follows:

Algorithm 1 CAF
Stage 1

1. Extend the raw physiological data, pulse $\{X_1,..., X_N\}$, with asymmetric extension to overcome boundary influence.
2. Perform Meyer wavelet decomposition and obtain its decomposition coefficients.
3. Reconstruct the wavelet approximation of the physiological signal from the decomposition coefficients and truncate it to the length of N.
4. Compute the ER of the raw physiological signal. If ER > threshold, Pulse1$\{X(1),..., X(N)\}$ is equal to raw signal pulse$\{X_1,..., X_N\}$ directly and go to stage 2. Otherwise go to (5).
5. Subtract the approximation of the physiological signal from the raw signal pulse$\{X_1,..., X_N\}$. This process enhances Pulse1$\{X(1),..., X(N)\}$ to a much higher ER.

Stage 2

1. Compute E1, the character points of signal Pulse1$\{X(1),..., X(N)\}$.
2. Take these character points as knots of the cubic spline estimation.
3. Compute E2, the cubic spline estimation of the baseline drift.
4. Obtain the corrected signal Pulse2 = Pulse1 − E2.

4.2.2 Detection Level of Baseline Drift Using ER

4.2.2.1 Why Detect ER

The baseline drift in pulse wave can be much or little. When there is little baseline drift, the wavelet filter may introduce some distortion. To demonstrate the distortion caused by unnecessary filter, we conducted a simulation using known baselines and clean pulse signals. Figure 4.6 illustrates the result using a wavelet filter to approximate the pulse's baseline when the baseline drift is at zero level; that is to say, the baseline drift does not drift. In Fig. 4.6, Baseline1 is the baseline estimated by the wavelet filter, and Baseline2 is the actual zero level baseline. Compared with Baseline2, Baseline1 caused extraneous distortions, i.e., the baseline drift is overfitted. This suggests that when there is little baseline drift, the wavelet approximation may cause some distortion. Spline estimation, however, can correct the baseline drift to zero position. Therefore, when the ER of a pulse waveform to its baseline

Fig. 4.6 The wavelet filtered result when the pulse's actual baseline drift is at the zero level. Baseline1 is the baseline drift estimated by wavelet filter and Baseline2 is the real baseline drift. That is to say, this actual pulse has no baseline drift, only the wavelet filter introduced some distortion

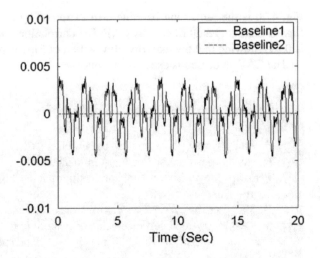

drift is sufficiently high, spline estimation corrects baseline drift more effectively than a wavelet filter.

On the other hand, when the ER of a pulse waveform to its baseline drift is low, wavelet filter corrects baseline drift more effectively than spline estimation. In Fig. 4.7, Baseline1 is the baseline drift extracted by wavelet filter, and Baseline2 is the baseline drift extracted by spline filter. Baseline is the real baseline, which is obtained by filtering a random noise with a low-pass filter at the cutoff frequency of 0.6 Hz. Figure 4.7a shows the baseline drift whose amplitude is low, while Fig. 4.7b shows the situation where the amplitude of the baseline drift is high. They are added separately to the same clean pulse signal. We can find that when the baseline drift is high, the wavelet filter performs better than cubic spline estimation. However, it is not the case when both the signal and the baseline drift are low. The simulated baseline drifts in Fig. 4.7a and c are the same, but the ER in Fig. 4.7a is 40 dB higher than that in Fig. 4.7c. In Fig. 4.7c, the wavelet filter performs better than cubic spline estimation. The result illustrated in Fig. 4.7c is similar to that in Fig. 4.7b. It is because the ER in Fig. 4.7c is the same as that in Fig. 4.7b. Shusterman has used the mean square error (MSE) as a criterion to judge whether the baseline drift was sufficiently low [21]; nevertheless, the MSE-based method only takes into account the amplitude of the baseline drift. As illustrated in Fig. 4.7c, you can find that when MSE is small and the physiological signal is too small, the wavelet filter can correct the baseline drift well because its baseline drift is still heavy compared with its physiological signal. This shows that the key to the performance of baseline drift removal is the ER of the signal's fluctuation to that of its baseline drift, not the amplitude of the baseline drift.

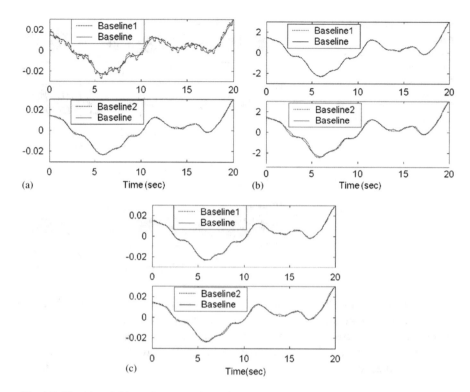

Fig. 4.7 The (**a**) and (**b**) are the comparison of spline and wavelet filters' performance on removing baseline drifts with different amplitudes. Baseline1 and Baseline2 are the baseline drifts estimated by the spline and wavelet filter, respectively. Baseline is the simulated baseline drift. In (**a**) and (**b**), the amplitudes of the baseline drifts are 0.02 and 2, respectively. Meanwhile, their clean pulses are the same pulse waveform with the amplitude being 10. (**a**) and (**c**) are the comparison of spline and wavelet filters' performance on pulse signals with same baseline drift but different energy ratios of clean pulse signal to baseline drift, the former one's ER being 40 dB higher than the latter one's. Baseline1 and Baseline2 are the baseline drift filtered by the spline and wavelet filter, respectively. Baseline is the simulated baseline drift

4.2.2.2   How to Compute the ER of Pulse Signal

The ER of pulse signal to its baseline drift is calculated through wavelet decomposition. In wavelet analysis, a signal is split into two parts: an approximation and details. The approximation is then split into a second-level approximation and further details. This process can be repeated. In this chapter, we choose the discrete Meyer wavelet and decompose the corrupted pulse signal several times. In our

Fig. 4.8 Contaminated pulse and its decompositions. Pulse is the contaminated pulse waveform; *A*1 and *A*7 are its coarse contents of wavelet decompositions at first and seventh scales

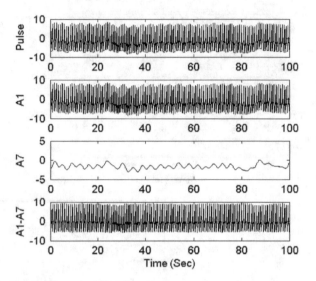

former work, we use the corrupted pulse signal's first-level approximation to its sixth-level approximation to compute the ER of the corrupted pulse signal [22]. For more accuracy, we use the corrupted pulse signal's first-level approximation and its seventh-level approximation to compute the ER of the corrupted pulse signal. The ER is computed as

$$\text{ER} = 20 \log_{10} \frac{\left\| A1 - A7 - d\text{mean}\left(A1 - A7\right)\right\|}{\left\| A7 - \text{mean}\left(A7\right)\right\|}, \tag{4.1}$$

where *A*1 is the first-level approximation content of a corrupted pulse signal and *A*7 is the seventh-level approximate content. ‖ ‖ means the two-order norm, and mean (*A*1 − *A*7) stands for the average of (*A*1 − *A*7).

In Fig. 4.8, Pulse is the corrupted pulse waveform; *A*1 and *A*7 are the approximations of the discrete Meyer wavelet at first and seventh scale decompositions. Here, we use *A*1 − *A*7 and *A*7 to approximate the pulse signal and its baseline drift, respectively.

The reason that we choose (*A*1 − *A*7) and *A*7 as the approximation of pulse signal and its baseline drift is based on the following assumptions and facts. The lowest pulse rate that can be processed is considered to be 48 beats per minute, while the highest is 180 beats per minute [23]. The pulse is assumed to be periodic. The first harmonics frequency of the pulse spectrum is greater than 0.8 Hz and less than 3 Hz. It is generally believed that the human's pulse rate is four to five times of the respiration rate [24]. The motion artifacts are also characterized by low-frequency components when the objects are quiet. Consequently, the main frequency component of the baseline drift is less than 0.68 Hz. The sampling rate of pulse data is 100 Hz, and the cutoff frequency of the seventh-level scale function is 0.78 Hz. The

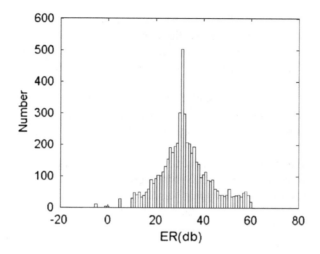

Fig. 4.9 ER distribution histogram of pulse waveforms in our pulse database

frequency content of the pulse waveform is less than 40 Hz [25]. Thus, $(A1 - A7)$ and $A7$ are used to approximate the pulse signal and its baseline drift, respectively. If the sampling rate of the physiological signal changes, the order of the wavelet approximate will change too.

Our pulse database contains 5395 clinical pulse data with the durations range from 1 to 10 min, sampled at a rate of 100 Hz. The more the pulse is corrupted by the baseline drift, the less its ER is. The ER of the clean pulse is more than 60 dB. We calculated the ERs of all pulses in our pulse database. Figure 4.9 illustrates the ER distribution of these 5395 pulse data. We find that the ERs of 8% real pulses are more than 50 dB and the ERs of 1.5% real pulses are less than 10 dB. Experiments have shown that ER = 50 dB is the best criterion for discerning whether to use the wavelet filter. This will be further discussed in Sects. 4.3 and 4.4.

4.2.3   The Discrete Meyer Wavelet Filter

4.2.3.1   Design of the Discrete Meyer Wavelet Filter

As a very promising technique for joint time-frequency analysis, wavelet transforms have been applied in diverse signal processing. A continuous wavelet transform (CWT) is defined as the integral of the signal multiplied by scaled, shifted versions of the wavelet function ψ (scale, position, t) as

$$C(\text{scale, position}) = \int_{-\infty}^{\infty} f(t)\psi(\text{scale, position}, t)dt \qquad (4.2)$$

In Eq. (4.2), the result of CWT is the wavelet coefficient C, which is a function of scale and position. The discrete wavelet transform (DWT) is much more efficient than the CWT. In 1988, Mallat developed an efficient way to implement this scheme through filters [26]. As a result, DWT has been widely applied in medical signal processing [27].

The wavelet's frequency resolution is higher at low frequencies than that at high frequencies. This chapter employs its frequency resolution in low frequencies to estimate the baseline drift and then subtract the baseline drift from the contaminated pulse signal.

To eliminate or reduce the baseline drift effectively, the approximation must have a narrow spectrum. In order to obtain both a good reconstruction and a decomposition of the signal in non-overlapping bands, we chose the discrete Meyer wavelet. Unlike the Daubechies wavelet, the Meyer wavelet, which is linear phase and orthogonal, has compact support character in the frequency domain. The Meyer function $\psi(w)$ is defined in the frequency domain, starting with an auxiliary function as follows [28]:

$$\psi(w) = \begin{cases} (2\pi)^{-1/2} \times e^{jw/2} \times \sin\left(\frac{\pi}{2} \times v\left(\frac{3}{2\pi}|w|-1\right)\right) \text{if } \frac{2\pi}{3} \le |w| \le \frac{4\pi}{3}, \\ (2\pi)^{-1/2} \times e^{jw/2} \times \cos\left(\frac{\pi}{2} \times v\left(\frac{3}{4\pi}|w|-1\right)\right) \text{if } \frac{4\pi}{3} \le |w| \le \frac{8\pi}{3}, \\ 0 \qquad\qquad\qquad\qquad\qquad \text{if } |w| \notin \left[\frac{2\pi}{3}, \frac{8\pi}{3}\right], \end{cases} \quad (4.3)$$

where the auxiliary function can be expressed as

$$v(a) = a^4 \times (35 - 84 \times a + 70 \times a^2 - 20 \times a^3), a \in [0,1]. \qquad (4.4)$$

The Meyer wavelet is infinitely differentiable and can decrease to zero faster than any inverse polynomial. Moreover, it does not produce aliasing errors or distortions. Conforto et al. have successfully used the Meyer wavelet to process myoelectric signals [29].

4.2.3.2   Performance of Discrete Meyer Wavelet Filter on Pulse Waveform

In this section, we will compare performance of the discrete Meyer wavelet filter with those of several typical filters. These typical filters are time-invariant frequency filter, time-variant frequency filter, Wiener filter, least mean square (LMS) adaptive filter, cubic spline estimation, and morphology filter. The pulse can be distorted greatly or slightly. Sometimes, it is distorted by respiration, sometimes it is distorted by motion artifact, and sometimes it is distorted by both respiration and motion artifact. The information on the baseline drift and pulse waveform is unable to

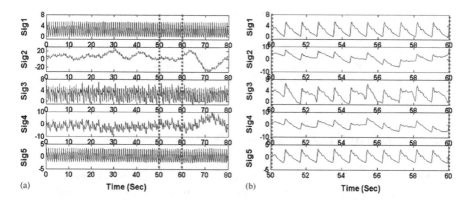

Fig. 4.10 Corrupted pulse wave and its filtered results by morphology filter, 600-order FIRLS, and Meyer wavelet, where (**b**) is the local enlargement of (**a**). Sig2 is attained by adding baseline drift to a clean pulse wave Sig1; Sig3, Sig4, and Sig5 are the results of Sig2 filtered with morphological filter, FIRLS, and discrete Meyer wavelet filter, respectively

obtain. Lacking reference signal, the adaptive LMS filter and Wiener filter cannot achieve high performance in removing pulse waveform's baseline drift. The time-variant filter proposed by Sörnmo et al. is level dependent or rhythm dependent. However, the pulse rate may not be easily detected when a pulse waveform has excessive baseline drift. Consequently, we only compare the performances of the morphology filter, the FIR filter, and the wavelet filter in removing the pulse's baseline drift in this chapter.

As shown in Fig. 4.10, Sig1 is the pulse waveform without baseline drift; Sig2 is the contaminated signal of Sig1 being added some baseline drift; Sig3 is the result of the morphological filter. This morphological filter first performs an opening operation and then a closing operation. The sampling rate of our pulse acquisition system is 100 Hz, and the pulse beat is about 900 ms. Therefore, we choose a disk-shaped sequence at the length of 50 sampling points as the structuring element sequence of this morphology filter. This filter's parameters are optimal for pulse signals, but it cannot filter the pulse's baseline drift satisfyingly.

Sig4 shows the result produced by the traditional linear-phase least-squares error FIR filter (FIRLS). It is a 600-order forward and reverse filter with a cutoff frequency of 0.6 Hz, but it was not effective in canceling the baseline drift and might cause Gibbs phenomenon [30].

Sig5 shows the result of Sig2 processed by the discrete Meyer wavelet. Figure 4.10b is the local enlargement of Fig. 4.10a. Compared with Sig1, Sig3 was greatly distorted, and Sig4s baseline drift was depressed a little. The discrete Meyer wavelet filter is better than morphological filter and FIRLS both in removing Sig2s baseline drift and in preserving Sig1s complex.

The morphological filter cannot filter the pulse's baseline drift satisfyingly; the traditional linear-phase FIRLS was not effective in canceling the baseline drift and might cause Gibbs phenomenon. The discrete Meyer wavelet filter is better than morphological filter and FIRLS both in removing baseline drift and in preserving diagnostic information. However, after filtered by Meyer wavelet, the signal still contains some baseline drift, so it is necessary to further rectify the distortion. Because the discrete Meyer wavelet filter greatly enhances the ER of a pulse waveform, spline estimation can satisfyingly correct baseline drift further.

4.2.4   Cubic Spline Estimation Filter

As the Meyer wavelet filter cannot reduce the baseline drift of a pulse to exactly zero, the remaining baseline drift is estimated using cubic spline. For the pulse with high ER, as discussed in Sect. 4.2.2, cubic spline is needed to estimate the baseline drift directly. We regard the onsets of pulse as the knots of spline for estimating the baseline drift. In this section, we first discuss the detection of the onset in each period of pulse waveform, and then we discuss the cubic spline estimation.

4.2.4.1   Detecting Pulse's Onsets

A pulse is composed of an ascending period and a descending period, and the slope of ascending is notable in both pulse waveform and its first central difference. We take the onsets of the pulse as the knots of the cubic spline estimation.

Many methods have been proposed for detecting the QRS complex of ECGs [31, 32]. Up to now, many algorithms on accurate detection of the intervals between blood pressure waveform's beats have been proposed [33–35]. However, for different physiological signals, the method of detecting onsets may differ. Having referred those methods, we proposed an approach to detect the onsets of pulse waveform based on pulse waveform's amplitude and derivatives. Let $\{X(1), X(2), \ldots, X(N)\}$ represent the sampling points of a pulse waveform. We compute its first derivative through the first central difference of pulse. The first derivative $Y(n)$ is calculated at each point of $X(n)$ as

$$Y(n) = \left[X(n+1) - X(n-1) \right] / 2, 2 < n < N-1, \tag{4.5}$$

$$Y(1) = Y(N) = 0. \tag{4.6}$$

Then $Y(n)$ is rectified as

$$Z(n) = \begin{cases} Y(n) & \text{if } Y(n) \geq 0, 1 < n < N, \\ 0 & \text{if } Y(n) < 0, 1 < n < N. \end{cases} \tag{4.7}$$

In Fig. 4.11a, the upper panel is a pulse waveform, and the middle panel is its first derivative. As Fig. 4.11a illustrated, the first derivative Signal1 has less baseline

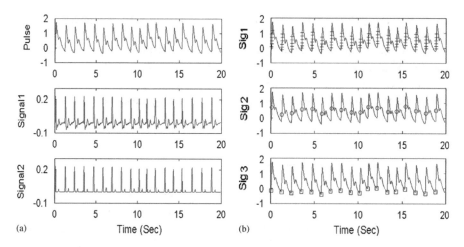

Fig. 4.11 The scheme for detecting the onset of pulse. In (**a**), Signal1 is Pulse's central difference, and Signal2 is the nonnegative processed signal of Signal1 and (**b**) the process for searching every period's onset of Pulse

drift than Pulse itself. In the lower panel of Fig. 4.11a, Signal2 is the rectified result of Signal1. We acquire pulse data at a sampling rate of 100 Hz; thus, 200 sampling points must include at least one entire pulse period. Applying the moving window with the size of 200 sampling points, we search for the maximum in the window from first central difference six times and get six maximums of its first derivative, $M_1, M_2, \ldots, M_6$.

Next, we calculate the threshold to detect the main peak in every period of pulse. Amplitude threshold is calculated as

$$\text{Amplitude threshold} = \left[\text{MIN} - \left(\text{MAX2} - \text{MIN2} \right) \right] \times 0.9, \qquad (4.8)$$

where

$$\text{MIN} = \min \left(M1, M2, \ldots, M6 \right), \qquad (4.9)$$

$$\text{MAX2} = \text{The second maximum among} \left(M1, M2, \ldots, M6 \right), \qquad (4.10)$$

$$\text{MIN2} = \text{The second minimum among} \left(M1, M2, \ldots, M6 \right). \qquad (4.11)$$

The threshold may vary with different pulse signals. When $Z(n) \geq$ amplitude threshold, the main peaks of the derivative must be included. In Fig. 4.11b, Sig1 illustrates the points whose first derivatives are bigger than threshold. Having detected the maximum in every period of the first derivative, shown in Sig2, we search backward 20 sampling points and find the local minimum point, which is the onset of every pulse period. These onsets are shown in Sig3, the lower panel of Fig. 4.11b.

Having used this approach to detect the onsets of 2000 clinical data and 1000 simulated pulse, we find that when ER > 10 dB and SNR > 15 dB, the accuracy is 99.7%. The approach for detecting the onsets of pulse waveform is simple, robust and accurate, which ensures the accuracy of estimating pulse baseline drift using cubic spline.

4.2.4.2 Cubic Spline Estimation

Estimation is a way of selecting an approximating function, based on experience. A simple way to approximate a function is to sample a large but limited number of points. The whole interval of a function to be estimated is divided into several sub-intervals by a set of points called knots, and usually the estimation function is a polynomial with a specified degree between knots. We prefer the cubic spline functions to the other methods when the signal's ER is high enough. Researchers in Shanghai University of traditional Chinese medicine applied the linear interpolation method to remove the baseline drift. However, the linear interpolation estimation will cause some distortion because the baseline drift produced by respiration and the body's motion has nonlinear and quasiperiodic contents. Assuming that $x \in [A,B]$ and $F(x)$ is the function to be estimated, the interval [A,B] is divided into suffi-ciently small intervals $[X_j, X_{j+1}]$, with $A = X_1 < \ldots < X_L = B$. In this way, within each subinterval, a cubic spline function $S(x)$ can provide a good approximation of $F(x)$. The piecewise cubic spline function $S(x)$ can be defined as

$$S(x) = \sum_{k=0}^{3} a_k x^k + \sum_{i=1}^{L} b_i (x - X_i)_+^3, \tag{4.12}$$

$$(x - X_i)_+^3 = \begin{cases} (x - X_i)^3 & (x \geq X_i) \\ 0 & (x < X_i) \end{cases}, \tag{4.13}$$

where a_k and b_i are the coefficients of the polynomial; $(X_i, F(X_i))$ is the knot of the cubic spline; $k = 0,1,2,3$ and $i = 1,\ldots,L$; L is the total number of knots.

From Eq. (4.12), we can deduce the second derivative of $S(x)$:

$$S''(x) = 2! \times a_2 + 3! \times a_3 \times x + 3! \times \sum_{i=1}^{L} b_i \times (x - X_i)_+. \tag{4.14}$$

From formula (4.14), we can find that, at every knot $(X_i, F(X_i))$, the second deriv-ative is continuous. The baseline drift is smooth, which means that the derivative of baseline must be continuous. The high-degree polynomial is smooth, but its conver-gence is unsatisfactory and may cause Runge phenomenon. Flexibility and linearity in parameters are the important properties of the spline functions. Furthermore, there is at most one inflexion in every interval between adjacent knots of a baseline drift. Consequently, the cubic spline estimation is satisfying.

The performance of pulse conditioning is judged by the extent of interference reduction and pulse distortion. In this study, algorithms are evaluated according to two parameters: the baseline correction ratio (BCR) and the pulse distortion ratio (PDR), which are defined as follows:

$$
\text{BCR} = \frac{\sum_{t=1}^{T} \left\| bw(t) - bw_o(t) \right\|}{\sum_{t=1}^{T} \left\| bw_o(t) \right\|},
\tag{4.15}
$$

$$
\text{PDR} = \frac{\sum_{t=1}^{T} \left\| p_0(t) - p(t) \right\|}{\sum_{t=1}^{T} \left\| p_0(t) \right\|},
\tag{4.16}
$$

where $\|\ \|$ stands for two-norm; T stands for the whole time duration; $bw_0(t)$, $t \in [1,T]$, is the baseline component in the original input signal; $bw(t)$ is the baseline drift extracted by the filtering algorithms; $p_0(t)$ is the clean pulse component in the input signal; and $p(t)$ is the filtered pulse. BCR is defined to measure the degree of baseline correction; and PDR is defined to measure the degree of pulse distortion after conditioning. The less the PDR and BCR, the better is the correction of the pulse baseline drift.

4.3   Simulated Signals: Experimental Results and Analysis

4.3.1   Experimental Results of the CAF for Different Baseline Drifts

In this section, we study the performances of CAF, morphology, FIRLS, and spline estimation using some simulated pulse signals. In these simulations, the morphology filter, FIRLS, and spline estimation are the same filters in Sect. 4.2.3. In order to quantitatively evaluate filters, firstly we corrupt a known clean pulse by adding a known baseline drift. We then apply those filters to filter the simulated pulse and compare the filter's BCRs and PDRs.

In these simulations, we use the periodic components to simulate the baseline drift results from respiration. The nonperiodic components of pulse baseline drift were simulated by the low-pass filtered random noise. The contaminated pulse signal can be modeled as

$$
cp(n) = p(n) + bw_1(n) + bw_2(n),
\tag{4.17}
$$

where $cp(n)$ is the corrupted pulse signal; $p(n)$ is a noise-free pulse (ER > 60 dB) selected from our pulse database; and $bw_1(n)$ and $bw_2(n)$ are the periodic part and nonperiodic part of baseline drift. As illustrated in Eqs. (4.18) and (4.19), $bw_1(n)$ is modeled by a sine signal; and $bw_2(n)$ is modeled by the low-pass filtered random noise with the cutoff frequency at 0.68 Hz:

$$bw_1(n) = a_1 \times \sin(2n \times f \times n), \tag{4.18}$$

$$bw_2(n) = a_2 \times \text{filtered\_random}(n), \tag{4.19}$$

where f is the frequency of the sinusoidal signal; $a1$ and $a2$ are the amplitude coefficients of the simulated baseline; and filtered_random(n) is the random signal filtered by low-pass filter.

After that, we add the simulated baseline drift to the noise-free pulse in different proportions and get the simulated contaminated pulses with known ERs. The corrupted pulse is passed through filters, and then its baseline drifts are estimated. To estimate the performances of removing baselines drifts, we compute the PDRs and BCRs of these filters through the noise-free pulse, the corrupted pulse, the corrected pulse, and the extracted baseline drift. Four cases are studied:

- Periodic baseline drifts with constant frequency and various ERs.
- Periodic baseline drifts with constant ER and various frequencies.
- Nonperiodic baseline drifts with various ERs.
- Baseline drifts with 0.1, 0.2, 0.4, and 0.6 Hz periodic components and the nonperiodic component integration in equal proportion under various ERs, i.e.,

$$bw(n) = a \times \left[\begin{array}{l} \sin(2\pi \times 0.1 \times n) + \sin(2\pi \times 0.2 \times n) + \sin(2\pi \times 0.4 \times n) \\ + \sin(2\pi \times 0.6 \times n) + \text{filtered\_random}(n) \end{array} \right]. \tag{4.20}$$

Figure 4.12 displays the PDRs and BCRs of the CAF, FIRLS, spline, and morphology filters with different ERs when the baseline drift is the periodic signal at the frequency of 0.1, 0.2, 0.4, and 0.6 Hz, respectively. The CAF works better than the other filters, while the performance of the morphology filter is the worst. Figure 4.12a, c, e, and g demonstrate the PDRs of the filters; and Fig. 4.11b, d, f, and h demonstrate their BCRs. In Fig. 4.12a, c, e and g, the CAF's PDRs is the least. In Fig. 4.12b, d, f and h, the upper panel and lower panel illustrate the BCRs of CAF, FIRLS, and spline estimation in different scales. The BCRs of the morphology filter are so high that the BCRs of FIRLS, CAF, and spline filter cannot be distinguished; thus, we have to demonstrate the BCRs in two panels. In the lower panel of Fig. 4.12b, it is notable that the BCR of CAF is the least. When the periodic baseline drift's frequency is not high, the performances of CAF and the FIRLS have little difference. However, when ER is more than 50 dB, the BCR of FIRLS is much big-

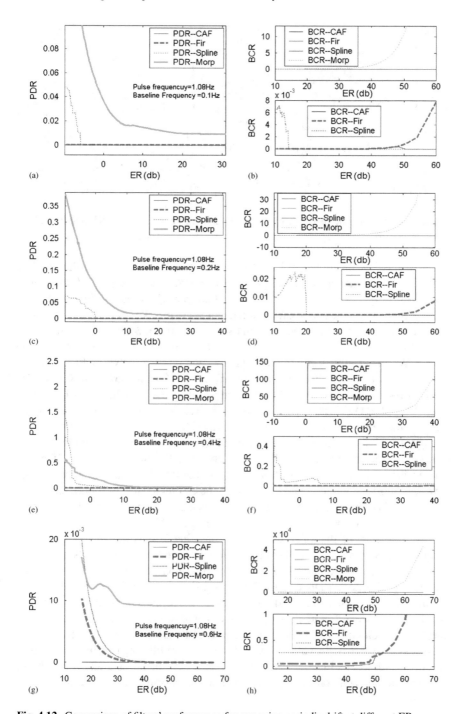

Fig. 4.12 Comparison of filters' performance for removing periodic drift at different ERs

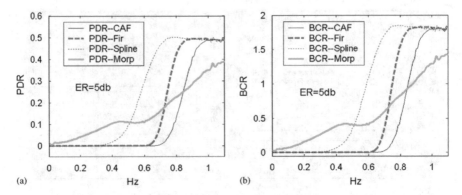

Fig. 4.13 Comparison of filter's performance for removing periodic drift of different frequencies when ER is 5 dB

ger than CAF as illustrated in Fig. 4.12b, d and h. Moreover, when the baseline drift's frequency increases, FIRLS performance degrades more quickly than that of CAF. From Fig. 4.12b, d, f, and h, we can find that when the baseline drift's frequency gets higher, the spline estimation becomes worse. The performance of cubic spline estimation degrades greatly when ER is less than 15, 20, 8, and 50 dB, respectively, to remove the periodic baseline drift at the frequency of 0.1, 0.2, 0.4, and 0.6 Hz. When baseline drift's frequency is low and its ER is between 40 and 50 dB, the BCR of the spline filter slightly outperforms CAF as illustrated in Fig. 4.12b, whereas the BCRs of CAF are less than those of spline filter in Fig. 4.12f and h. When the pulse's ER is more than 50 dB, the BCRs and PDRs of the CAF and spline filter are the same because in this condition the CAF is equal to spline filter.

Figure 4.13 shows the filters' PDRs and BCRs against various periodic baseline drift's frequencies when the ER is 5 dB. The characteristics of BCR and PDR are similar. When the baseline's frequency is less than 0.68 Hz, the CAF is satisfying. However, morphology filter and the cubic spline estimation can introduce enormous distortion when the frequency of baseline drift is higher than 0.1 and 0.4 Hz, respectively. The FIRLS's performance is also worse than CAF as ER increases.

The frequency of the pulse waveform's baseline drift is full of low-frequency nonperiodic contents. Figure 4.14a and b demonstrate the filters' PDRs and BCRs against various nonperiodic baseline drifts of the filters during different ERs. The morphological filter's PDR and BCR are the biggest, while those of CAF are the smallest. Figure 4.14c and d illustrate the filters' performances when the baseline is composed of several frequencies (0.1, 0.2, 0.4, and 0.6 Hz), periodic contents, and nonperiodic contents with same amplitudes during various ERs. Apparently, when ER is less than 10 dB, the CAF outperforms greatly in filtering baseline drift. Thus, the simulation results illustrate that the proposed CAF achieves the better trade-off between the preservation of important diagnostic information and the removal of baseline drift.

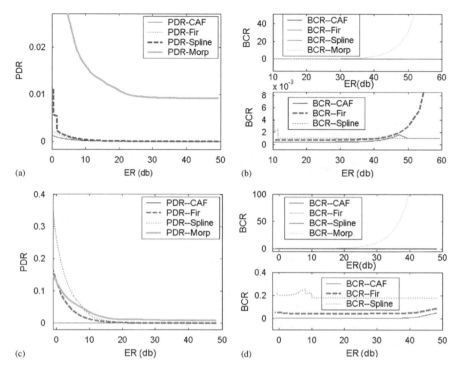

Fig. 4.14 Comparison of filters' performance of removing baseline drifts with periodic contents and nonperiodic contents during various ERs: (**a**) the PDRs of different filters in removing nonperiodic baseline drift with different ERs; (**b**) the BCRs of different filters in removing nonperiodic baseline drift with different ERs; (**c**) the PDRs of different filters in removing baseline drift with periodic and nonperiodic contents integration during different ERs; and (**d**) the BCRs of different filters in removing baseline drift with periodic and nonperiodic contents integration during different ERs

4.3.2 Experimental Results for Different ER Thresholds

The ER threshold of CAF can be different for removing the baseline drift of different kinds of physiological signals. In this section, we compare the PDRs and BCRs of the CAF at different ER thresholds. The baseline drifts are simulated by the integrations of periodic and nonperiodic signals, which are the same as those in Sect. 4.3.1. Figure 4.15 demonstrates the PDRs and BCRs of CAFs at different ER thresholds. In Fig. 4.15a, the X-, Y-, and Z-axis are, respectively, the ERs of the different simulated signals and the different ER thresholds of the CAFs and the PDRs, while in Fig. 4.15b, the X-, Y-, and Z-axis are, respectively, the ERs of the different simulated signals and the different ER thresholds of the CAFs and the BCRs. When the ER threshold is small, the CAF can cause great PDR and BCR. It is because the

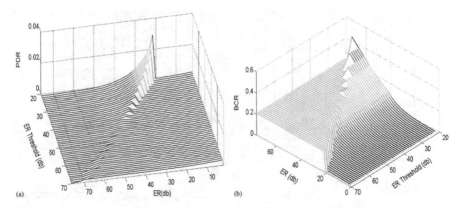

Fig. 4.15 The performance of CAF with different ER thresholds in removing baseline drifts. The baseline drifts are simulated by the integration of periodic and nonperiodic components: (**a**) the PDRs of CAF with different ER thresholds in removing baseline drifts of pulse signals and (**b**) the BCRs of CAF with different ER thresholds in removing baseline drifts of pulse signals

performance of spline estimation degrades greatly at low ER. When the ER threshold is 50 dB, the CAF has the optimum performance. However, for removing the baseline drift of different physiological signals, the ER threshold should be selected again carefully.

4.3.3   Experimental Results for Several Typical Pulses

Section 4.3.1 demonstrated the character of CAF through the simulated periodic and nonperiodic drifts. However, there are several types of pulses distinctive in morphologies. We might wonder whether this CAF can perform satisfyingly in removing the baseline drifts of those typical pulses or not. To further analyze this performance, we mixed five typical pulses with ten real baseline drifts at different ERs. In order to accurately acquire the signal of a subject's respiratory and body's motion artifacts, we attached our pulse sensor to the wrist near the radial artery. The baseline drift acquired by the transducer was amplified and conditioned in the same way as the pulse signal acquired by the transducer.

From our pulse database, we selected 50 clean pulses from five typical pulses such as taut pulse, smooth pulse, normal pulse, slow pulse, and rapid pulse, each including ten clean pulse waveforms. The reasons that we choose these five types of pulses are these pulses have typical morphology or rhythms. The rapid pulse's rate ranges from 110 to 120 pulse beats per minute. The slow pulse's rate ranges from 49 to 53. The other three pulses' rates range between 62 and 85. All the ten baseline drifts were acquired from the ten volunteers in supine or sitting positions. Having mixed the 50 clean pulses with the 10 baseline drifts at several ERs, we choose the maximum among the 10 PDRs. These PDRs are listed in Table 4.1 to illustrate the

Table 4.1 PDRs of the CAF in filtering several typical pulses distinct in morphology and rhythm

	ER(dB)	10	5	0	−5	−10	−15	−20
PDR	Taut pulse	0	0	0.0001	0.0003	0.001	0.003	0.003
	Smooth pulse	0.0008	0.0008	0.001	0.0013	0.002	0.005	0.007
	Normal pulse	0.001	0.001	0.001	0.002	0.004	0.006	0.007
	Slow pulse	0.005	0.005	0.006	0.008	0.01	0.014	0.014
	Rapid pulse	0.0001	0.0002	0.0002	0.0004	0.001	0.003	0.003

CAF performance. We find that the PDR of the CAF is still small even when the ER is less than −10 dB. The performance of CAF degraded only when we corrected the slow pulse, which is usually from patients with the long-term cardiac diseases. These bradycardic pulse waveforms are of poor quality, which degrades the performance of the CAF.

4.4 Experimental Results for Actual Pulse Records

The above experiments are the simulated results. They demonstrate CAF's performance quantitatively. This section testifies the CAF using actual records through visual observation. We randomly choose 500 pulse data from our pulse database and filter them using the CAF. The CAF was also tested in actual records using visual observation of experts in TCPD. Three experts in TCPD were asked to visually diagnose these 500 raw pulse waves and their processed pulse waves whose baseline drift was removed by this CAF. After CAF filtering, the accuracy of visual diagnosis rose from 67% to 83%, demonstrating the effectiveness of the CAF. Figure 4.16 illustrates some results in this testifying, demonstrating the performance of this CAF.

In Fig. 4.16a, Sig1 is a 600 s pulse chosen from 8 h sleep monitoring pulse database; Sig2 is the baseline extracted from Sig1; Sig3 is the corrected pulse. After removing the baseline of this long-term pulse, we can accurately analyze the variability of the pulse during sleep. The baseline itself, which contains motion and respiration interference of the pulse during sleep, can also be analyzed.

In Fig. 4.16b, Sig1 is the actual contaminated pulse; Sig2 is the pulse corrected by the CAF; Sig3, Sig4, and Sig5 are the pulse corrected by the spline estimation, the symmetric forward and reverse 600-order FIRLS, and the morphology filter. Sig2 has less visual distortion than others.

The performance of this CAF does not degrade as the pulse waveform varies with time. In Fig. 4.16c, we find that the pulse may vary considerably with time. This pulse, which changes from smooth pulse to normal pulse, was acquired from a healthy, sleeping person. The variability of the pulse waveform arises from the changes of the subject's body position.

Intuitively, all the filtered results of 500 real pulses by the CAF are satisfying. Nor does it stop here; Fig. 4.16d illustrates the result of ECG baseline drift removal

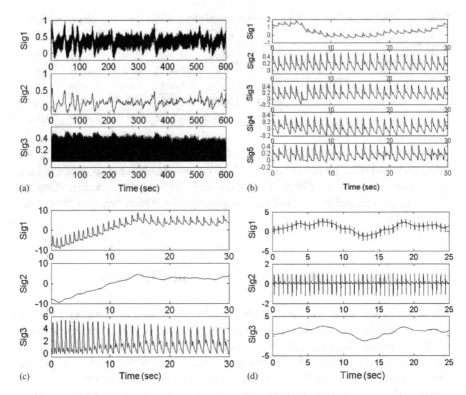

Fig. 4.16 Actual pulses and their results filtered by the CAF: (**a**) 600 s pulse and the result filtered by CAF, (**b**) comparison of filter's performances in preserving the useful information of pulse waveform, (**c**) the type-changing pulse filtered by CAF, and (**d**) the corrupted ECGs filtered by CAF

using the CAF. The result illustrates that this CAF is useful for removing the baseline drift of other physiological signals. Here, the sampling rate of ECG is 200 Hz. We selected first- and eighth-level decomposition to estimate its ER and set 45 dB as the ER threshold.

4.5   Summary

This chapter firstly proposed the ER-based method to detect the baseline drift level of pulse waveform and then described a two-step cascaded filter to remove the baseline drift. According to the level of pulse baseline drift, we took different strategies to remove the baseline drift. If the ER is more than a given threshold, the baseline drift can be removed only by cubic spline estimation; otherwise it must be filtered by, in sequence, a discrete Meyer wavelet filter and the cubic spline estimation.

The CAF's two tuning parameters, the order of the wavelet filter and the ER threshold, need to be selected according to the characteristics of the physiological signal. The order of the wavelet filter depends on the sampling rate of the physiological signal. The ER threshold of CAF can be optimized through simulation.

Four different filters, morphological filter, FIRLS, cubic spline estimation, and the CAF, were compared by means of a set of experimental trials using synthetic pulse signals. The simulation demonstrated that the CAF performs better both in removing baseline drift and in preserving diagnostically useful information. We also used the CAF on 500 real pulses and found it was efficient and robust in filtering various baseline drifts of pulse waveforms. This CAF is very useful in preprocessing pulse waveforms based on both TCPD and Western medicine. The CAF is also effective to the baseline drift of other physiological signals.

References

1. Q. Bian, The Classic of Difficulties (Nan Jing), Tianjing Technology Press, 1979.
2. O.R. Michael, D.F. Edward, "Pulse pressure: is this a clinically useful risk factor?" Hypertension (1999) 372–374.
3. Y.W. Ling, "Frequency distribution of human pulse spectra," IEEE Trans. Biomed. Eng. 32 (1985) 245.
4. W.A. Lu, Y.Y. Wang, W.K. Wang, "Pulse analysis of patients with severe liver problems," IEEE Eng. Med. Biol. 18 (1) (1999) 73–75.
5. J. Ling, D.C. Winter, B.L. Robey, "Cardiac output monitor using fuzzy logic blood pressure analysis," U.S. Patent No. 6007491, December 1999.
6. Inukai, et al., "System and method for evaluating the autonomic nervous system of a living subject," U.S. Patent No. 5830148, November 1998.
7. M.F. O'Rourke, R.P. Kelly, "Wave reflection in the systemic circulation and its implications in ventricular function," J. Hypertension 11 (1993) 327–337.
8. M.F. O'Rourke, J. Lei, D.E. Gallagher, A.P. Avolio, "Determination of the ascending aortic pressure wave augmentation from the radial artery pressure pulse contour in humans," Circulation 92 (1995) 745.
9. Y.Z. Yoon, M.H. Lee, K.S. Soh, "Pulse type classification by varying contact pressure," IEEE Eng. Med. Biol. November/December (2000) 106–110.
10. L.S. Xu, K.Q. Wang, D. Zhang, "Modern researches on traditional Chinese pulse diagnosis," Eur. J. Oriental Med. 4 (5) (2004) 46–54.
11. S.Z. Li, Pulse Diagnosis, Paradigm Press, 1985.
12. L. Li, Z.Z. Wang, "Study on interval variability of arterial pulse," Proceedings of 21st Annual Conference and the 1999 Annual Fall Meeting of the Biomedical Engineering Society BMES/EMBS Conference, vol. 1, 1999, p. 223.
13. J. Allen, A. Murray, "Variability of photoplethysmography peripheral pulse measurements at the ears, thumbs and toes," A. Science, Measurement and Technology, IEE Proceedings, vol. 147, November 2000, pp. 403–407.
14. C.R. Meyer, H.N. Keiser, "Electrocardiogram baseline noise estimation and removal using cubic spline and state space computing techniques," Comput. Biomed. Res. 10 (1977) 459–470.
15. Y. Sun, K.L. Chan, S.M. Krishnan, "ECG signal conditioning by morphological filtering," Comput. Biol. Med. 32 (2002) 465–479.
16. Sörnmo, "Time-varying filtering for removal of baseline wander in exercise ECGs," Computers Cardiology Proceedings, 1991, pp. 145–148.

17. P. Strobach, K.A. Fuchs, "Event-synchronous cancellation of the heat interference in biomedical signal," IEEE Trans. Biomed. Eng. 41 (4) (1994) 343–350.
18. N.V. Thakor, Y.S. Zhu, "Application of adaptive filtering to ECG analysis: noise cancellation and arrhythmia detection," IEEE Trans. Biomed. Eng. 38 (8) (1991) 785–794.
19. L. Pablo, J. Raimon, P. Caminal, "The adaptive linear combiner with a periodic-impulse reference input as a linear comb filter," Signal Process. 48 (3) (1996) 193–203.
20. C.C. Chiu, S.J. Yeh, "A tentative approach based on Wiener filter for the reduction of respiratory effect in pulse signals," Proceedings of 19th International Conference of IEEE/EMBS, October 1997, pp. 1394–1397.
21. V. Shusterman, S.I. Shah, A. Beigel, et al., "Enhancing the precision of ECG baseline correction: selective filtering and removal of residual error," Comput. Biomed. Res. 33 (2000) 144–160.
22. L.S. Xu, D. Zhang, K.Q. Wang, "Wavelet-based cascaded adaptive filter for removing baseline drift in pulse waveforms," IEEE Trans. Biomed. Eng. 52 (11) (2005) 1973–1975.
23. J.A. Van, T.S. Schilder, "Removal of baseline wander and power-line interference from the ECG by an efficient FIR filter with a reduced number of taps," IEEE Trans. Biomed. Eng. 32 (12) (1985) 1052–1060.
24. W. Huh, Y.B. Park, H.K. Kim, et al., "Development of pulse rate detection system for oriental medicine," Proceedings of 19th International Conference-IEEE/EMBS, October 1997, pp. 2406–2408.
25. B.H. Wang, J.L. Xiang, "Detecting system and power spectral analysis of pulse signals of human body," Proceedings of ICSP 1998, 1998, pp. 1646–1649.
26. S. Mallat, "A theory for multiresolution signal decomposition: the wavelet representation," IEEE Pattern Anal. Mach. Intell. 11 (7) (1989) 674–693.
27. M. Unser, A. Aldroubi, "A review of wavelets in biomedical application," Proc. IEEE 84 (1996) 626–638.
28. I. Daubechies, Ten Lectures on Wavelets, SIAM, Philadelphia, PA, 1992.
29. S. Conforto, T. D'Alessio, S. Pignatelli, "Optimal rejection of movement artifacts from myoelectric signals by means of a wavelet filtering procedure," J. Electromyography Kinesiol. (1999) 47–57.
30. A.J. Jerri, "The Gibbs Phenomenon in Fourier Analysis," Splines and Wavelet Approximations, Kluwer Academic Publishers, Dordrecht, 1998.
31. G.M. Friesen, T.C. Jannett, M.A. Jadallah, et al., "A comparison of the noise sensitivity of nine QRS detection algorithms," IEEE Trans. Biomed. Eng. 37 (1990) 85–98.
32. B.U. Kohler, C. Hennig, R. Orglmeister, "The principles of software QRS detection," IEEE Eng. Med. Biol. Mag. 21 (1) (2002) 42–57.
33. M.A. Navakatikyan, C.J. Barrett, G.A. Head, J.H. Ricketts, "A real-time algorithm for the quantification of blood pressure waveforms," IEEE Trans. Biomed. Eng. 49 (7) (2002) 662–670.
34. G. Gratze, J. Fortin, A. Holler, K. Grasenick, G. Pfurtscheller, P. Wach, J. Schonegger, P. Kotanko, F. Skrabal, "A software package for noninvasive, real-time beat-to-beat monitoring of stroke volume, blood pressure, total peripheral resistance and for assessment of autonomic function," Comput. Biol. Med. 28 (1998) 121–142.
35. K.G. Belani, J.J. Buckley, M.O. Poliac, "Accuracy of radial artery blood pressure determination with the vasotrac," Canad. J. Anesthesiol. 46 (1999) 488–496.

Chapter 5
Detection of Saturation and Artifact

Abstract During the pulse signal acquisition, corruptions would be inevitably introduced such as high-frequency noise, baseline drift, saturation, and artifact. Some of the corrupted pulse signals can be recovered via preprocessing, but several types of corrupted pulse signals would be difficult to recover and should be removed from the pulse signal dataset. Therefore, low-quality pulse signal detection plays an important role in computational pulse diagnosis especially in the real-time pulse monitoring. In this work, we focus on the detection of two common pulse corruption types, i.e., saturation and artifact. For the detection of saturation, we use two criteria from its definition. For the artifact detection, we transform the pulse signal into a complex network and detect the artifact by measuring the connectivity of the network. The experimental results show that the saturation and artifact detection method can both achieve better detection accuracy and better time resolution.

5.1 Introduction

Pulse diagnosis has played an important role in oriental medicine for thousands of years [1–3]. Generally, wrist pulse signal is produced by cardiac contraction; moreover it is also affected by the characteristic of blood and the vessel, which make it effective for analyzing both cardiac and non-cardiac diseases.

However, pulse diagnosis is a subjective skill which needs years of training and practice to master, and the diagnosis result relies on the personal experience of the practitioner [4]. For different practitioners, the diagnosis results may be inconsistent. To overcome these limitations, computational pulse diagnosis has recently been studied to make pulse diagnosis objective and quantitative. Several devices have been reported for pulse signal acquisition [5–9]. In the diagnosis research, connection of pulse signals with several certain diseases has been verified [10–17].

During the pulse signal acquisition, interference and other factors may introduce corruptions in pulse signals, e.g., high-frequency noise, baseline drift, saturation, and artifact are some common errors. Part of these corruptions can be mended by some preprocessing methods such as denoising [18–23] and baseline drift removal [22–25]. However, not all the pulse signal with corruptions can be recovered; some

© Springer Nature Singapore Pte Ltd. 2018
D. Zhang et al., *Computational Pulse Signal Analysis*,
https://doi.org/10.1007/978-981-10-4044-3_5

of the corruptions is hard to remove due to the loss of information or the overlapped frequency band of the interference and pulse signal such as saturation and artifact. These errors will make the pulse dataset contain outliers and affect the performance of feature extraction and classification. Thus, dealing with these errors is an important work in computational pulse diagnosis especially in real-time pulse monitoring for sleep studies, intensive care, sports, and so on, since manual detection is impossible in those cases.

In this chapter, we focus on the detection on two common corruptions, i.e., the saturation and artifact. For saturation detection, two criteria were presented according to its definition. For artifact detection, most of the current methods are based on the statistical analysis which set thresholds on the statistics such as the mean value, the standard derivation, and the sample entropy [26, 27]. Since the empirical mode decomposition (EMD) method can isolate the high-frequency component which may contain most of the artifact dynamics, the EMD method is usually used in the artifact detection [28, 29]. However, most of these methods can only detect the existence of artifact but cannot provide the accurate corrupted position. To detect the corrupted position, one needs to divide the pulse signal into multiple segments (usually each segment contains 5~10 s pulse signal) and apply the detection method on each segment to get a detection with time resolution of 5~10 s. In this work, we intend to provide a more accurate artifact detection method with the time resolution around 0.7 s (the time of a pulse cycle) by considering the similarity between pulse cycles. To achieve this, we develop a detection method which transforms the pulse signal from time domain into network domain according to the similarity between pulse cycles and detects the artifact by measuring the connectivity of a complex network.

The remainder of the chapter is organized as follows. Section 5.2 briefly introduces saturation and artifact. Section 5.3 provides the detail of the detection method. Section 5.4 provides experimental results to demonstrate the effectiveness of the presented method. Finally, Sect. 5.5 gives several concluding remarks.

5.2 Saturation and Artifact

In this section, we will give a brief introduction of saturation and artifact; the reason of these corruptions was discussed, and we also provide some example signals with saturation and artifact.

5.2.1 Saturation

Saturation is a pulse signal with amplitude that exceeds the system limit and will result in the pulse signal which has many flat peak or flat valley. Some of the useful information was lost in the saturated signal because part of the signal was not

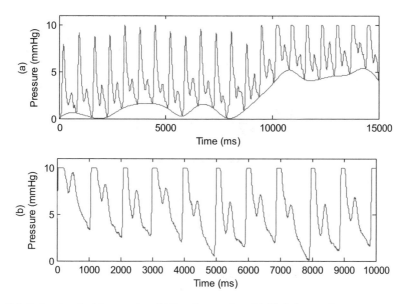

Fig. 5.1 Pulse signal with saturation. (**a**) Local saturation. (**b**) Global saturation

recorded correctly. We can divide the saturation into local saturation and global saturation by their statured percent. Figure 5.1 shows two examples of saturated pulse signals; pulse signal in Fig. 5.1a and b belongs to local saturation and global saturation, respectively. One can see that in Fig. 5.1a, the pulse signal was lifted by the baseline drift which led to saturation, and in Fig. 5.1b, all of the pulse cycles have a flat peak. Local saturation is usually caused by large baseline drift such as the baseline drift caused by body movement. Global saturation is usually caused by improper gain settings or hold-down pressure. Saturated signal is hard to recover because part of the information was lost.

5.2.2 Artifact

Artifact is an undesired irregular segment in the pulse signal; similar as saturation, we also divide artifact into local artifact and global artifact. Figure 5.2 shows two examples of pulse signals with artifact; pulse signal in Fig. 5.2a and b belongs to local artifact and global artifact, respectively. In Fig. 5.2a the segment with local artifact was marked with a box; one can see the local artifact is a small fraction of confusing parts in the pulse signal. In Fig. 5.2b we can barely see the heart rhythm in the signal. The reason of the local artifact may be because of the instability of the sampling system or the quick body movement such as arm twitching or the power supply noise generated by other medical equipment present in the patient care environment. Global chaos artifact is mainly caused by inaccurate sensor position.

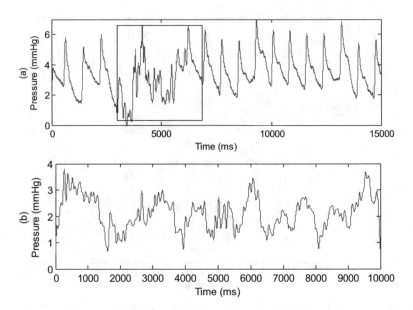

Fig. 5.2 Pulse signal with local artifact. (**a**) Local artifact. (**b**) Global artifact

Moreover, for a minority of patients, their radial arterial vessel is not very close to the skin of his wrist; this will increase the difficulties of finding the good sampling position and result in inaccurate sensor position. Artifact is a serious interference, and the pulse signal with artifact usually is hard to recover if we only have the corrupted pulse signal.

5.3   The Detection of Saturation and Artifact

In this section the preprocessing and their priority were discussed, and the detailed methods for the detection of saturation and artifact were provided.

5.3.1   The Preprocessing and the Priority

In this subsection we provide a brief introduction of some preprocessing process, i.e., denoising and baseline drift removal. Moreover, the priority between preprocessing, saturation detection, and artifact detection was discussed.

Denoising High-frequency noise is the sparkle noise coupled with sampled pulse signal. It is a common interference from the power line, and the frequency band of the power line interference is around 50 Hz or 60 Hz in most of the countries. The frequency band of pulse signal is usually below 30 Hz. Thus their frequency bands are not overlapped, and the noise can be removed by low-pass filters. The low-pass filter can either be a FIR filter or wavelet filter. FIR filter is stable and easy to be implemented for real-time denoising; the wavelet denoising can eliminate the noise while preserving the sudden changes; thus, it was commonly used in non-real-time pulse denoising [18–23].

Baseline Drift Removal Baseline drift is a low-frequency fluctuation in the pulse signal which causes the start points of a pulse signal not in a straight line. It is an inevitable interference which is caused by breathing and body movement. Baseline drift can be removed by filtering method or fitting method. Filtering method [30] assumes that the baseline is mostly composed by breathing, and the frequency bands are lower than that of pulse signal. Thus, the baseline drift can be removed using high-pass filter. Fitting method [31] assumes that the start points of each cycle are on the baseline; thus, fitting the start point using a spline curve may roughly get the baseline, and by subtracting the baseline, we can get a pulse signal with aligned start point.

Both filtering and fitting method have some shortcomings. For filtering method, after the baseline drift removal, these start points of each pulse cycles may not exactly be in a straight line. For fitting method, the baseline was estimated from these sparse start points which may not close to the real baseline. Thus, it is better to combine the two methods where we can remove the baseline according to its frequency property first and then using curve fitting to align these start points [25].

Priority Since the preprocessing processes and the detection process may interact with each other, the priority between these processes may influence the process results.

For the priority between preprocessing processes, since denoising may reduce these sparkle noises which are helpful for start point detection, usually the priority of denoising is higher than baseline drift removal especially when fitting method was used in the baseline removal. For the priority between preprocessing processes and detection processes, since generally the preprocessing can increase the quality of the pulse signal which is helpful in increasing the accuracy of detection processes, thus usually the preprocessing would have the higher priority.

For artifact detection, as the previous discussion after the denoising and baseline drift removal, pulse cycles were aligned and contain less noise which is helpful in the detection of artifact; thus, the artifact detection has lower priority than the preprocessing process. However, the saturation detection would be influenced by filtering or fitting method, and the denoising and baseline drift removal may increase the difficulty of saturation detection. For example, Fig. 5.3a is a saturated signal, and Fig. 5.3b is an enlarged view of the saturated segment. Figure 5.3c and d are the results of noise removal by FIR filter and wavelet filter, respectively. One can see that after the noise removal, these flat saturated segments become a fluctuant segment and more difficult to detect. Figure 5.4 is signal in Fig. 5.2a after baseline drift removal; one can see that the statured segment was pulled down the flat saturated

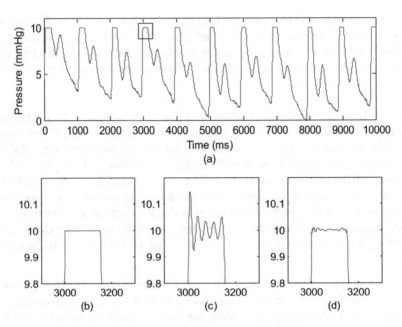

Fig. 5.3 Statured signal after denoising: (**a**) the raw pulse signal. (**b**) The enlarged view of the raw pulse signal. (**c**) The enlarged view of the pulse signal after being filtered by Fourier low-pass filter. (**d**) The enlarged view of the pulse signal after wavelet denoising

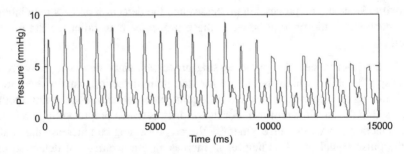

Fig. 5.4 Pulse signal coupled with baseline drift and saturation

segment and becomes a slope segment; moreover the position of segment also changed which increases the difficulty of the saturation detection. Thus, in this work the saturation detection has higher priority than preprocessing processes, and pre-processing processes have higher priority than artifact detection. The sequence of these processes was shown in Fig. 5.5. We use yellow and orange to represent pre-processing processes and detection processes, respectively, and use the greed bars with different depths to represent pulse signal with different conditions as illustrated in the Fig. 5.5.

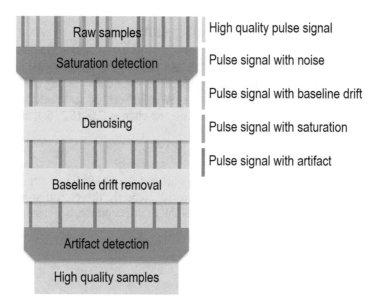

Fig. 5.5 Priority of saturation and artifact detection and common preprocessing processes

5.3.2 Saturation Detection

The saturation detection method is simple; saturation can be detected by two criteria from its definition. The first one is if pulse signal X is saturated at the position i, x_i should equal to the maxima (or the minima) of X. The second one is if X is saturated at the position i, the derivative of X at i should be zero. For example, to detect saturation at the upper part of pulse cycles, we can verify if x_i satisfy the following condition:

$$\max(X) - x_i = 0, \tag{5.1}$$

$$\text{diff}(X)\big|_{x=x_i} = 0. \tag{5.2}$$

In most of the time, Eq. (5.1) is not very robust to the fluctuations in the power supply. We use a more relaxed form as Eq. (5.3) to increase the robustness:

$$\max(X) - x_i \leq \varepsilon, \tag{5.3}$$

where ε in Eq. (5.3) can be set to a small positive number (usually two or three times the minimal resolution). In this work we set ε to 0.0007. We also correspondingly change Eq. (5.2) to the following criterion:

$$\left| \text{diff}\left(X\right)\right|_{x=x_i} \le \varepsilon. \tag{5.4}$$

To avoid the interference from the highest peak in the pulse signal, we further request if x_i is a saturated point; its neighborhood should also satisfy the Eqs. (5.3) and (5.4). In this work we set the radius of the neighborhood to 10 ms.

To detect the saturation at the bottom, we can change Eqs. (5.3, 5.4, and 5.5):

$$x_i - \min\left(X\right) \le \varepsilon. \tag{5.5}$$

The detection result was given by the start and the end indices of the saturated segment; a saturation segment is taken to be correctly detected if it is detected within 20 ms of the annotation time; thus the time resolution is the sampling frequency of the pulse signal.

5.3.3 Artifact Detection

The existing artifact detection method usually divides the pulse signal into multiple segments of 5~10 s pulse signal and extracts the mean value, standard derivation, or sample entropy from these segments. Then set thresholds on these features to detect the artifact [26, 27]. In previous studies, the empirical mode decomposition (EMD) method was used to isolate the high-frequency component [28, 29]. However, these methods did take the similarity between pulse cycles of same pulse signal into consideration which may greatly increase both the detection accuracy and time resolution. In this work we present a new detection method based on the similarity between pulse cycles.

Before the artifact detection, the pulse signal was first preprocessed and segmented. For segmentation we segment the pulse signal to pulse cycles according to the start points of each cycle. In TCPD the start point of a pulse cycle is the valley before the main peak, and usually it is the lowest point in the pulse cycle. The start point can be located by finding the position that the difference changes its sign or by finding the local minimum in a sliding window. Usually we need some limitations to exclude some false detection introduced by the dicrotic notch and some noise. Limitations can be introduced based on the average cycle length, e.g., if we use the local minimum to find the start point, we can set the size of the sliding window between half of the average cycle length and the average cycle length. The average cycle length can be estimated by finding the major frequency from the Fourier frequency spectrum of the pulse signal. If the pulse signal is a pulse signal with global artifact and is a nonperiodic signal, we use the average cycle length of most human (0.7 s in this work) as its average cycle length.

To illustrate the proposed method, we use the signal in Fig. 5.2 a as an example. Figure 5.6 is the signal in Fig. 5.2 a after denoising, baseline drift removal, and segmentation. One can see pulse signal is a quasiperiodic signal composed by

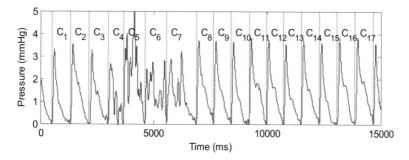

Fig. 5.6 Preprocessed and segmented pulse signal

multiple pulse cycles, for clarity we marked the pulse cycles as C_1, C_2, C_3, etc. In these cycles we found that the normal cycles are similar to each other; however, the cycles with artifact (C_4, C_5, C_6, C_7) are the abnormal part in the pulse signal which are neither similar to these normal cycles nor other artifact cycles. We noted that pulse cycles in pulse signal with good quality also have some difference between each other; however, it is much smaller than the difference between the normal pulse cycles and cycles with artifact. Thus, the artifact can be detected by comparing the similarity between pulse cycles.

In artifact detection we construct a network according to the similarity of pulse cycles. We use vertexes to represent the pulse cycles and use edges to represent the similarity of two cycles. We connect similar cycles with edges and not add edges between cycles not look alike. Then the pulse signal was transformed from time domain into network domain. Since the normal cycles are similar to each other, they should be connected with each other, and the cycles with artifact are not similar to other cycles; they should be isolated points in the network, and thus, we can detect the artifact by analyzing the connectivity of the network.

To measure the similarity between pulse cycles, we can use the Euclidean distance or the correlation coefficient. Two similar pulse cycles, C_i and C_j, should be close in Euclidean space, and the closer the two cycles, the smaller the Euclidean distance. The correlation coefficient is another metric of the similarity between pulse cycle C_i and C_j; the closer the two cycles, the larger the coefficient. In fact, these metrics are essentially equivalent in measuring the similarity of two pulse cycles [32].

If we use the phase distance, the similarity can be calculated as:

$$D_{ij} = \min_{l=0,1,\dots,|l_j - l_i|} \frac{1}{\min(l_j, l_i)} \sum_{k=1}^{\min(l_j, l_i)} \|X_k - Y_{k+l}\|, \tag{5.6}$$

where D_{ij} is the phase space distance of pulse cycle C_i and C_j in time domain, X_k and Y_k are the kth point of pulse cycle C_i and C_j, and l_i and l_j are the lengths of pulse cycle C_i and C_j.

If we use the correlation coefficient, the similarity can be calculated as:

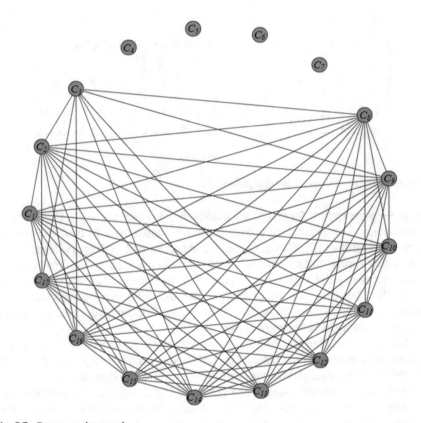

Fig. 5.7 Constructed network

$$\mathrm{Cor}_{ij} = \max_{l=0,1,\dots,l_j-l_i} \frac{\mathrm{cov}\left[C_i\left(1:l_i\right),C_j\left(1+l:l_i+l\right)\right]}{\sqrt{\mathrm{Var}\left[C_i\left(1:l_i\right)\right]}\sqrt{\mathrm{Var}\left[C_j\left(1+l:l_i+l\right)\right]}}, \qquad (5.7)$$

where Cor_{ij} is the correlation coefficient of pulse cycle C_i and C_j, Cov is the covariance operator, and Var is the variance operator. In this work we use the correlation coefficient because it is more robust to interferences.

When constructing the network, we first apply a fully connected network by connecting every vertex and use the similarity as the weight of these edges. Then, we set a threshold on these weights; if the weight is smaller (or larger if we use Euclidean space distance) than the threshold, we remove the corresponding edges from the fully connected network. Finally, we remove all of the weights to get a binary network. Figure 5.7 is a constructed network of signal in Fig. 5.1. One can see that cycles with artifact (C_4, C_5, C_6, C_7) were isolated and these normal cycles are connected with each other. By finding the maximal connected subgraph, we can get all the normal cycles, and the left isolated cycles are these artifact cycles. The

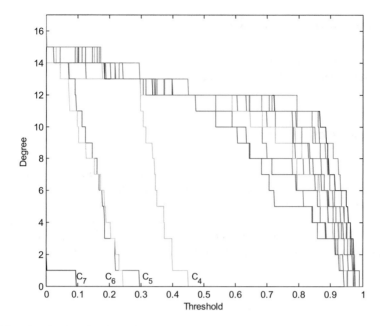

Fig. 5.8 Pulse signal and pulse cycles

cycle number will indicate the position of the artifact; since the pulse segment was divided into pulse cycles, the time resolution of the detection is similar to the average cycle length and usually around 0.7 s.

Since the normal cycles also have some small variations, the maximal connected subgraph may not be a fully connected network like the subgraph in Fig. 5.7. For artifact detection, we only need these normal cycles in a connected subgraph rather than a fully connected subgraph

Finding an effective threshold which can isolate these cycles with artifact while keeping the normal cycle in a connected subgraph is an important work. Actually, the distance between artifact cycles and normal cycles is large, an effective threshold can be selected from a wide interval, and all the thresholds in the optimal interval can isolate the artifact cycles and keep normal cycles connected.

Figure 5.8 shows that the degree of pulse cycles in Fig. 5.6 changes with the increase of the threshold. The trend of the degree variance of each cycle was represented in different colors. From Fig. 5.8 one can see that the degree drops with increasing of the threshold, which is because larger threshold removes more edges from the fully connected networks. Moreover, one can see that the degree of these cycles with artifact decreases faster than that of normal cycles, and for this pulse signal, the effective interval is 0.45 ~ 0.94. In most of the time, a threshold around 0.9 can achieve a better performance, and in this work a series of thresholds was tested, and threshold with best performance was used.

5.4 Experimental Results

In this section, we presented some experiment to validate the presented saturation detection method and artifact detection method.

5.4.1 Saturation Detection

In the saturation detection experiment, we construct a dataset with 161 saturated pulse signals. These pulse signals were sampled in a large hold-down pressure and a large gain. Each pulse signal was labeled by two independent experts. A saturation segment is taken to be correctly detected if it is detected within 20 ms of the annotation time. In the experiment the detection accuracy is 100%; all of the saturated segment was correctly detected, and no false detection occurred.

5.4.2 Artifact Detection

In the artifact detection experiment, two datasets were used to evaluate the effectiveness of the detection method. Firstly, we use a simulated dataset to analyze the performance of detecting artifact with different frequencies, amplitudes, and lengths. Then we use a real dataset to evaluate the performance of real circumstance.

The simulated pulse signals were generated from 200 high-quality pulse signals by adding white noise in different frequency bands, lengths, and amplitudes. We intend to analyze the performance in detecting artifact in different frequencies, lengths, and amplitudes. The frequency band of the simulated samples includes 0~15 Hz, 15~30 Hz, and 30~45 Hz. 0~15 Hz is completely overlapped with pulse signal frequency band, 15~30 Hz is partially overlapped with pulse signal frequency band, and 30~45 Hz is little overlapped with pulse signal frequency band. Since the time resolution of the detecting method is the same to the length of pulse cycles thus in the simulated dataset, artifact with the length of 0.2, 0.4, 0.8, 2, and 5 times the length of the pulse cycles was generated and added to the high-quality pulse signal. The amplitude of the artifact includes 0.2, 0.4, 0.8, and 1.2. (In the artifact detection, the amplitude of pulse signal was normalized.)

In the experiment, statistics-based method was used for comparison. We apply the statistics-based method on pulse cycles to achieve the same time resolution as the proposed method. In the statistics-based method, we extract the mean value, standard derivation, and sample entropy from pulse cycles and set thresholds on these metrics to detect the artifact. Since the EMD-based method may introduce phase shift and usually need at least 5 s of pulse signal which is much longer than a pulse cycle, we do not take the EMD-based detection method in comparison.

For threshold selection in the proposed method, thresholds which varied from 0 to 1 at intervals of 0.005 were tested and the best threshold was selected. For the statistics method, we have three statistics features, and thus, we have three different thresholds. We let each threshold vary from 0 to 1 at intervals of 0.005; all of the combinations were tested, and the best combination was selected. In most of the time, a pulse signal has more normal cycles than artifact cycles; thus, in the experiment the sensitivity and specificity were used for parameter optimization and performance evaluation. Sensitivity is defined as the percentage of artifact cycles which are correctly identified, specificity was defined as the percentage of normal cycles which are correctly identified, and detection accuracy is defined as the percentage of all the correctly identified pulse cycles [33]. The threshold (or threshold combination for statistics-based method) with highest detection accuracy which the difference between the sensitivity and specificity is smaller than 5% was selected. If none of the result has this difference smaller than 5%, the result with the smallest difference between sensitivity and specificity was used.

The detection results on simulated dataset using statistics-based method are listed in Table 5.1, and the detection results using proposed method are listed in Table 5.2. In Tables 5.1 and 5.2, the ACC is short for the detection accuracy, the SEN is short for sensitivity, and the SPE is short for specificity, and the result was listed in percentage. From Tables 5.1 and 5.2, we found that the long artifacts with high frequency and large amplitude are relatively easy to detect, both the proposed method and statistics-based method can achieve good detection result. The short artifacts with low frequency and small amplitude are relatively difficult to detect, and the result is worse than the detection on long artifacts with high frequency and large amplitude. This may be because the artifact with lower frequency has a similar frequency band with the pulse signal, and short artifacts with small amplitude have a relatively small impact to the correlation coefficient or the statistics. From the result, we can see that the proposed method can achieve better performance than the statistics-based method especially in the detection of short artifact with small amplitude and low frequency.

The second dataset contains 113 pulse signals with real artifact. The detection result was shown in Table 5.3. From the result one can see the proposed detection method can also achieve a much better performance than the statistics-based method.

5.5 Summary

In this chapter, new methods were developed for the detection of saturation and artifact. For the detection of saturation, we develop two criteria from its definition and achieve 100% detection accuracy with the time resolution the same as the sampling frequency. For the artifact detection considered that the similarity should be an effective feature to detect the artifact, we transform the pulse signal into a complex network according to the similarity between pulse cycles and detect the artifact by measuring

Table 5.1 Detection result on simulated dataset using statistics-based method

Frequency band		0.2			0.4			0.8			2			5		
		ACC	SEN	SPE	ACC	SEN	SPE	ACC	SEN	SPE	ACC	SEN	SPE	ACC	SEN	SPE
0–15	0.2	40.1	38.0	40.2	25.4	22.0	25.6	15.1	11.5	15.3	45.5	41.5	45.9	54.8	54.2	54.9
	0.4	44.0	45.5	43.9	43.7	40.5	43.9	33.7	31.0	33.9	52.8	52.0	52.8	61.5	60.8	61.7
	0.8	50.8	47.5	51.0	51.0	52.0	51.0	53.9	49.5	54.2	62.7	61.3	62.8	64.6	63.9	64.8
	1.2	57.0	54.0	57.1	60.8	57.0	61.0	60.9	58.0	61.0	68.0	64.3	68.4	64.7	63.7	65.0
15~30	0.2	50.8	47.0	51.0	40.3	41.0	40.2	37.5	38.0	37.5	90.5	86.8	90.9	96.0	92.3	97.2
	0.4	60.8	57.0	61.0	69.5	65.5	69.7	78.8	75.0	79.0	99.3	96.3	99.7	99.3	97.8	99.8
	0.8	69.4	65.0	69.7	80.7	77.5	80.9	90.3	86.0	90.6	99.6	97.3	99.9	99.6	98.8	99.9
	1.2	72.5	70.0	72.7	82.7	81.5	82.7	95.6	91.5	95.8	99.7	98.3	99.9	99.7	99.1	99.9
30–45	0.2	57.2	58.5	57.1	54.1	52.5	54.2	60.9	58.5	61.0	98.3	94.0	98.9	99.2	97.5	99.7
	0.4	72.6	72.0	72.7	82.7	81.0	82.7	92.7	88.0	92.9	99.9	99.8	99.8	99.9	99.9	99.9
	0.8	76.6	74.5	76.7	91.2	86.5	91.4	98.2	94.0	98.4	99.9	100	99.9	100	100	99.9
	1.2	82.6	79.0	82.7	94.0	89.5	94.2	99.7	97.0	99.9	99.9	100	99.9	99.9	100	99.9

Table 5.2 Detection result on simulated dataset using proposed method

Frequency band		0.2			0.4			0.8			2			5		
		ACC	SEN	SPE	ACC	SEN	SPE	ACC	SEN	SPE	ACC	SEN	SPE	ACC	SEN	SPE
0–15	0.2	64.1	76.0	63.5	88.3	81.0	88.6	99.8	98.5	99.9	99.9	99	100	99.9	99.5	100
	0.4	64.2	79.5	63.5	88.0	76.5	88.5	99.7	97.0	99.9	100	99.8	100	99.7	99.2	99.9
	0.8	64.5	85.5	63.5	88.4	86.5	88.5	99.7	97.0	99.9	100	100	100	99.8	99.3	100
	1.2	88.0	76.0	88.6	88.5	88.5	88.5	99.7	95.5	99.9	99.9	99.3	100	99.9	99.9	99.9
15~30	0.2	64.3	81.0	63.5	88.1	79.5	88.6	99.8	96.0	100	100	100	100	100	100	100
	0.4	64.5	84.5	63.5	88.5	88.0	88.5	99.9	98.5	100	100	100	100	100	100	100
	0.8	88.0	77.5	88.5	95.9	94.0	96.0	100	100	100	100	100	100	100	100	100
	1.2	88.2	81.5	88.5	96.0	94.5	96.1	100	100	100	100	100	100	100	100	100
30–45	0.2	64.4	82.0	63.5	88.1	80.0	88.5	99.8	99.0	99.9	100	100	100	100	100	100
	0.4	87.5	65.0	88.5	88.7	91.0	88.5	99.9	97.5	100	100	100	100	100	100	100
	0.8	88.2	82.5	88.5	95.9	92.5	96.0	100	99.0	100	100	100	100	100	100	100
	1.2	88.6	89.0	88.6	98.7	94.5	98.9	100	100	100	100	100	100	100	100	100

Table 5.3 Artifact detection result on real dataset

	ACC	SEN	SPE
Proposed method	99.54	95.58	99.73
Statistics-based method	80.51	76.11	80.73

the connectivity of the network; the result of artifact detection shows that the proposed method can achieve better performance than statistics-based method. In the real artifact detection, we achieve the detection accuracy of 99.54% with the sensitivity and specificity of 95.58% and 99.73%, respectively. The time resolution of artifact detection is around 0.7 s which is more precise than the current detection method.

References

1. S. Walsh and E. King, Pulse Diagnosis: A Clinical Guide. Sydney Australia: Elsevier, 2008.
2. V. D. Lad, Secrets of the Pulse. Albuquerque, New Mexico: The Ayurvedic Press, 1996.
3. E. Hsu, Pulse Diagnosis in Early Chinese Medicine. New York, American: Cambridge University Press, 2010.
4. R. Amber and B. Brooke, Pulse Diagnosis: Detailed Interpretations For Eastern & Western Holistic Treatments. Santa Fe, New Mexico: Aurora Press, 1993.
5. H. Sorvoja, V. M. Kokko, R. Myllyla, and J. Miettinen, "Use of EMFi as a blood pressure pulse transducer," IEEE Transactions on Instrumentation and Measurement, vol. 54, pp. 2505–2512, 2005.
6. E. Kaniusas, H. Pfutzner, L. Mehnen, J. Kosel, C. Tellez-Blanco, G. Varoneckas, et al., "Method for continuous nondisturbing monitoring of blood pressure by magnetoelastic skin curvature sensor and ECG," IEEE Sensors Journal, vol. 6, pp. 819–828, Jun 2006.
7. H.-T. Wu, C.-H. Lee, and A.-B. Liu, "Assessment of endothelial function using arterial pressure signals," Journal of Signal Processing Systems, vol. 64, pp. 223–232, 2011.
8. C.-S. Hu, Y.-F. Chung, C.-C. Yeh, and C.-H. Luo, "Temporal and Spatial Properties of Arterial Pulsation Measurement Using Pressure Sensor Array," Evidence-Based Complementary and Alternative Medicine, vol. 2012, pp. 1–9, 2012.
9. P. Wang, W. Zuo, and D. Zhang, "A Compound Pressure Signal Acquisition System for Multichannel Wrist Pulse Signal Analysis," Instrumentation and Measurement, IEEE Transactions on, vol. 63, pp. 1556–1565, 2014.
10. Y. Chen, L. Zhang, D. Zhang, and D. Zhang, "Wrist pulse signal diagnosis using modified Gaussian Models and Fuzzy C-Means classification," Medical Engineering & Physics, vol. 31, pp. 1283–1289, Dec 2009.
11. Y. Chen, L. Zhang, D. Zhang, and D. Zhang, "Computerized wrist pulse signal diagnosis using modified auto-regressive models," Journal of Medical Systems, vol. 35, pp. 321–328, Jun 2011.
12. L. Liu, W. Zuo, D. Zhang, N. Li, and H. Zhang, "Combination of heterogeneous features for wrist pulse blood flow signal diagnosis via multiple kernel learning," IEEE Transactions on Information Technology in Biomedicine, vol. 16, pp. 599–607, Jul 2012.
13. L. Liu, W. Zuo, D. Zhang, N. Li, and H. Zhang, "Classification of wrist pulse blood flow signal using time warp edit distance," Medical Biometrics, vol. 6165, pp. 137–144, 2010.
14. D. Y. Zhang, W. M. Zuo, D. Zhang, H. Z. Zhang, and N. M. Li, "Wrist blood flow signal-based computerized pulse diagnosis using spatial and spectrum features," Journal of Biomedical Science and Engineering, vol. 3, pp. 361–366, 2010.

15. Q. L. Guo, K. Q. Wang, D. Y. Zhang, and N. M. Li, "A wavelet packet based pulse waveform analysis for cholecystitis and nephrotic syndrome diagnosis," in IEEE International Conference on Wavelet Analysis and Pattern Recognition, Hong Kong, China, 2008, pp. 513–517.
16. S. Charbonnier, S. Galichet, G. Mauris, and J. P. Siche, "Statistical and fuzzy models of ambulatory systolic blood pressure for hypertension diagnosis," IEEE Transactions on Instrumentation and Measurement, vol. 49, pp. 998–1003, 2000.
17. H.-T. Wu, C.-H. Lee, C.-K. Sun, J.-T. Hsu, R.-M. Huang, and C.-J. Tang, "Arterial Waveforms Measured at the Wrist as Indicators of Diabetic Endothelial Dysfunction in the Elderly," IEEE Transactions on Instrumentation and Measurement, vol. 61, pp. 162–169, 2012.
18. L. Jing, S. Hao, G. Yinjing, and S. Hongyu, "Pulse Signal De-Noising Based on Integer Lifting Scheme Wavelet Transform," in International Conference on Bioinformatics and Biomedical Engineering, WuHan, China, 2007, pp. 936–939.
19. S. Su, Q. Yan-Yan, and Q. Jun-Fei, "Research on de-noising of pulse signal based on fuzzy threshold in wavelet packet domain," in International Conference on Wavelet Analysis and Pattern Recognition, Beijing, China, 2007, pp. 103–106.
20. G. Rui, W. Yiqin, Y. Jianjun, L. Fufeng, and Y. Haixia, "Wavelet based De-noising of pulse signal," in IEEE International Symposium on IT in Medicine and Education, Xiamen, China, 2008, pp. 617–620.
21. C. Fengxiang, H. Wenxue, Z. Tao, J. Jung, and L. Xulong, "Research on Wavelet Denoising for Pulse Signal Based on Improved Wavelet Thresholding," in International Conference on Pervasive Computing Signal Processing and Applications, Harbin, China, 2010, pp. 564–567.
22. D. Wang and D. Zhang, "Analysis of pulse waveforms preprocessing," in International Conference onComputerized Healthcare, HongKong, 2012, pp. 175–180.
23. H. Wang, X. Wang, J. R. Deller, and J. Fu, "A Shape-Preserving Preprocessing for Human Pulse Signals Based on Adaptive Parameter Determination," IEEE Transactions on Biomedical Circuits and Systems, vol. 8, pp. 594–604, 2013.
24. G. Zheng-Gang, G. Yun, L. Li-Yan, and C. Chen, "Pulse wave signal baseline wander elimination using morphology," in IEEE International Conference on Signal Processing Beijing, China, 2010, pp. 74–77.
25. L. Xu, D. Zhang, and K. Wang, "Wavelet-based cascaded adaptive filter for removing baseline drift in pulse waveforms," IEEE Transactions on Biomedical Engineering, vol. 52, pp. 1973–1975, Nov 2005.
26. J. Havlik, Z. Martinovska, J. Dvorak, and L. Lhotska, "Detection of artifacts in oscillometric pulsations signals," in Biomedical and Health Informatics (BHI), 2014 IEEE-EMBS International Conference on, 2014, pp. 709–711.
27. D. Migotina, A. Calapez, and A. Rosa, "Automatic Artifacts Detection and Classification in Sleep EEG Signals Using Descriptive Statistics and Histogram Analysis: Comparison of Two Detectors," in Engineering and Technology (S-CET), 2012 Spring Congress on, 2012, pp. 1–6.
28. L. Jinseok, D. D. McManus, S. Merchant, and K. H. Chon, "Automatic Motion and Noise Artifact Detection in Holter ECG Data Using Empirical Mode Decomposition and Statistical Approaches," IEEE Transactions on Biomedical Engineering, vol. 59, pp. 1499–1506, 2012.
29. L. Shaopeng, H. Qingbo, R. X. Gao, and P. Freedson, "Empirical mode decomposition applied to tissue artifact removal from respiratory signal," in Annual International Conference of the IEEE Engineering in Medicine and Biology Society, Vancouver, Canada, 2008, pp. 3624–3627.
30. C. Dianguo, L. Liu, and W. Peng, "Removing Baseline Drift in Pulse Waveforms by a Wavelet Adaptive Filter," in International Conference on Bioinformatics and Biomedical Engineering, Shanghai, China, 2008, pp. 2135–2137.
31. Y. Lin, Z. Song, L. Xiaoyang, and Y. Yimin, "Removal of Pulse Waveform Baseline Drift Using Cubic Spline Interpolation," in International Conference on Bioinformatics and Biomedical Engineering, Chengdu, China, 2010, pp. 1–3.
32. J. Zhang, X. Luo, and M. Small, "Detecting chaos in pseudoperiodic time series without embedding," Physical Review E, vol. 73, pp. 1–5, 2006.
33. A. G. Lalkhen and A. McCluskey, "Clinical tests: sensitivity and specificity," Continuing Education in Anaesthesia, Critical Care & Pain, vol. 8, pp. 221–223, 2008.

Chapter 6
Optimized Preprocessing Framework for Wrist Pulse Analysis

Abstract Since wrist pulse signals collected by the sensors are often corrupted by artifacts in real situations, many approaches on the wrist pulse preprocessing including pulse denoising and baseline drift removal are introduced for more accurate wrist pulse analysis. However, these scattered methods are incomplete with some limitations when used to preprocess our special pulse data for the clinical applications. This chapter presents a robust signal preprocessing framework for wrist pulse analysis. The cascade filter based on frequency-dependent analysis (FDA) is first introduced to remove the high-frequency noises and to select the significant intervals. Then the curve fitting method is developed to adjust the direction and the baseline drift with minimum signal distortion. Last, the period segmentation and normalization is applied for the feature extraction. The effectiveness of the proposed framework is validated through experiments on actual pulse records with biochemical markers. Both quantitative and qualitative results are given. The results show that the proposed pulse preprocessing framework is effective in extracting more accurate pulse features and practical for wrist pulse analysis.

6.1 Introduction

Wrist pulse contains rich information of the human body. It has been applied to health diagnosis in Traditional Chinese Medicine (TCM) since ancient times [1]. The Chinese medicine practitioners used to feel the pulsations by placing three fingers at the radial artery to judge the health status of patients. Thus, the pulse diagnosis depends heavily on the subjective analysis of practitioners and turns out to be unreliable and inconsistent [2]. With the advances in sensor technology, a number of pulse acquisition platforms are developed to collect the computation wrist pulse waveforms for more objective and accurate pulse diagnosis recently [3–6].

We design a novel wrist pulse acquisition platform with multichannel and fusion sensors. The pulsations at the wrist are first detected by the sensor arrays and then transformed into the digital voltage outputs through the analog and digital circuit. Since the wrist pulses are weak vibrations inside the human body, they are often noised by disturbances from environments. Three dominant artifacts present in our

© Springer Nature Singapore Pte Ltd. 2018
D. Zhang et al., *Computational Pulse Signal Analysis*,
https://doi.org/10.1007/978-981-10-4044-3_6

wrist pulse signals are (1) high-frequency noise caused by 50 Hz power line interferences and artifact motions acting on the sensors, (2) baseline drift caused by
respiration, and (3) cycle deviation that may be due to the chaos phenomenon. These
artifacts badly influence the wrist pulse analysis accuracy and should be removed to
avoid false-positive classification.

It is well known that the wrist pulse is a periodic physiological signal with each
single period representing a heartbeat cycle as electrocardiogram (ECG). The two
physiological signals are both driven by the heart and somewhat reflect the health
status of heart [7, 25]. Thus, ECG has been widely used for the heart monitoring and
arrhythmia checkup [8]. The heart rhythms can be accurately obtained from the
periods of these two signals. Compared with ECG, the wrist pulse waveform flows
a long way from the heart. As a result, it is not only influenced by the heart conditions but also affected by the conditions of the nerves, muscles, skin, arterial walls,
and blood parameters (volume, contents, viscosity, pressure, and velocity) [9].
Therefore, the wrist pulse contains more information than ECG due to the interac-
tions of inside organs [10]. And the methods for ECG preprocessing could not be
used to preprocess the wrist pulse directly.

A number of methods have been proposed for the wrist pulse preprocessing, but
to data all have been flawed for our wrist pulse database. In summary, the former
researches on pulse preprocessing can be divided into two categories, pulse denoising and baseline drift removal. For the pulse denoising, Ciaccio and Drzewiecki
[11] propose a differential steepest descent (DSD) adaptive noise cancellation
method. However, there is a large shift in the baseline level. Xia et al. [12] introduce
a zero-phase filtering on pulse trend, which processes the input pulse data in both
forward and reverse directions to overcome the phase shift. But the evaluation criterion of the filter is not verified by the wrist pulse analysis. Empirical mode decomposition (EMD) is introduced for the pulse denoising by Wu and Lee [13]. However,
the experiment is conducted by adding a white noise series to the targeted data
under simulated environments. And it is not suitable for our actual pulse records
collected under real environments. As a result of the baseline drift, the wrist pulse
has a relatively low-frequency component throughout the entire signal. This kind of
distortion also appears in ECG and other physiological signals [14, 15]. Approaches
from frequency view, including FIR filter, Kalman filter, and wavelet cascade filter,
are applied to remove the baseline drift [15–19]. They all attempt to suppress the
baseline drift with high-pass filter, which would introduce nonlinear phase distortion as well as the key-knot displacement caused by time domain convolution.
Besides, the wrist pulse signals in these experiments are corrupted by adding the
drift manually, which is not convincing for practical application.

Besides the two conventional preprocessing methods, we add the pulse period
segmentation into the framework for the first time. The period segmentation plays
an important role in pulse analysis to extract the intra-class information. Xia et al.
[12] propose a period segmentation and estimation method to represent the pulse
trend. Chen et al. [20] introduce a period segmentation for pulse analysis by using
modified Gaussian models. However, both of the two methods choose the average

single-period pulse from the entire signal after the period segmentation, resulting in the loss of detail information.

In this chapter, our focus is on building a robust signal preprocessing framework for wrist pulse analysis. We first introduce the proposed pulse acquisition platform and specify the inherent properties of the coarser pulse data. Then, a cascade filter based on frequency-dependent analysis is proposed for the wrist pulse denoising. Next, the interval selection is performed to remove the distortion sections. For the baseline drift in our database, the direction correction and curve fitting method is employed to adjust the baseline driftings. Last, the pulse normalization is developed for feature extraction.

Besides the description of the wrist pulse preprocessing algorithms and the related theoretical derivations, in this chapter, much attention is paid on comparisons of the methods through the quantitative and qualitative evaluations. We do experiments using the real wrist pulse records with definite labels, which are acquired from the volunteers of Prince of Wales Hospital, Hong Kong. The experiment results indicate that the classification accuracy is increased significantly by using the proposed preprocessing framework. And the experimental studies also demonstrate that the proposed pulse preprocessing framework outperforms the previous methods, especially for the wrist pulse analysis. The contributions of this work lie in two aspects. First, we introduce the novel algorithms in pulse signal enhancement. Second, the preprocessing framework is applied to extract the intraclass features for wrist pulse analysis.

The remainder of this chapter is organized as follows. In Sect. 6.2, we introduce the pulse acquisition platform and the characteristics of the original pulse database from both time domain and frequency domain. The preprocessing framework and the comparisons of the preprocessing methods are outlined in Sects. 6.3 and 6.4, respectively. Finally, a conclusion is given in Sect. 6.5.

6.2 Description of Pulse Database

6.2.1 Data Acquisition

In TCM, the practitioners took pulse by feeling the pulsations at *Cun*, *Guan*, and *Chi* three adjacent positions of the wrist with proper pressures (deep, middle, and superficial). The pressures and positions yield the concept of nine indicators. The health status of specific internal organs could be obtained from the relationships between nine indicators and the internal organs [21]. The relations are based on the *Mai Jing* (*The Pulse Classic*) compiled by Wang Shuhe, which is the first extant book specializing in sphygmology. Thus, for the pulsations from "*Cun*", "*Guan*" and "*Chi*" three parts should be collected completely for the pulse diagnosis.

In our work, a USB-based pulse acquisition platform with multichannel and fusion sensor array is developed to collect the wrist pulse signals from *Cun*, *Guan*,

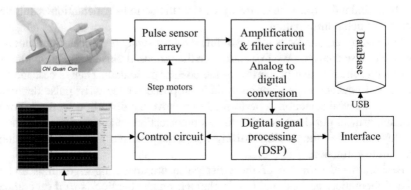

Fig. 6.1 A brief flowchart of the proposed pulse system

and *Chi* simultaneously (see Fig. 6.1). The proposed system is composed of three parts, pulse sensor array, circuit, and interface. And the three independent channels correspond to the *Cun*, *Guan*, and *Chi* positions. Each channel contains a pulse sensor array to transform the physical beatings into weak voltage outputs. Then, the millivolt voltages are processed by the amplification and filtering module. The amplified voltages from the sensor array are converted into digital signals simultaneously using a 12-bit data acquisition card at a sample rate of 500 Hz. Next, the micro digital signal processing module is applied to control the static contact pressures. Finally, the digital wrist pulse signals are sent to a PC for real-time monitoring through a universal serial bus interface and stored in Microsoft Database (MDB) format.

Figure 6.2 shows the proposed pulse acquisition platform. All measurements were undertaken in a quiet indoor environment. When taking the subject's pulse, we first search the rough positions of the wrist pulse by feeling the pulsations at the radial artery. Then the transducer is put around the wrist with the sensor array covering the right corresponding regions. Next, the contact pressure is subtly controlled by the step motors at the top to obtain optimal pulse waveforms. Once stable pulses with high amplitudes appear, we pause the pressure adjustment and preview the waveforms for a moment. Last, the wrist pulse signals are recorded for more than 60 s for each volunteer.

6.2.2 Time Domain Characteristic

Figure 6.3a shows a typical pulse waveform collected by the pulse acquisition platform. It can be seen that wrist pulse is a periodic signal similar to ECG. The periods are correlated with the cardiac rhythm. And the baselines often wander due to the respiration and artifact motions. The difference between the two physiological signals is that the shape of each single-period pulse varies with each other in the detail points.

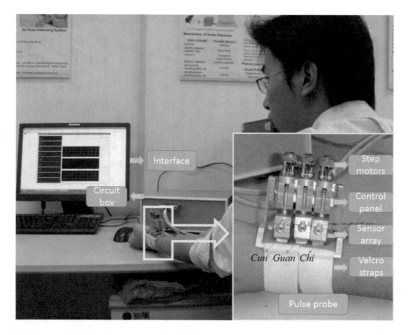

Fig. 6.2 The proposed pulse acquisition platform

Figure 6.3b presents a local enlargement of the single-period pulse signal. It is composed of an ascending limb and a descending limb. A tidal wave and a dicrotic wave often exist in the descending limb, which make up the characteristic points of pulse shape along with the percussion wave. Many methods such as auto-regressive (AR) model [22], Gaussian model [20], and spatial parameters [9] are proposed to extract the time domain pulse features.

6.2.3   Frequency Domain Characteristic

In general, the heart rate is around 30~90 beats per minute in an adult human being. The basic period of the pulse is, therefore, the same as heart rhythm. And the frequency components of the characteristic points are above the cardiac rhythm. A scientific way of studying the pulse should be to analyze its frequency spectrum distribution [10].

Figure 6.4 shows the frequency spectrum of the pulse waveform in Fig. 6.2a. The sampling rate is set to 500 Hz to cover the frequency bands of the pulsations. According to the Nyquist sampling theorem, the frequency range of the acquired pulse waveform is from 0 to 250 Hz. Figure 6.4a shows the global frequency distribution. The frequency spectrum is concentrated in the bands below 20 Hz. The high-frequency components at around 50 and 100 Hz belong to the power line inter-

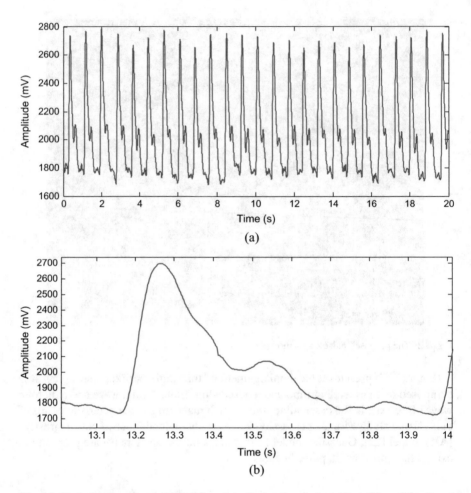

Fig. 6.3 Typical wrist pulse signal: (**a**) the original pulse signal of a subject; (**b**) partial enlarged view of the single-period pulse signal

ference. Figure 6.4b shows the frequency spectrum details from 0 to 20 Hz. The frequency component with the highest amplitude at around 1 Hz denotes to the basic period. Components with frequency lower than the period are caused by uncontrollable artifacts and respiration activities.

Based on the frequency distribution, we propose a frequency-dependent analysis (FDA) method to analyze pulse properties in frequency domain. Wavelet transform is a mature algorithm that has been widely applied to signal decomposition. By using the wavelet decomposition, the wrist pulse signals are divided into several frequency bands. We select the wavelets "*sym8*" as the basic component and the decomposition is processed at level eight. Figure 6.5 shows the wavelet decomposi-

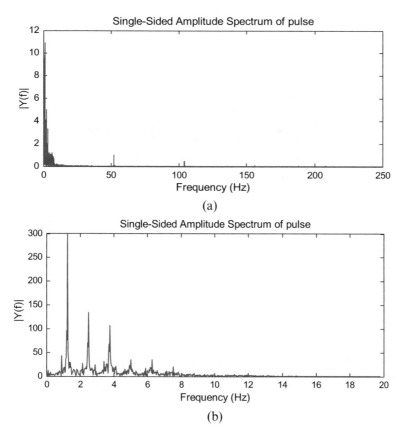

Fig. 6.4 The diagram of pulse frequency spectrum: (**a**) global frequency distribution of the pulse waveform; (**b**) local enlarged view of frequency bands of 0~20 Hz

tion coefficients of a typical wrist pulse. A partial enlargement view of the wavelet coefficients of band *CD1* to *CD4* is placed in the center.

Table 6.1 shows the relationship between the divided frequency bands and the levels of wavelet decomposition. According to the energy distribution properties, we separate them into four groups: noise, details, structure, and baseline. The pulse information is mainly contained in the bands from *CD4* to *CD8*, which covers the frequency spectrum range from 1 to 20 Hz. Because the energies decrease rapidly above 20 Hz, which belongs to the power line interference section, we simply ignore this range in the pulse analysis. The energy at the band *AD8* reflects the DC component and the baseline drift, and this band can be discarded. The pulse denoising and baseline drift removal are performed in the *CD1~CD4* bands and *CA8* band, respectively.

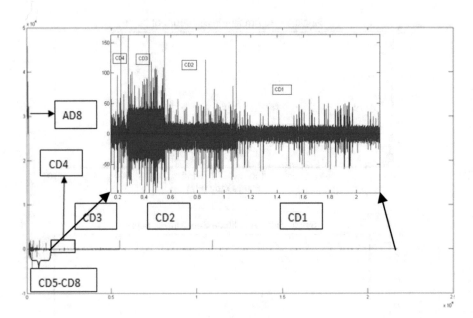

Fig. 6.5 Pulse decomposition at N = 8 by wavelets "sym8" (Redraw)

Table 6.1 The definition of the frequency component

Frequency bands	Description
CD1–CD3(30~250 Hz)	Power frequency interference noise
CD4 (16~30 Hz)	Power frequency interference noise
CD5 (8~16 Hz)	
CD6 (4 ~8 Hz)	Detail features of pulse waveform
CD7 (2~4 Hz)	
CD8 (1~2 Hz)	Structure of pulse waveform
CA8 (0~1 Hz)	Baseline of pulse waveform

6.3 Proposed Pulse Preprocessing Method

The wrist pulse waveforms collected by electronic sensing elements bring in noise, inevitably. And the pulse baseline drift varies with each individual. Besides, distortions, inversions, and period variances exist in the pulse database. These interferences should be removed to perform accurate pulse analysis. Figure 6.6 shows the proposed preprocessing framework for wrist pulse analysis, which consists of four stages in sequence: pulse denoising, interval selection, baseline drift removal, and period segmentation and normalization.

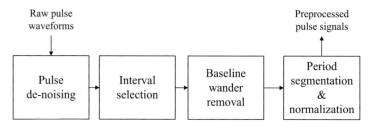

Fig. 6.6 The flowchart of the proposed pulse preprocessing method

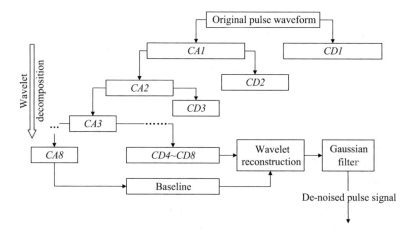

Fig. 6.7 The proposed cascade filter for pulse denoising

6.3.1 Pulse Denoising

The wrist pulse is easily noised by micro disturbance such as the 50 Hz power line interference, tiny jitter, and talking. In addition, the circuit itself also brings in white Gaussian noise and high-frequency noise at the analog to digital conversion module. According to the FDA theory, the useful pulse information is contained below 20 Hz. Consequently, we first design an Equiripple FIR low-pass filter with pass-band frequency at 12 Hz and stop-band frequency at 16 Hz to eliminate the high-frequency noise caused by power line interference and the AD conversion module. It removes the burrs and keeps the trends. However, the low-pass filter brings distortions to the denoised pulse signals due to the errors between the desired filter and ideal filter. And the dramatic subtle ups and downs in the pulse waveforms are restrained owing to the filtering effect. These disadvantages motivate us to find a more accurate pulse denoising method.

We design a cascade denoising method by combining the wavelet transform with the Gaussian filter. Figure 6.7 presents the diagram of the proposed denoising method. First, the original pulse waveform is divided into eight bands based on wavelet decomposition. According to the FDA theory, the pulse information is mainly contained in the bands from *CD4* to *CD8*. In band *CA8*, the coefficients approximate the pulse baseline. Then, the coefficients of these bands are used to reconstruct the pulse waveform by using the inverse wavelet transform. Finally, the reconstructed signals are smoothed by the Gaussian filter.

6.3.2 Interval Selection

Although body movements, hysterical emotions, talking, and coughing are forbidden during the pulse collecting, the pulse waveforms are often corrupted by unconscious jitters, coughing, or uncontrollable movements of the patient's arm. Besides, signal magnitudes maybe exceed the quantization range and lead to truncations in certain pulse samples. These distortions are still reserved after the pulse denoising procedure.

Figure 6.8a illustrates a pulse waveform disturbed by a sudden body movement. Figure 6.8b presents a typical truncated pulse waveform owing to the saturation effect, and the corresponding value distribution is shown in Fig. 6.8c. The values of normal pulse waveforms are distributed evenly over the whole range. Conversely, the outlying observations such as the truncated and abnormal values lie in the two ends of the histogram. These two kinds of distortion cannot be recovered as critical information is missing. Therefore, we propose an adaptive thresholding method to eliminate the pulse intervals with the unrecoverable distortions. The interval selection algorithm is defined by the formula below:

$$p(t) = \begin{cases} 1, \{t \,|\, s(t) - E(s) \le \theta_1^* \delta_1(s) + \theta_1' \delta_1'(s) \} \\ 0, \text{otherwise} \end{cases}, \tag{6.1}$$

$$u(t) = s(t) * p(t)$$

$$q(t) = \begin{cases} 1, \left\{ t \,\middle|\, \left| \dot{u}(t) - E\left(\dot{u}\right) \right| \le \theta_2^* \delta\left(\dot{u}\right) \right\} \\ 0, \text{otherwise} \end{cases}. \tag{6.2}$$

$$y(t) = q(t) * u(t)$$

First, we calculate the global standard deviation $\delta_1(s)$ and the local standard deviation $\delta_1'(s)$ of the pulse waveform, which are used to eliminate the intervals with abnormal values. Since the normal pulse waveforms change gradually during the sampling period, then the first-order derivation which measures the gradient is extracted to eliminate the intervals with drastic changes. The weighted parameters θ_1, θ_1', and θ_2 are set to 0.5, 2, and 1.5 based on the experience. In order to guarantee

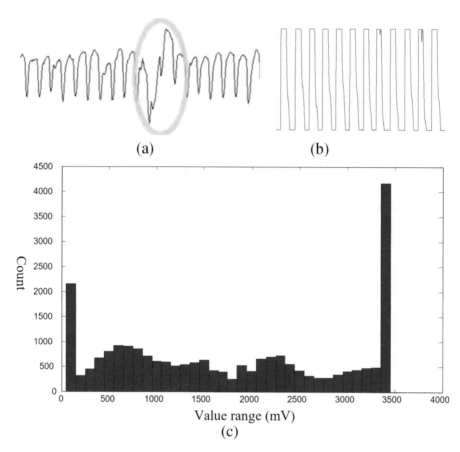

(a)   (b)

(c)

Fig. 6.8 Two types of signal distortion in pulse and the distribution histogram: (**a**) pulse signal noised by sudden movements; (**b**) pulse signal with saturation effect; (**c**) value distribution of truncated pulse

that all segmented waveforms contain several complete pulse periods, the length of the selected intervals is required to have at least four cycle periods.

6.3.3   Baseline Drift Removal

Figure 6.9 presents the procedure of the pulse baseline drift removal. It consists of three steps. First, the pulse direction is adjusted to the same standard. Next, the consecutive local minimums of each period are extracted for the cubic spline interpolation. Finally, the drift is removed by subtracting the estimated drift curve.

Direction adjustment is performed before baseline estimation. As a result of the influence of the wrist skin, the direction of the wrist pulse collected by the proposed

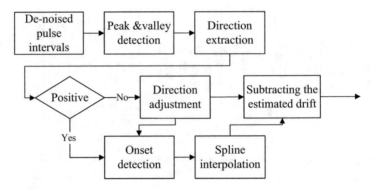

Fig. 6.9 A flowchart of the pulse baseline drift adjustment

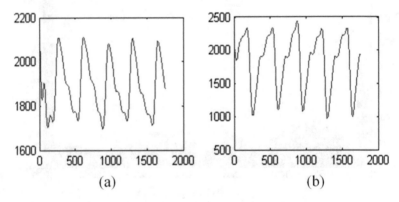

Fig. 6.10 Pulse waveforms with positive and negative directions: (**a**) positive; (**b**) negative

system presents two kinds of state. Figure 6.10 gives the typical pulse signals with opposite directions. Figure 6.10a shows the normal pulse waveform with positive direction. Figure 6.10b presents the variant pulse signal with negative direction.

In order to reduce the variety in directions, we need to adjust the pulse waveforms to the same standard. In the experiments, we set the pulse waveform with a shorter length ascending branch as the standard direction. Meanwhile, the onset point of the first cycle is regarded as the pulse zero-phase. Peak and valley detection is employed to compare the length of ascending and descending branch. And the pulse direction is determined by the length of the two branches. An adaptive sliding window method is adopted to obtain the peak and valley points in the signals (see Fig. 6.11). The whole algorithm is described as follows:

Step 1.   Perform the Fourier transform to find out the basic frequency f_p basic period is calculated as $T_p = 1/f_p$.

Step 2.   Detect peak and valley points of the pulse signal within initial window $[0, T_P]$. Peak is the maximum point and valley is the minimum. The corresponding positions at timing axis are p_1 and v_1, respectively.

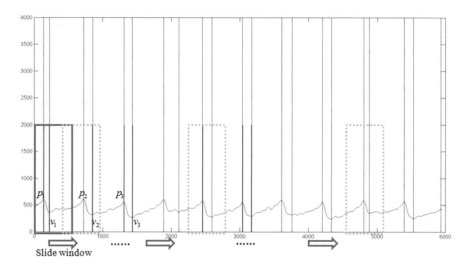

Fig. 6.11 Peak and valley detection based on slide window

Step 3.   Slide the window step-by-step to update the information. The second extreme points p_2 and v_2 are detected in time interval $[p_1 + (T_p/2), p_1 + (3T_p/2)]$.

Step 4.   Repeat the procedure steps 2 and 3 till the window moves to the end. Check up the missing valleys and peaks by the rules of one-to-one correspondence.

Assuming that x stands for a pulse signal, the time sets of pulse peaks and valleys are given by $p(x) = [p_1, p_2, \ldots, p_m]$ and $v(x) = [v_1, v_2, \ldots, v_m]$, respectively. They meet the condition $v_1 < p_1 < v_2 < p_2 < \ldots < v_m < p_m$, and m is the length of the pulse cycle. The pulse direction is given by the following formulas:

$$D(x) = \mathrm{sgn}\left[\frac{1}{m-1}\sum_{i-1}^{m-1}(v_{i+1} - p_i) - \frac{1}{m}\sum_{i=1}^{m}(p_i - v_i)\right].$$

$$p_i \in p(x), v_i \in v(x)$$

(6.3)

Then the algorithm of pulse direction adjustment is given by the formula below:

$$y(t) = D(x)x(t) + \frac{1 - D(x)}{N}\sum_{i=1}^{N}x(i), t = 1, 2, \cdots, N.$$

(6.4)

If the pulse waveform is negative, the peaks will be turned into valleys after the direction adjustment. The time sets of pulse valleys $v(x) = [v_1, v_2, \cdots, v_m]$ are used for baseline estimation.

The cubic spline is selected as the interpolation curve. Since the baseline drift caused by respiration has nonlinear contents and the linear estimation will bring

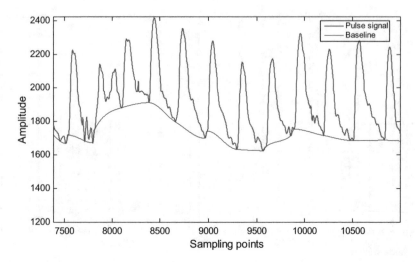

Fig. 6.12 Baseline drift in the pulse waveform

distortions if used, we thus prefer the cubic spline functions to the linear interpolation in baseline drift estimation. Figure 6.12 shows the baseline estimation result. The pulse waveforms are then corrected by subtracting the estimated remaining drift.

6.3.4   Period Segmentation and Normalization

Pulse is a periodical physiological signal driven by the heart and flows along the artery through the internal organs. It is not a determinate process that can be expressed by a mathematic function. Although the rough structures of each period in one sample are almost the same, the details vary from cycle to cycle. The traditional period selection and average single-period pulse extraction both ignore the intra-class information. Thus, the period segmentation methods are necessary to extract the intra-class distance among cycles for pulse analysis.

The period segmentation is developed following the baseline drift removal module. From an overall point of view, each cycle can be regarded as the basic element of pulse waveforms. Consequently, pulse samples are segmented into a set of the single-period signals. Different segmentations are employed in this module, since the segmentation performance is affected by the strategies. To obtain the optimal segmented single-period pulse sets, we propose six segmentation strategies to ensure the split points as below:

Encoding valley detection (EVD): The pulse value is encoded using the integer function to remove the interferences caused by small extreme points. Then, the valley of each cycle is set as the onsets.

Encoding peak detection (EPD): The encoding method is the same as FPD and the
  peak of each cycle is set as the onsets.
Local minimum (LM) The standard methods by using the local minimum value of
  each cycle as the onsets without encoding and the baseline drift removal.
Local minimum slope (LMS): Onsets are determined by the local minimum slope of
  the ascending limb at each cycle.
Wander correction (WC): Baseline drift removal and encoding are used to ensure
  the onsets.
First derivation (FD): The original pulse waveforms are mapped into derivation
  space and the local minimum is detected as the onsets.

The performance comparisons on the segmentation strategies are discussed in
Sect. 6.4.2.

Due to the variances of heart rhythm, the pulse periods vary from individual to
individual. Therefore, the segmented single-period pulse signals always have
unequal lengths. The amplitude, which is influenced by static contact pressure and
pulse energy, also differs. Additionally, the onsets and ending points of each single-
period pulse are not in a horizontal line, which leads to the pulse rotation.
Consequently, the pulse normalization is essential to preprocess the pulse data from
various operational and environmental conditions. It consists of three stages, pulse
rotation transformation, downsampling, and amplitude normalization.

The rotation transformation aims to rotate the wrist pulse to be horizontal. The
angle between the horizontal line and the line connecting the onset and end point of
the single-period pulse is defined as the rotation angle θ. The adjusted pulse is
obtained by using the transformation formula below:

$$\left[t', y\left(t' \right) \right] = \left[t, x\left(t \right) \right] \begin{bmatrix} \cos\theta & -\sin\theta \\ \sin\theta & \cos\theta \end{bmatrix}. \tag{6.5}$$

Downsampling and amplitude normalization are applied to obtain equal single-
period pulse points and to scale the value magnitude to a proper range, respectively.
Let the single-period pulse be a time series $y(i)$. Where, N_1 stands for the number of
original single-period points and N_2 for the resampled single-period points. Linear
interpolation is used to calculate the value of pulse point $y(i + \Delta t)$ between points
$y(i)$ and $y(i + 1)$. The downsampling procedure is accomplished by the following
equations to get the resampled signal $z(i)$:

$$\underset{i=1,\cdots,m}{z(i)} = y\left(1 + \left(i - 1 \right) \times \frac{N-1}{m-1} \right). \tag{6.6}$$

$$y\left(i + \Delta t \right) = \left(1 - \Delta t \right) \cdot y\left(i \right) + \Delta t \cdot y\left(i + 1 \right). \tag{6.7}$$

The amplitude scale normalization is given by the formula below:

$$\overline{z}(i) = \frac{z(i) - \min\limits_{i=1,\cdots,m} z(i)}{\max\limits_{i=1,\cdots,m} z(i) - \min\limits_{i=1,\cdots,m} z(i)} \times A, \tag{6.8}$$

where A is the predetermined rescaled amplitude and max $(\cdot)$ and min $(\cdot)$ denote the maximum value and the minimum value of the pulse data series, respectively.

6.4   Experiments on Actual Pulse Database

6.4.1   Comparison of Pulse Denoising

In the first experiment, we study the performances of the proposed cascade denoising filter, wavelet filter, FIR low-pass filter, and moving average filter by using actual pulse records. We randomly choose 300 pulse data from our database and pass the coarse pulse data series through the filters. Figure 6.13 illustrates the results, demonstrating the performance of the proposed filter. In Fig. 6.13a, Sig1 is the clean pulse waveform and Sig2 is the noised pulse waveform. Sig3, Sig4, Sig5, and Sig6 are the denoised pulse signals of Sig2 by using wavelet filter, FIR low-pass filter, moving average filter, and the proposed cascade filter, respectively. Figure 6.13b is the local enlargement of Fig. 6.13a.

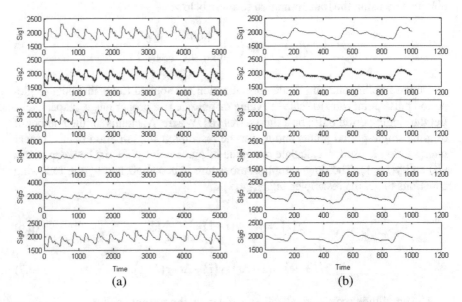

Fig. 6.13 Comparisons of pulse denoising by using four different methods: (**a**) the overall view; (**b**) local enlarged view

Table 6.2 The denoising performance

Method	Mean error	Std error	Smooth
Wavelet	0.0157	0.0049	1.6555
FIR filter	0.0644	0.0346	1.1689
Moving average	0.0158	0.0068	1.3481
Proposed cascade filter	0.0157	0.0012	0.9804

Three parameters are used to quantitatively evaluate the quality of the denoised pulse signals, i.e., percentage mean error (PME), percentage standard deviation error (PSDE), and percentage smoothness (PS). The PS parameter is to measure the smoothness of the denoised pulse waveform in contrast to the noised pulse, and it correlated with continuity of the derivative. The parameters of PME, PSDE, and PS are defined, respectively, as:

$$\text{PME} = \frac{\bar{m} - m}{m}, \bar{m} = \frac{1}{N}\sum_{i=1}^{N}\bar{x}(i), m = \frac{1}{N}\sum_{i=1}^{N}x(i), \tag{6.9}$$

$$\text{PSDE} = \frac{\bar{x} - \bar{m}_2 - x - m_2}{x - m_2}, \tag{6.10}$$

$$\text{PS} = (x - \bar{x})'_2 / x'_2, \tag{6.11}$$

where $\bar{x}(i)$ represent the denoised pulse signal, N denotes the number of points of the pulse waveform, and m and $\bar{m}$ are the mean values of original and denoised pulse, respectively. x' represents the first-order derivation vector and is calculated by using the function $f = [f_2 - f_1, f_3 - f_2, \cdots, f_N - f_{N-1}]$. The smaller the evaluation parameters, the better is the pulse denoising performance.

The evaluation result is listed in Table 6.2. It can be seen that the parameters of the denoised signals by using the proposed cascade filter are the smallest. The FIR filter brings much distortions to the shape components around the cutoff frequency. The wavelet filter and the moving average filter both have shortcomings in keeping continuous. The experimental result illustrates that the proposed denoising filter outperforms the others in keeping details of the pulse signals and preserving the smoothness.

6.4.2   Optimal Segmentation Strategy

In the second experiment, the proposed period segmentation strategies are compared to select the optimal algorithm. The collected pulse signals are authentic and original in the truest sense. And the pulse from healthy subjects and diabetic patients are chosen as two classes. The labels of the healthy subjects are determined according to the recent health check. The diabetic patients are confirmed by comparing their blood levels with standard clinical blood markers. The period segmentation is introduced to extract the interclass distance information for the pulse analysis. An optimal period segmentation guarantees that the variance should be small within the class and the distance between classes should be distinguishable. Thus, the interclass distance and intra-class distance are employed as the evaluation criterions.

In total, we collect 125 healthy and 125 diabetic samples. All patients are volunteers from the Hong Kong Hospital. For each subject, the pulse denoising, interval selection, and baseline drift correction are applied to the wrist pulse before the period segmentation module. Six criterions are then developed to find the optimal algorithm. The interclass distance and intra-class distance of the segmented single-period pulse signals are given by the formulas below:

$$m_i = \frac{1}{N_i}\sum_{x \in \phi_i} x, i = 1, 2, \cdots, N, \qquad (6.12)$$

$$M_j = \sum_{m_i \in P_j} m_i, j = 1, 2. \qquad (6.13)$$

In the above equation, x stands for the single-period pulse signal segmented from the sample ϕ_i and m_i denotes the average waveform. The pulses from healthy subjects and diabetic patients are divided into two classes P_j and M_j which is the center of class. Thus, the interclass distance S_b can be obtained by the formula below:

$$S_b = (M_1 - M_2)(M_1 - M_2)^T. \qquad (6.14)$$

The intra-class scatter matrix S_i is calculated in each sample ϕ_i, and the total intra-class scatter matrix S_w is defined by the formula below:

$$S_i = \sum_{x \in \phi_i} (x - m_i)(x - m_i)^T, \qquad (6.15)$$

$$S_w = \sum_i S_i. \qquad (6.16)$$

And the intra-class distance is given by the formula below:

$$l = tr(S_w)/N, \qquad (6.17)$$

where $tr()$ denotes the trace of a matrix. The intra-class distance l describes the pulse self-similarity and the pulse stability.

The segmentation comparison result is shown in Fig. 6.14. The average single-period pulse and the standard deviation of the two classes are presented in different

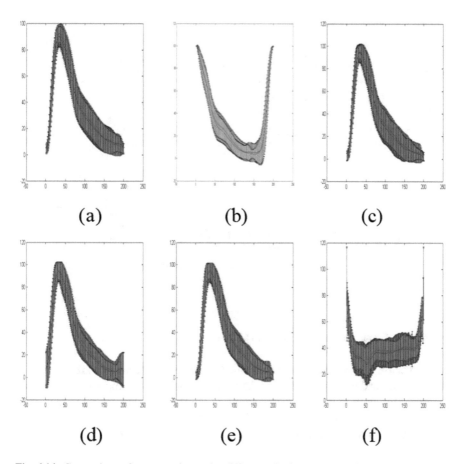

Fig. 6.14 Comparison of segmentation under different criterions: (**a**) encoding valley detection; (**b**) encoding peak detection; (**c**) local minimum; (**d**) local minimum slope; (**e**) drift removal before peak detection; (**f**) first derivation

colors. The red line stands for the healthy class and the blue line for the diabetes. Error bars show the confidence intervals of the deviation at each point. Figure 6.14a and b displays the segmentation results by using valley and peak detection with encoding. Figure 6.14c shows the original method by detecting the local minimum points in the valleys. Figure 6.14d gives the single-period pulse waveforms by using the local minimum slope as the onsets. Figure 6.14e shows the segmentation strategy with the baseline drift correction module. Figure 6.14f presents the segmented results based on first derivation method.

The evaluation result of the proposed segmentation strategies is shown in Table 6.3. The first derivation segmentation (FDS) has the smallest intra-class distance and the largest interclass distance among the six strategies. The intra-class distance of the signals reflects the segmentation quality, and the small intra-class distance is preferred. The interclass distance measures the separability from the

Table 6.3 Evaluation of the criterions

Segmentation criterion	Interclass distance (S_w)	Intra-class distance (S_b)
EVD	23.17	2.41×10^4
EPD	21.62	1.95×10^4
LM	18.39	5.93×10^4
LMS	19.61	2.77×10^4
WC	24.51	2.40×10^4
FDS	25.80	1.34×10^4

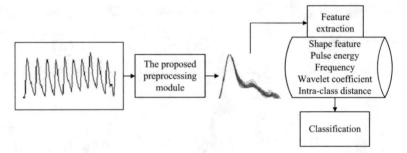

Fig. 6.15 A diagram of the pulse waveform analysis.

center vector. The encoding and baseline drift correction strategies are superior to the original local minimum strategy. And the peak detection is superior to the valley detection in the time domain space owing to the stability. The single-period pulse signals segmented in derivation space have the most distinguishable state. Thus, the FDS strategy is finally selected in the period segmentation module.

6.4.3 Preprocessing for Pulse Diagnosis

In the third experiment, we intend to compare the proposed pulse preprocessing with other methods on diabetes diagnosis. In the former pulse analysis researches, the pulse waveforms were considered as a determinate periodic signal. As a result, one cycle from the pulse was manually selected for the feature extraction. In this chapter, we take the wrist pulse waveforms as a complicated set with variances from cycle to cycle. The pulse features are extracted from the entire signal. The experiment is performed on pulse database which contains 125 healthy samples and 125 diabetic samples. Thus, there are 250 samples in total, in which 150 are for training and the others for testing.

Figure 6.15 shows the flowchart of pulse analysis. The raw pulse waveforms are first successively processed by the proposed preprocessing framework, which consists of pulse denoising, interval selection, baseline drift adjustment, and period segmentation and normalization. After preprocessing, the single-period pulse set of

Table 6.4 Performance of preprocessing

Preprocessing	Classifier	Feature	Accuracy
Deviation normalization	SVM	AR model [22]	82.3%
Pulse denoising and period segmentation	Fuzzy clustering	Gaussian model [20]	85.9%
Amplitude normalization and period segmentation	SVC	Wavelet feature [23]	85.6%
Pulse denoising and baseline drift removal	Multiple kernel	Heterogeneous features [24]	66.89%
Without preprocessing	KSVM	Fusion feature	61.2%
Proposed preprocessing	KSVM	Fusion feature	91.6%

each pulse sample is obtained. Then, the characteristic points, amplitudes, periods, pulse width, intra-class distance, and wavelet coefficients are extracted as the pulse fusion features. At last, the support vector machine (SVM) with Gaussian kernel is employed to construct a proper classification hyperplane and distinguish the diabetic samples from the healthy samples.

Three comparison pulse preprocessing techniques and the related features are also used for diabetes diagnosis. Chen et al. [22] proposed an AR model to extract the disease-sensitive features. The AR model deals with the entire signal. In order to normalize the measured data with respect to varying operational and environmental conditions, each wrist pulse signal $f(t)$ is normalized prior to fitting an AR model by the formula below:

$$\tilde{f}(t) = \frac{f(t) - m_f}{\delta_f}. \tag{6.18}$$

where, m_f and δ_f are the mean and standard deviation of $f(t)$, respectively. Table 6.4 gives the classification results. An accuracy of 82.3% is obtained by using the AR features.

Gaussian model [20], which is similar to the AR model, is also developed to match the pulse waveforms. Nevertheless, the Gaussian model deals with the single-period pulse signals. Both the low-frequency baseline drift and the high-frequency noise are reduced simply by using a 7-level 'db6' wavelet transform. Then a single-period pulse signal is selected and expressed by a two-term Gaussian function with an offset. The fitting parameters of the model are taken as the feature inputs to the fuzzy clustering classifier. The accuracy reaches 85.9% by using the Gaussian model features with denoising and period segmentation preprocessing.

Zhang et al. [23] introduce a wavelet-based method for wrist pulse analysis. Before feature extraction, the amplitudes of the pulse signals are first normalized to the same scale. Then, the wavelet coefficient features are extracted by using the wavelet decomposition at each level. A maximal margin support vector classifier is used for the pattern recognition. The classification rate reaches 85.6% for diabetes diagnosis. Liu et al. [24] select a stable segment of 1200 points from entire pulse signals to extract heterogeneous features for wrist pulse diagnosis. The classification accuracy reaches 66.89% for classifying healthy persons and patients with three kinds of diseases by using multiple kernel learning method.

The performances between pulse analysis with preprocessing and without preprocessing are also developed. For pulse signals without preprocessing procedure, we extract the fusion features of shape, energy, frequency, and wavelet coefficient, except the intra-class distance. And the features are classified by using the kernel SVM classifier. In the condition without preprocessing, an accuracy of 61.2% is obtained for diabetes diagnosis. And the classification rate reaches 91.6% by using the proposed pulse preprocessing framework. A ratio of 30% increase is obtained. It demonstrates that the proposed pulse preprocessing framework is necessary for pulse analysis. The experimental result also implies that the single-period pulse signals from different cycles bring complementary information.

It is evident in Table 6.4 that the classification accuracy of the fusion feature by using the proposed pulse preprocessing is much higher than the other methods on diabetes diagnosis. An increase of 5.7% and 6.0% is obtained compared to the Gaussian model method and the wavelet method, respectively. The wrist pulse preprocessing of AR model and multiple kernel learning only considers the deviation normalization and denoising for a segment of entire pulse, respectively. The accuracy is lower than the methods with period segmentation. And the wrist pulse diagnosis without any preprocessing gains the worst performance.

By this experiment, we can draw a conclusion that the performance of the proposed preprocessing framework is effective and superior to the previous researches. The preprocessing framework is robust under various conditions, and it is also practical for wrist pulse analysis.

6.5 Summary

Pulse preprocessing influences the pulse analysis. The idea and theory proposed in this chapter enrich the pulse preprocessing. A robust signal preprocessing framework for wrist pulse analysis comes into being. As a comparison, an outstanding advantage of the proposed preprocessing is that the increase of feature dimension is obtained after period segmentation. Thus, on the one hand, the intra-class variance is saved in the process of subsequent classification; on the other hand, the periodicity of the pulse is acquired from the period segmentation. The experiments on healthy and diabetic pulse database indicate that the recognition accuracy is increased significantly under the proposed preprocessing framework. What is more, the experimental results demonstrate that the proposed period segmentation feature is better than the AR model and Gaussian model for diabetes diagnosis.

References

1. S. Lukman, Y. He, and S.-C. Hui, "Computational methods for Traditional Chinese Medicine: A survey," Computer Methods and Programs in Biomedicine, vol. 88, pp. 283–294, 12, 2007.
2. L. Xu, K. Wang, D. Zhang, Y. Li, Z. Wan, and J. Wang, "Objectifying researches on traditional Chinese pulse diagnosis," in Informatica Medica Slovenica, 2003, pp. 56–63.
3. H. Sorvoja, V. M. Kokko, R. Myllyla, and J. Miettinen, "Use of EMFi as a blood pressure pulse transducer," Instrumentation and Measurement, IEEE Transactions on, vol. 54, pp. 2505–2512, 2005.
4. M. Nitzan, "Automatic noninvasive measurement of arterial blood pressure," Instrumentation & Measurement Magazine, IEEE, vol. 14, pp. 32–37, 2011.
5. C.-H. Luo, Y.-F. Chung, C.-S. Hu, C.-C. Yeh, X.-C. Si, D.-H. Feng, Y.-C. Lee, S.-I. Huang, S.-M. Yeh, C.-H. Liang, "Possibility of quantifying TCM finger-reading sensations: I. Bi-Sensing Pulse Diagnosis Instrument," European Journal of Integrative Medicine, vol. 4, pp. e255-e262, 9, 2012.
6. P. Wang, W. Zuo, and D. Zhang, "A Compound Pressure Signal Acquisition System for Multichannel Wrist Pulse Signal Analysis," Instrumentation and Measurement, IEEE Transactions on , vol.63, no.6, pp.1556,1565, June 2014
7. M. Aboy, J. McNames, T. Tran, D. Tsunami, M. S. Ellenby, and B. Goldstein, "An automatic beat detection algorithm for pressure signals," Biomedical Engineering, IEEE Transactions on, vol. 52, pp. 1662–1670, 2005.
8. H. M. Haqqani, J. B. Morton, and J. M. Kalman, "Using the 12-Lead ECG to Localize the Origin of Atrial and Ventricular Tachycardias: Part 2—Ventricular Tachycardia," Journal of cardiovascular electrophysiology, vol. 20, pp. 825–832, 2009.
9. D.-Y. Zhang, W.-M. Zuo, D. Zhang, H.-Z. Zhang, and N.-M. Li, "Wrist blood flow signal-based computerized pulse diagnosis using spatial and spectrum features," Journal of Biomedical Science and Engineering, vol. 3, p. 361, 2010.
10. C. T. Lee and L. Y. Wei, "Spectrum analysis of human pulse," Biomedical Engineering, IEEE Transactions on, pp. 348–352, 1983.
11. E. J. Ciaccio and G. M. Drzewiecki, "Tonometric Arterial Pulse Sensor with Noise Cancellation," Biomedical Engineering, IEEE Transactions on, vol. 55, pp. 2388–2396, 2008.
12. C. Xia, Y. Li, J. Yan, Y. Wang, H. Yan, R. Guo, et al., "A practical approach to wrist pulse segmentation and single-period average waveform estimation," in BioMedical Engineering and Informatics, 2008. BMEI 2008. International Conference on, 2008, pp. 334–338.
13. H.-T. Wu, C.-H. Lee, A.-B. Liu, W.-S. Chung, C.-J. Tang, C.-K. Sun, et al., "Arterial stiffness using radial arterial waveforms measured at the wrist as an indicator of diabetic control in the elderly," Biomedical Engineering, IEEE Transactions on, vol. 58, pp. 243–252, 2011.
14. M. Blanco-Velasco, B. Weng, and K. E. Barner, "ECG signal denoising and baseline wander correction based on the empirical mode decomposition," Computers in biology and medicine, vol. 38, pp. 1–13, 2008.
15. M. Mneimneh, E. Yaz, M. Johnson, and R. Povinelli, "An adaptive Kalman filter for removing baseline wandering in ECG signals," in Computers in Cardiology, 2006, 2006, pp. 253–256.
16. L. Xu, D. Zhang, and K. Wang, "Wavelet-based cascaded adaptive filter for removing baseline drift in pulse waveforms," Biomedical Engineering, IEEE Transactions on, vol. 52, pp. 1973–1975, 2005.
17. K. Wang, L. Xu, L. Wang, Z. Li, and Y. Li, "Pulse baseline wander removal using wavelet approximation," in Computers in Cardiology, 2003, 2003, pp. 605–608.
18. D. Wang and D. Zhang, "Analysis of pulse waveforms preprocessing," in Computerized Healthcare (ICCH), 2012 International Conference on, 2012, pp. 175–180.
19. L. Xu, D. Zhang, K. Wang, N. Li, and X. Wang, "Baseline wander correction in pulse waveforms using wavelet-based cascaded adaptive filter," Computers in Biology and Medicine, vol. 37, pp. 716–731, 5, 2007.

20. Y. Chen, L. Zhang, D. Zhang, and D. Zhang, "Wrist pulse signal diagnosis using modified Gaussian models and Fuzzy C-Means classification," Medical engineering & physics, vol. 31, pp. 1283–1289, 2009.
21. A. D. S. Ferreira, "Resonance phenomenon during wrist pulse-taking: A stochastic simulation, model-based study of the 'pressing with one finger' technique," Biomedical Signal Processing and Control, vol. 8, pp. 229–236, 5, 2013.
22. Y. Chen, L. Zhang, D. Zhang, and D. Zhang, "Computerized Wrist Pulse Signal Diagnosis Using Modified Auto-Regressive Models," Journal of Medical Systems, vol. 35, pp. 321–328, 2011.
23. D. Zhang, D. Zhang, and Y. Zheng, "Wavelet based analysis of Doppler ultrasonic wrist-pulse signals," in BioMedical Engineering and Informatics, 2008. BMEI 2008. International Conference on, 2008, pp. 539–543.
24. L. Liu, W. Zuo, D. Zhang, N. Li, and H. Zhang, "Combination of heterogeneous features for wrist pulse blood flow signal diagnosis via multiple kernel learning," Information Technology in Biomedicine, IEEE Transactions on, vol. 16, pp. 598–606, 2012.
25. R. J. Martis, U. R. Acharya, and L. C. Min, "ECG beat classification using PCA, LDA, ICA and Discrete Wavelet Transform," Biomedical Signal Processing and Control, vol. 8, pp. 437–448, 9, 2013.

Part IV
Pulse Signal Feature Extraction

Chapter 7
Arrhythmic Pulse Detection

Abstract This chapter proposes a novel approach to the detection of arrhythmic pulses using the Lempel-Ziv complexity analysis. Four parameters, one lemma, and two rules, which are the results of heuristic approach, are presented. This approach is applied on 140 clinic pulses for detecting 7 pulse patterns, not only achieving a recognition accuracy of 97.1% as assessed by experts in TCM but also correctly extracting the periodical unit of the intermittent pulse.

7.1 Introduction

The quantification and analysis of physiological signals have become more important recently. The research on traditional Chinese pulse diagnosis (TCPD) is relatively new in this area. Usually, practitioners of TCPD use pulse sensors to acquire patients' pulse waveforms of the wrists and then investigate the patients' pulse waveforms [1–7]. Presently, the long-term monitoring of pulse waveforms is becoming more popular. The automatic analysis and recognition of pulse waveforms are useful in reducing the heavy burden on practitioners of observing and analyzing pulse waveforms.

Many pattern recognition methods have been applied to the automatic recognition and classification of pulse waveforms. For example, Lee et al. applied fuzzy theory to analyze several cases of pulse waveforms and got good results [8]; Yoon et al. introduced three characteristics to describe a pulse: its position, its size, and its strength [9]; Stockman et al. used structural pattern recognition to identify the shape of carotid pulse waveforms [10]; Wang et al. proposed an improved dynamic time warping algorithm for recognizing five pulse patterns that are distinct in their shapes [11]. Wang and Xiang applied a three-layer artificial neural network in order to recognize seven types of pulse patterns [12]. In all of these researches, only pulse patterns' features of position or shape are analyzed. We cannot find the research into differentiating pulse patterns according to their rhythms, yet the rhythm is a useful feature for identifying pulse patterns. The arrhythmic pulse patterns, which have distinctive rhythms, are difficult to recognize using their linear features. This chapter presents an approach to the differentiation of the seven pulse patterns according

© Springer Nature Singapore Pte Ltd. 2018
D. Zhang et al., *Computational Pulse Signal Analysis*,
https://doi.org/10.1007/978-981-10-4044-3_7

to their rhythms. Four parameters were proposed to discriminate between rhythmic and arrhythmic pulses. We then applied the Lempel-Ziv complexity analysis in order to identify arrhythmic pulse patterns, achieving a total accuracy of 97.1%.

This chapter is organized as follows. Section 7.2 analyzes pulse rhythms. Section 7.3 proposes an approach based on Lempel-Ziv complexity analysis in order to recognize the characteristic rhythms of the seven pulse patterns. Section 7.4 discusses the experimental results. Section 7.5 offers conclusion.

7.2   Clinical Value of Pulse Rhythm Analysis

TCPD recognizes that there are seven pulse patterns which have distinctive rhythms: four patterns are rhythmic and three patterns are arrhythmic. The four rhythmic pulse patterns are called swift pulse, rapid pulse, moderate pulse, and pulse. The three arrhythmic pulses are called running pulse, knotted pulse, and intermittent pulse. Figure 7.1a–g illustrates these pulses. In each figure, the first panel is the pulse waveform and its onsets and the second panel is its pulse interval series. Pulse interval (PI) is the interval between two consecutive onsets of pulse waveform.

Just as the heart rhythms identified using ECGs are important in Western medicine, these seven pulse patterns are important in TCPD [13]. They relate to syndromes identified in traditional Chinese medicine (TCM) and their specific behaviors closely guide diagnosis [14]. Swift pulse often occurs in severe acute febrile disease or consumptive conditions. Rapid pulse usually indicates the presence of heat. Moderate pulse reflects a normal condition of the body. Slow pulse often relates to endogenous cold. The running pulse feels rapid but loses a beat at irregular intervals, indicating blood stasis or the retention of phlegm. The knotted pulse feels leisurely but loses a beat at irregular intervals. The irregularity and slowness of this pulse are due to the obstruction of blood. The intermittent pulse, comparatively relaxed and weak, stops at regular intermittent intervals. It often occurs in exhaustion of viscera organs, severe trauma, or moments of fright. The intermittent pulse periodically loses a beat after several but less than six normal PIs. Otherwise, the arrhythmic pulse may be either running or knotted pulse [13].

7.3   The Approach to Automatic Recognition of Pulse
Rhythms

In Sect. 7.3.1, we will first outline the basic idea of Lempel-Ziv complexity analysis. After that, we will introduce the definitions of four parameters, one lemma, and two rules in Sect. 7.3.2. Finally, we will describe our approach to recognize the seven pulse patterns according to the different rhythms in Sect. 7.3.3.

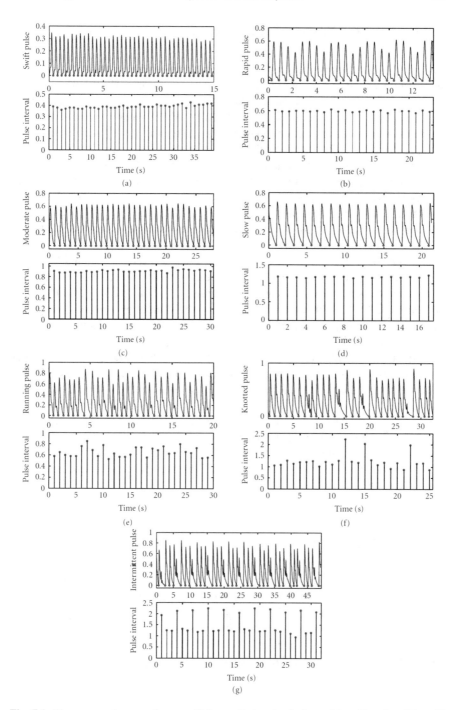

Fig. 7.1 The seven pulse waveforms, which are distinct in rhythms: (**a**) swift pulse; (**b**) rapid pulse; (**c**) moderate pulse; (**d**) slow pulse; (**e**) running pulse; (**f**) knotted pulse; (**g**) intermittent pulse

7.3.1   Lempel–Ziv Complexity Analysis

Lempel-Ziv complexity analysis is an approach to evaluating the randomness of finite sequences. It is closely related to information entropy [15–18]. The Lempel-Ziv complexity measures the rate at which new patterns are generated in a symbolized sequence. It is based on a coarse-graining of the measurement, that is, the signal to be analyzed is transformed into a sequence made up of just a few symbols. Lempel-Ziv complexity measures the number of steps in a self-delimiting production process by which a given sequence is presumed to be generated. The complexity counter $c(n)$ measures the number of distinct patterns contained in a given sequence. Briefly, a sequence $S = s_1s_2s_3 \cdots s_n$ (where s_1, s_2, etc. denote symbols, e.g., "0" or "1") is scanned from left to right letter by letter, and the $c(n)$ is increased by one unit when a new pattern of consecutive characters is encountered [19, 20].

The process of Lempel-Ziv complexity analysis is as follows. Let Q and R denote, respectively, subsequences of the sequence $S = s_1s_2s_3 \ldots s_n$, and let QR be the concatenation of Q and R, while subsequence QRD is derived from QR after its last character is deleted (D means the operator to delete the last character in a sequence). Let L (QRD) denote the lexicon of all different patterns of QRD. In the beginning, $c(n) = 1$, $Q = s_1$, and $R = s_2$; therefore, $QRD = s_1$. Now assume that $Q = s_1s_2s_3 \ldots s_i$, and $R = s_{i+1}$, then $QRD = s_1s_2s_3 \ldots s_i$. If $R \in L(QRD)$, that is, R is a subsequence of QRD, then R is not a new pattern. At this time, Q need not change and renew R to be $s_{i+1}s_{i+2}$. After that, we judge whether R belongs to L(QRD) and continue until $R \notin L(QRD)$. If $R = s_{i+1}s_{i+2} \ldots s_{i+j}$ is not a subsequence of $QRD = s_1s_2s_3 \ldots s_{i+j-1}$, increase $c(n)$ by one. Thereafter, combine Q with R and renew Q to be $s_1s_2s_3 \ldots s_{i+j}$. At the same time, renew R to be s_{i+j+1}. Repeat these processes until R is the last character in the sequence S. Thus, the number of different patterns is $c(n)$, that is, the measure of complexity. Ziv and Lempel insert slashes into the sequence S at the position where a new pattern occurs. Thus, they divided the sequence S into $c(n)$ blocks using those slashes.

7.3.2   Definitions and Basic Facts

To recognize pulse patterns with different rhythms, we first extract four parameters defined in Definitions 1 and 2. The parameters in Definition 1 are extracted from PI series and are used to judge if the pulse waveform is arrhythmic. If the pulse waveform is arrhythmic, we need to symbolize its PI series. The parameters in Definition 2 are extracted from symbolized pulse intervals (SPIs), which are obtained by the coarse-graining technique, and then they are used to judge if the pulse waveform is an intermittent pulse.

7.3.2.1   Definitions

Assume that $T = $ "$t_1, t_2, \ldots , t_N$" is a *PI* series. To judge whether its corresponding pulse is arrhythmic or not, define two parameters.

Variation Range (VR)   VR is the difference between the maximum element and minimum element of T, that is,

$$VR = \max(T) - \min(T) \tag{7.1}$$

Variation Coefficient (VC)   VC is the ratio between standard deviation and the average of this series T:

$$VC = \frac{SD}{\bar{t}} \times 100\%, \tag{7.2}$$

where:

$$\bar{t} = \frac{1}{N}\sum_{i=1}^{N} t_i, SD = \sqrt{\frac{\sum_{i-1}^{N}(t_i - \bar{t})^2}{N-1}}. \tag{7.3}$$

Assume that $S = $ "$s_1 s_2 \cdots s_N$" is a *SPI* sequence. To determine whether an arrhythmic pulse is an intermittent pulse or not, define two parameters as follows.

Minimum Recurrent Unit (MRU)   MRU is the subsequence that is the minimum periodic unit of the sequence S.

Recurrent Degree (RD)   RD is the recurrent time of a finite sequence S. The RD = $\lfloor L/L_r \rfloor$, where L_r is the length of its MRU; L is the length of the sequence S. That is to say RD is the largest integer, which does not exceed the value of L divided by L_r.

For example, the sequence "1,234,005" is a nonperiodic sequence, whose MRU is itself "1,234,005" and whose RD = $\lfloor 7/7 \rfloor$ = 1; the sequence "1,212,121" is a periodic sequence, whose MRU is "12" and whose RD = $\lfloor 7/2 \rfloor$ = 3.

7.3.2.2   Rules

To differentiate pulse rhythms, we offer two rules which combine the experience of experts in TCPD with the Lempel-Ziv complexity analysis. According to Rule 1, the rhythmic pulses and arrhythmic pulses can be differentiated. According to Rule 2, the intermittent pulse can be differentiated from the running pulse and the knotted pulse.

Given the VC and VR of a PI series, it is possible to determine whether the pulse is arrhythmic according to Rule 1. If the pulse is arrhythmic, we need to symbolize the PI series using coarse-graining method. We then extract the subsequences from SPI series and simplify those subsequences further (the simplification process will be discussed in Sect. 7.3.3.4).

The intermittent pulse periodically has one pause after several normal beats. The number of consecutive normal beats must be less than 6 and constant. Thus, we scan the SPI sequence from leftmost to rightmost and extract several subsequences that begin with first symbol "1" and end at symbol "1" which has at least six continuous "0" s on its right or is the rightmost symbol "1" of this whole sequence. For example, "0000100100000010000010010100010000000000001000" is a symbolized pulse interval series. The extraction of its subsequences can be "0000#1001$000000#100 0001001010001$0000000000#1$000." The symbols "#" and "$" stand for the beginning and the end of the subsequence we extracted, respectively. Here, Subsequence1 = "1001," Subsequence2 = "1000001001010001," and Subsequence3 = "1."

Rule 1 If the VC of a PI series is greater than 20% or the VR of a PI series is more than the second minimum of this PI series, the pulse corresponding to this PI series is an arrhythmic pulse.

Rule 2 After the coarse-graining, subsequence extraction, and simplification processes, we can obtain the symbolized subsequences of the original PI series. If the RD of a symbolized subsequence is equal to or more than three, its corresponding pulse is an intermittent pulse [13].

Rule 2 requires that the symbolized subsequences of an intermittent pulse be periodic and contain at least three periods because just having two periods could be a random phenomenon and should not be taken as regularity. Consequently, the problem of differentiating the intermittent pulse from the knotted pulse and the running pulse is equivalent to judging whether a subsequence S_{sub} is a periodic subsequence with at least three periods. This kind of periodic symbolized subsequences has special characteristics described in the following lemma:

7.3.2.3 Lemma

Lemma 1 Assume that a periodic symbolized subsequence $S_{sub} = s_1 s_2 \cdots s_N$ contains at least three periods and the length of its MRU is P. Ziv and Lempel insert delimiters into the subsequence to be analyzed using the two rules they defined [15, 16]. These delimiters divide a subsequence into several blocks. In Fig. 7.2, insert "◆" to divide the subsequence into k blocks. It will be proved that the Lempel-Ziv complexity analysis result of periodic subsequence S_{sub}, which contains at least three periods, must satisfy the following five inequalities:

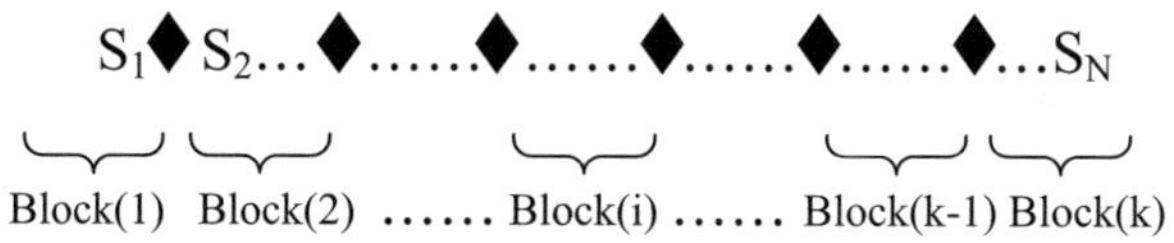

$$S_1 \blacklozenge S_2 \ldots \blacklozenge \ldots \ldots \blacklozenge \ldots \ldots \blacklozenge \ldots \ldots \blacklozenge \ldots \ldots \blacklozenge \ldots S_N$$

Block(1) Block(2) ...... Block(i) ...... Block(k-1) Block(k)

Fig. 7.2 Result of the Lempel-Ziv complexity analysis of one sequence. We insert "♦" where a new pattern emerges according to the Lempel-Ziv complexity analysis. Here, the k "♦"'s divide the sequence "$S_1S_2 \cdots S_N$" into k blocks

$$P \le \frac{1}{3}\sum_{i=1}^{k}\left|\text{Block}(i)\right|, \tag{7.4}$$

$$P > \sum_{i=1}^{k-2}\left|\text{Block}(i)\right|, \tag{7.5}$$

$$P \ge \left|\text{Block}(i)\right|, \ i = 1,\ldots,k-1, \tag{7.6}$$

$$2P > \sum_{i=1}^{k-1}\left|\text{Block}(i)\right| \ge P, \tag{7.7}$$

$$\left|\text{Block}(k)\right| > P, \tag{7.8}$$

where |Block (i)| is the length of the ith block. In the following, these five inequalities (7.4, 7.5, 7.6, 7.7, and 7.8) will be proved.

Proof Equation (7.4) According to the premise, the subsequence S_{sub} is periodic and contains at least three periods. Thus, $\sum_{i=1}^{k}\left|\text{Block}(i)\right| \ge 3P$, that is, $P \le (1/3)\sum_{i=1}^{k}\left|\text{Block}(i)\right|$.

Equation (7.5) If $\sum_{i=1}^{k-2}\left|\text{Block}(i)\right| \ge P$, the former $k-2$ blocks must contain at least one MRU. Then, *Block(k − 1)* and *Block(k)* must repeat the former patterns because subsequence S_{sub} is a periodic subsequence which contains three periods at least. Thus, Block($k - 1$) and Block (k) cannot be segmented into two blocks according to Lempel-Ziv complexity analysis. Therefore, $P > \sum_{i=1}^{k-2}\left|\text{Block}(i)\right|$.

Equation (7.6) According to Eq. (7.5), we know that $P \ge$ |Block(i)|,$i = 1, \ldots, k - 2$. Thus, we only need to prove $P \ge$ |Block($k - 1$)|. Assume that $P <$ |Block($k - 1$)|, then Block ($k - 1$) contains more than one MRU. In (7.5), $P > \sum_{i=1}^{k-2}\left|\text{Block}(i)\right|$, the first P symbols of Block ($k - 1$) must be a new pattern, which is different from the first $k - 2$ blocks. Therefore, Block ($k - 1$) must be divided into several blocks according to Lempel-Ziv complexity analysis. However, Block($k - 1$) is the $k - 1$ th block. Thus, $P \ge$ |Block(i)|, $i = 1, \ldots, k - 1$.

Equation (7.7) If $P > \sum_{i=1}^{k-1}\left|\text{Block}(i)\right|$, the first P − 1 symbols of Block(k) must be a new pattern; otherwise the length of the MRU of S is less than P, contradicting

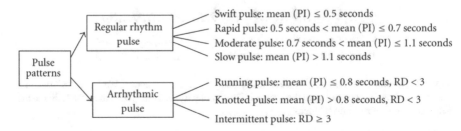

Fig. 7.3 The characteristics of seven pulse patterns, which differ in rhythm. PI is the abbreviation of pulse interval. The mean (PI) stands for the average of PI series. RD is the abbreviation of recurrent degree

the assumption. Thus, $\sum_{i=1}^{k-1}\left|\text{Block}(i)\right| \geq P$. According to Eq. (7.5), if $\sum_{i=1}^{k-1}\left|\text{Block}(i)\right| \geq 2P$, the length of Block($k - 1$) must be larger than P. However, the first $P - 1$ symbols of Block($k - 1$) must be a new pattern, that is, the length of Block($k - 1$) should be less than $P - 1$, contradicting Eq. (7.6). Therefore, we draw the conclusion that $2P > \sum_{i=1}^{k-1}\left|\text{Block}(i)\right| \geq P$.

Equation (7.8). According to Eq. (7.4) and (7.7), that is, $\sum_{i=1}^{k}\left|\text{Block}(i)\right| \geq 3P$ and $\sum_{i=1}^{k-1}\left|\text{Block}(i)\right| < 2P$, we can prove that|Block(k)| > P.

7.3.2.4   The Seven Pulse Patterns' Characteristics in Rhythms

Figure 7.3 illustrates the rhythmic characteristics of these seven pulse patterns. The swift, rapid, moderate, and slow pulses are rhythmic pulses and are differentiated by the average of their PIs. The knotted, running, and intermittent pulses are arrhythmic pulses, and their SPIs have different RDs. The intermittent pulse has periodic arrhythmia, and the RD of the symbolized intermittent pulse interval sequence is higher than 2. The RDs of both the knotted pulse and the running pulse are less than 3. Additionally, the PI average of the knotted pulse is longer than that of the running pulse.

7.3.3   Automatic Recognition of Pulse Patterns Distinctive in Rhythm

Essentially, TCM practitioners identify pulse rhythms in three steps. First, they identify the average of PI series. Second, they identify the variation of PI series and judge if the pulse is arrhythmic or not. Finally, if the pulse is arrhythmic, they must ascertain whether the irregular rhythm is periodic. Figure 7.4 outlines our approach to the automatic recognition of these seven pulse patterns. The pulse waveform,

Fig. 7.4 Our approach to
the differentiation of the
seven rhythmically distinct
pulse patterns

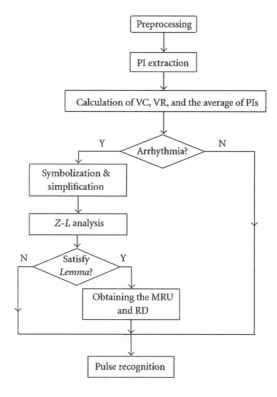

which is easy to be distorted by noise and baseline drift, must be preprocessed
firstly. We then extract the PI series and calculate the VC, VR, and the average of
this PI series and judge if this PI series is arrhythmic. The PI series will be symbolized and the subsequences that contain the abnormal PI will be extracted. After that,
we simplify the extracted subsequences. Next, the Lempel-Ziv complexity analysis
method is used to analyze the extracted symbolized subsequences. Finally, we judge
if the symbolized subsequences are periodic according to the lemma and Rule 2.
Thus, the seven pulse patterns can be automatically differentiated.

7.3.3.1   Preprocessing the Pulse Waveform

The pulse waveform should be preprocessed before being analyzed because noise,
respiration, and artifact motion can be introduced during pulse waveform acquisition. It is important to remove the pulse waveform's baseline drift and attenuate
noise before the automatic analysis of pulse waveforms. First, we filtered the pow-
erline interference at 50 Hz and then applied wavelet approximation to estimate the
baseline drift of pulse waveform [21]. After that, the signal-to-noise ratio of the
pulse waveform is greatly enhanced; thus, the accurate extraction of PI series in the
following step is assured.

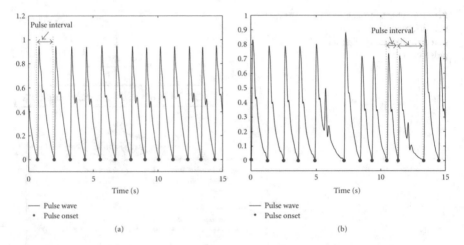

Fig. 7.5 Pulse onsets and PI series: (**a**) the pulse waveform with normal rhythm; (**b**) the pulse waveform with abnormal rhythm

7.3.3.2   Pulse Interval Extraction and Calculation of its VC and VR

In order to analyze the rhythm of the pulse waveform, we first extract the PI series of pulse waveform and then calculate its VC and VR. Many algorithms have been previously proposed for the accurate detection of the intervals between the beats of a blood pressure waveform [22–24]. Here, we use the method in [25] to detect the onsets of pulse waveform.

In order to further explain the calculation of the VC, VR, and Rule 1, we take Figs. 7.5 and 7.6 as examples. Figure 7.5a shows a slow pulse, whose VR = (1.41–1.12) < 1.20 s and VC = 8% < 20% (where the maximum, the minimum, the second minimum, and the average of PI series are 1.41, 1.12, 1.20, and 1.26 s, respectively). In Fig. 7.5b, the pulse is arrhythmic and its VR = (1.92–0.90) > 0.96 s (where the maximum, the minimum, and the second minimum of PI series are 1.92, 0.90, and 0.96 s, respectively). Figure 7.7 shows the 157 PIs of the 200-second pulse waveform in Fig. 7.6. Its VR = 2.25–0.86 = 1.39 > 0.91, and its VC is 25%, illustrating that this 200-second pulse is arrhythmic according to Rule 1 (where the maximum, the minimum, and the second minimum of PI series are 2.25, 0.86, and 0.91 s, respectively).

7.3.3.3   Symbolizing Pulse Interval Series and Subsequence Extraction

To classify the pulse pattern of an arrhythmic pulse, we analyze the distribution of the PI series and then symbolize this PI series according to its distribution. It can be imagined that the histogram of an arrhythmic PI series must contain two peaks with a valley between them: the first peak corresponds to the normal interval and the second corresponds to the abnormal interval. We define T_a as the PI corresponding

Fig. 7.6 Arrhythmic pulse of 200 s (157 pulse periods)

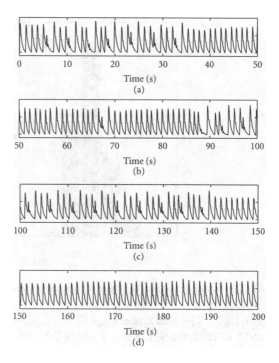

Fig. 7.7 Pulse intervals of a 200-second arrhythmic pulse; Tsym = 1.67

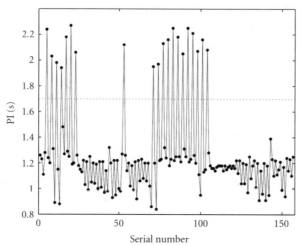

to the first peak in the leftmost of the PI histogram and T_b as the PI corresponding to the second peak of the PI histogram. We then define T_{sym} as $(T_b + T_a)/2$. If the PI is higher than T_{sym}, it is symbolized as "1"; otherwise it is symbolized as "0." Fig. 7.8 shows the histogram of the PIs extracted from the pulse waveform in Fig. 7.6. Here,

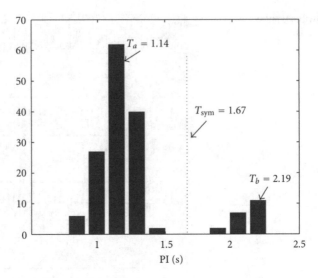

Fig. 7.8 Histogram of PIs. Ta, Tb, and Tsym are also demonstrated here

$T_a = 1.14$ s, $T_b = 2.19$ s, and $T_{sym} = (Tb + Ta)/2 = 1.67$ s, as demonstrated in Figs. 7.7 and 7.8. Thus, the SPI of Fig. 7.6 is as follows:

$$SPI =$$
$$00001001001001001001001000000000000000000000$$
$$0000000010000000000000000001001001001001001001001001001001. \qquad (7.9)$$
$$10010010010010010000000000000000000000000000$$
$$00000000000000000000000000 \left(length = 157 \right)$$

Usually, the PIs are normal. Abnormal PIs occur only occasionally but should receive considerable attention in automatic pulse rhythm analysis because they are related to the disorder of cardiovascular system. we search the SPI sequence from left to right and then extract the subsequences that start from the first symbol "1" and end at the symbol "1" which is followed by at least six continuous "0" s or is the rightmost "1" of the sequence. This process is repeated until the whole sequence has been searched.

Equation (7.10) illustrates the extraction result of the SPI in Fig. 7.6. The symbols "#" and "$" stand for the start and the end of the subsequence we extracted, respectively:

$$SPI =$$
$$0000\#1001001001001001001\$000000000000000000$$
$$0000000000\#1\$00000000000000000\#1001001001001.\qquad(7.10)$$
$$001001001001001001001\$000000000000000000000$$
$$00000000000000000000000000000000000\,(\text{length} = 157)$$

From Eq. (7.10), we extracted three subsequences illustrated in Eqs. (7.11), (7.12), and (7.13):

$$\text{Subsequence1} = 1001001001001001001,\qquad(7.11)$$

$$\text{Subsequence2} = 1,\qquad(7.12)$$

$$\text{Subsequence3} = 1001001001001001001001001001001.\qquad(7.13)$$

7.3.3.4   Arrhythmic Pulse Recognition Based on Lempel–Ziv Complexity Analysis

Intermittent pulse is a special kind of arrhythmic pulse because its arrhythmia is periodical. Thus, after symbolizing the PI series and extracting subsequences of the SPI sequence, the recognition of the intermittent pulse is equivalent to judging if the symbolized subsequences are periodic subsequences that contain at least three periods. Hence, we can differentiate intermittent pulse using the string-matching method. The MRU of an intermittent pulse might be in the (a) basic form, 10^i (0^i represents i consecutive 0's), $0 \le i \le 5$; (b) composite form, combinations of the basic forms, such as $10^i 10^j$ ($0 \le i \le 5$, $0 \le j \le 5$, and $j \neq i$); and so on. For example, "10" is the MRU of sequence "101,010,101"; "100" is the MRU of sequence "1,001,001,001,001"; "10,100" is the MRU of sequence "101,001,010,010,100,101,001." However, Lempel-Ziv analysis can split the basic form 10^i. Thus, it will cause damage to the actual purpose of searching MRU.

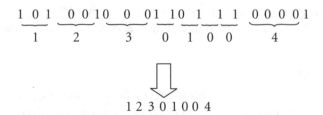

Fig. 7.9 An example of simplification. The new simplified sequence denotes the number of "0"s between two nearest "1"s. For sequence "10^i1" ($0 \le i \le 5$), we denote it as "i." If two "1"s are consecutive, there is no "0" between these two "1"s. Thus, we denote "0." In this figure, we scan the SPI "10100100011011100001" from left to right. Between the first "1" and the second "1," there is one zero; between the second "1" and the third "1," there are two zeros. Repeat this procedure until the last "1." We can simplify the SPI into "12301004"

Simplification of Symbolized Pulse Interval Sequence To prevent from splitting the basic form 10^i, we further simplify the binary SPI subsequences. We denote the basic form of the recurrent unit numerically by letting i denote 10^i1, $0 \le i \le 5$. That is to say, i denotes the number of successive "0"s between the two nearest "1"s. If two nearest "1"s are conjoint, the number of successive "0"s between these two nearest "1"s is 0. Thus, the original sequence can be simplified into a new sequence constituted by these "i"s. For example, the sequence "10100100011011100001" can be expressed as "12301004" illustrated in Fig. 7.9.

Thus the Subsequence1 and Subsequence3 in Eqs.. (7.11) and (7.13) can be simplified as:

$$\begin{aligned} \text{Subsequence1} &= 222222 \\ \text{Subsequence3} &= 22222222222 \end{aligned} \tag{7.14}$$

The Subsequence2 in (7.12) is only one symbol "1," whose RD = 1 is obvious.

Lempel-Ziv Complexity Analysis of Simplified Pulse Interval Sequence Assume a sequence $S = s_1 s_2 \cdots s_N$. To indicate a substring of S that starts at position i and ends at position j, we denote it as $S(i, j)$, $i \le j$. Q is called a prefix of S if there exists an integer i such that $Q = S(1, i)$, $1 \le i < N$.

One simple method for determining whether a symbolized subsequence is a periodic sequence that contains at least three periods is to assume that each of the prefixes of S is the MRU and then to match it with the remaining part of S. We call this method naive matching. If S is a periodic sequence with at least three periods, this method requires $O(n)$ time, where n represents the length of the sequence S. If S is not a periodic sequence with at least three periods, this method requires $O(n^2)$ time to make the conclusion, which is time consuming.

Considering the time consuming of naive matching, we proposed a matching method based on Lempel-Ziv complexity, which generally requires $O(n)$ time to make the conclusion whether S is a periodic sequence with at least three periods or not. Having simplified the expression of the SPI sequence, we analyze Subsequence1 and Subsequence3 in Eq. (7.14) using Lempel-Ziv complexity analysis. During the analysis, when a new pattern emerges, the symbol "♦" is inserted after it. The complexity analysis result of Subsequence1 is as follows.

- The first character is always a new pattern. Therefore, the first pattern is 2♦.
- The second character is "2" and this is identical to the first pattern. In this case, the old pattern also contains "2" so it is not a new pattern. The analysis result is 2♦2.
- The third character is "2." The current pattern is "22." The previous patterns are "2" and "22" so "22" still is not a new pattern and can be marked as 2♦22.
- Repeating this process, this sequence is segmented into two blocks:

$$\text{Subsequence1} = 2♦22222♦. \tag{7.15}$$

The complexity analysis of Subsequence3 is similar to the analysis of Subsequence1. Its Lempel-Ziv complexity analysis result is "2♦2222222222♦."

Judging Whether the Arrhythmic Pulse is an Intermittent Pulse Having analyzed the Lempel-Ziv complexity of the SPI series, we must judge whether the subsequence is a periodic subsequence which contains at least three periods. Our approach consists of two phases.

Phase 1.   Exclude the subsequences that could not satisfy the lemma. The Lempel-Ziv complexity analysis separates S_{sub} into k blocks. If the Block (k) is a new pattern, this subsequence must be nonperiodic. Furthermore, the length of each block ($|\text{Block }(i)|, 1 \leq i \leq k$) is obtained. If the Block (k) is not a new pattern, replace the variables in Eqs. (7.4), (7.5), (7.6), (7.7), and (7.8) of the lemma with the actual values to see whether the inequalities can be met simultaneously. If the answer is yes, continue the steps described in the second phase; otherwise, S_{sub} is not a periodic subsequence with at least three periods.

Phase 2.   Further determine whether the subsequences that satisfy the lemma are the periodic subsequences with at least three periods. In Phase 2, we first estimate the range of the MRU's length P according to Eqs. (7.4), (7.5), (7.6), (7.7), and (7.8). According to Rule 2, we then further judge if this subsequence is a periodic subsequence with at least three periods. If the answer is yes, we will extract the MRU of this subsequence and compute its RD. Assume that $S_{sub} = s_1 s_2 \ldots s_N$, the algorithm of the second phase is shown in Algorithm 7.1.

Algorithm 7.1 MRU Extraction
Input: Blocks of pulse sequence
Output: MRU and RD

$$\min P = \max\left(\sum_{1}^{k-2}\left|\texttt{Block}(i)\right|+1, \left|\texttt{Block}(k-1)\right|\right)$$

$$\max P = \min\left(\sum_{i=1}^{k-1}\left|\texttt{Block}(i)\right|, \left|\texttt{Block}(k)\right|-1, \left\lfloor\sum_{i=1}^{k}\left|\texttt{Block}(i)\right|/3\right\rfloor\right)$$

```
For  P = MinP… MaxP do:
        temp S1 = s₁s₂···sₚ
        temp S = {repeat temp S1 until the length reaches N};
            like temp S = s₁s₂···sₚ······s₁s₂···sₚs₁···s_q
        If  S_sub = temp S
            MRU = temp S₁;
            RD = ⌊N/P⌋;
            If  RD ≥ 3
                    Break;
            End If
        End If
End For
If RD ≥ 3
        S is a periodic subsequence with at least three
periods;
Else
        S is not a periodic subsequence with at least three
periods;
End If
```

In Algorithm 7.1, we first compute the range of the MRU's length P according to (7.4, 7.5, 7.6, 7.7, and 7.8). In the "For" loop, several periodic sequences are generated, with each one corresponding to a possible value of P, and these periodic sequences are matched with S_{sub}. In this process, the MRU and RD can be obtained at the same time. If RD < 3, S_{sub} is not a periodic subsequence with at least three periods and its corresponding pulse is not an intermittent pulse.

From the Lempel-Ziv analysis results of Subsequence1 and Subsequence3, we find that the Subsequence1 and Subsequence3 satisfy the inequalities of the lemma. Thus, we use the algorithm in Phase 2 to obtain the MRU and RD. The MRU of both Subsequence1 and Subsequence3 is "100." The length of Subsequence1 and Subsequence3 are 19 and 34, respectively. The RDs of Subsequence1 and Subsequence3

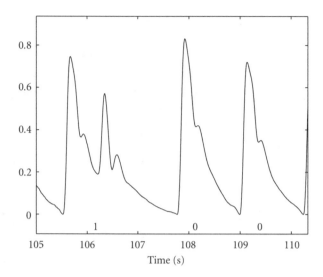

Fig. 7.10 The MRU of the arrhythmic pulses in Fig. 7.6

are $\lfloor 19/3 \rfloor = 6$ and $\lfloor 34/3 \rfloor = 11$, respectively. Thus, we can offer a conclusion that this pulse is an intermittent pulse, whose MRU is demonstrated in Fig. 7.10.

Our Lempel-Ziv-complexity-based matching method is faster than the naive matching method. The Lempel-Ziv complexity analysis is $O(n)$ time algorithm [26]. After the Lempel-Ziv complexity analysis, we exclude many subsequences that could not satisfy the inequalities in the lemma. Thus, our approach takes nearly the same time as Lempel-Ziv complexity analysis. If S_{sub} cannot be excluded, this subsequence can be further analyzed in Phase 2. Our approach usually needs to match only two or three times after estimating the range of the MRU's length. Thus, no matter whether S_{sub} is a periodic subsequence or not, our approach takes $O(n)$ time to judge whether S_{sub} is a periodic subsequence with at least three periods or not. Table 7.1 compares the matching times using the Lempel-Ziv analysis method and the naive matching method. We compared 100 SPI sequences, which are periodic or nonperiodic sequences with different lengths. The naive matching method requires 1.43 s, while our Lempel-Ziv based matching method requires just 1.07 s. Furthermore, the longer of the symbolized sequence is, the more time the Lempel-Ziv-based matching method can save.

7.4 Experiments

We applied our approach to 140 pulses with different rhythms: swift pulse (20 pulses), rapid pulse (20 pulses), moderate pulse (20 pulses), slow pulse (20 pulses), knotted pulse (20 pulses), running pulse (20 pulses), and intermittent pulse (20 pulses). The overall accuracy of the approach is 97.1%. Error arises because the

Table 7.1 Comparison of matching times of Lempel-Ziv analysis-based matching method and naive matching method

	Symbolized sequence	MinP	MaxP	Times of matching	
				Lempel-Ziv	Naive
RD ≥ 3	$(1)^{10}$	1	1	1	1
	$(12)^{10}$	2	2	1	2
	$(123)^{10}$	3	3	1	3
	$(1234)^{10}$	4	4	1	4
	$(4131123)^{10}$	7	7	1	7
RD = 2	11121112	3	2	0	$\lfloor 8/3 \rfloor = 2$
	111211121	3	3	1	$\lfloor 9/3 \rfloor = 3$
	1112111211	3	3	1	$\lfloor 10/3 \rfloor = 3$
	11121112111	3	3	1	$\lfloor 11/3 \rfloor = 3$
RD = 1	$1234(1)^6$	5	3	0	$\lfloor 10/3 \rfloor = 3$
	$1234(12)^{22}$	5	7	3	$\lfloor 48/3 \rfloor = 16$
	$(123)^7 1234$	21	0	0	$\lfloor 25/3 \rfloor = 8$
	$12(1)^{10}13$	10	0	0	$\lfloor 14/3 \rfloor = 4$
	$(123)^{10}13$	28	0	0	$\lfloor 32/3 \rfloor = 10$

average of PI varies with sex and age. For example, the PI of a healthy female is less than that of healthy male and the PI of a healthy young person is less than that of a healthy old person. In this chapter, we do not attempt to account for these influences, but it certainly is the case that the relationship of PI's average to age and sex must be studied in the future research in order to render more accurate classifications. The 20 intermittent pulses in our pulse database exhibit 15 kinds of rhythm variations. Our approach correctly extracts all the MRUs of the 20 intermittent pulses.

In this section, we take five pulses as examples to illustrate the performance of our approach. Figure 7.11 shows these five pulses and their SPI sequences. Pulse1 is a knotted pulse; Pulse2, Pulse3, Pulse4, and Pulse5 are all intermittent pulses. Their symbolization and subsequences extraction results are as follows:

$$\text{SPI}(\text{Pulse1}) =$$
$$0000\#1001\$000000\#1000001001010001\$000000000, \quad (7.16)$$
$$000000000000000000000\#1\$0000$$

$$\text{SPI}(\text{Pulse2}) =$$
$$\#100001000010000100001000010000100001000100, \quad (7.17)$$
$$0010000100001\$0000$$

$$\text{SPI}(\text{Pulse3}) =$$
$$00\#1001001001001001001001001001001001001010010, \quad (7.18)$$
$$01001001\$00$$

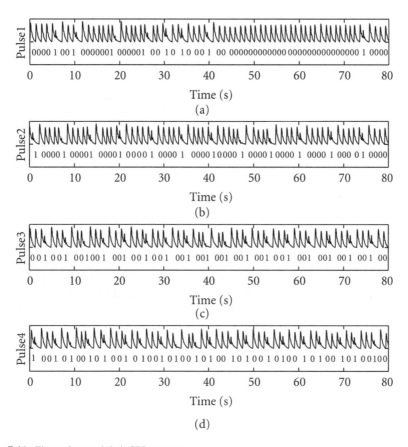

Fig. 7.11 Five pulses and their SPI sequences

$$SPI(Pulse4) =$$
$$\#1001010010100101001010010100101001010010100,$$ (7.19)
$$101001\$00$$

$$SPI(Pulse5) =$$
$$0\#1010101010101010101010101010101010101\$00.$$ (7.20)
$$000000000$$

Table 7.2 lists the Lempel-Ziv analysis results. The subsequence of Pulse1 is nonperiodic and its pulse rate is slow (the average of PIs is 1.25 s). We recognize Pulse1 as a knotted pulse. The other four examples, Pulse2, Pulse3, Pulse4, and Pulse5, are all intermittent pulses, each containing different MRUs.

Table 7.2 Results of Lempel-Ziv complexity-based matching approach

Pulse	Lempel-Ziv analysis result	Satisfy the lemma?	MRU	RD
Pulse1	"2"	No	"1000001001010001"	1
	"5♦2♦1♦3♦"	No	"1001"	1
	"1"	No	"1"	1
Pulse2	"4♦4444444444♦"	Yes	"10000"	11
Pulse3	"2♦222222222222222♦"	Yes	"100"	16
Pulse4	"2♦1♦21212121212121♦"	Yes	"10010"	9
Pulse5	"1♦11111111111111111♦"	Yes	"10"	19

7.5   Summary

This chapter proposes a Lempel-Ziv complexity analysis-based approach to the classification of seven pulse patterns that exhibit different rhythms and achieves an accuracy of 97.1%. The parameters of VR and VC are first extracted from PI series of pulse waveform and then are used to judge whether the pulse is arrhythmic or not according to Rule 1. If it is arrhythmic, the PI series should be symbolized and simplified. Combining with Rule 2 and the lemma, the Lempel-Ziv complexity analysis also makes it quite easy to identify the arrhythmic pulse patterns: running pulses, knotted pulses, and intermittent pulses. The automatic analysis of pulse rhythms relieves practitioners of the routine work of observing and diagnosing pulse data. Our approach can also be applied to the analysis of the rhythms of other physiological signals.

References

1. L. I. Hammer, Chinese Pulse Diagnosis: A Contemporary Approach, Eastland Press, Vista, Calif, USA, 2001.
2. J. H. Laub, "New non-invasive pulse wave recording instrument for the acupuncture clinic," American Journal of Acupuncture, vol. 11, no. 3, pp. 255–258, 1983.
3. B. Michael and M. Michael, "Instrument-assisted pulse evaluation in acupuncture, " American Journal of Acupuncture, vol. 14, no. 3, pp. 255–259, 1986.
4. H. Seng, "Objectifying of pulse-taking," Japanese Journal of Oriental Medicine, vol. 27, no. 4, p. 7, 1977.
5. K.-Q. Wang, L.-S. Xu, Z. Li, D. Zhang, N. Li, and S. Wang, "Approximate entropy based pulse variability analysis," in Proceedings of 16th IEEE Symposium on Computer-Based Medical Systems (CBMS '03), pp. 236–241, New York, NY, USA, June 2003.
6. W. K. Wang, T. L. Hsu, Y. Chiang, and Y. Y. Lin Wang, "Study on the pulse spectrum change before deep sleep and its possible relation to EEG, " Chinese Journal of Medical and Biological Engineering, vol. 12, pp. 107–115, 1992.
7. L. Y. Wei and P. Chow, "Frequency distribution of human pulse spectra, " IEEE Transactions on Biomedical Engineering, vol. 32, no. 3, pp. 245–246, 1985.

8. H.-L. Lee, S. J. Suzuki, Y. Adachi, and M. Umeno, "Fuzzy theory in traditional Chinese pulse diagnosis," in Proceedings of International Joint Conference on Neural Networks (IJCNN '93), vol. 1, pp. 774–777, Nagoya, Japan, October 1993.

9. Y.-Z. Yoon, M.-H. Lee, and K.-S. Soh, "Pulse type classification by varying contact pressure," IEEE Engineering in Medicine and Biology Magazine, vol. 19, no. 6, pp. 106–110, 2000.

10. G. K. Stockman, L. N. Kanal, and M. C. Kyle, "Structural pattern recognition of Carotid pulse waves using a general waveform parsing system, " Communications of the ACM, vol. 19, no. 12, pp. 688–695, 1976.

11. L. Wang, K.-Q. Wang, and L.-S. Xu, "Recognizing wrist pulse waveforms with improved dynamic time warping algorithm, " in Proceedings of the 3rd International Conference on Machine Learning and Cybernetics (ICMLC '04), vol. 6, pp. 3644–3649, Shanghai, China, August 2004.

12. B. H. Wang and J. L. Xiang, "ANN recognition of TCM pulse states, " Journal of Northwestern Polytechnic University, vol. 20, no. 3, pp. 454–457, 2002.

13. S. L. Huang and M. Y. Sun, The Study of Chinese Pulse Image, Chinese People's Sanitation Press, Beijing, China, 1995.

14. L. S. Zhen, Pulse Diagnosis, Paradigm Publications, Brookline, Mass, USA, 1985.

15. A. Lempel and J. Ziv, "On the complexity of finite sequences," IEEE Transactions on Information Theory, vol. 22, no. 1, pp. 75–81, 1976.

16. J. Ziv, "Coding theorems for individual sequences, " IEEE Transactions on Information Theory, vol. 24, no. 4, pp. 405–412, 1978.

17. R. Nagarajan, "Quantifying physiological data with Lempel-Ziv complexity-certain issues," IEEE Transactions on Biomedical Engineering, vol. 49, no. 11, pp. 1371–1373, 2002.

18. L. Y. Huang, Q. X. Sun, and J. Z. Cheng, "Novel method of fast automated discrimination of sleep stages," in Proceedings of the 25th Annual International Conference of the IEEE Engineering in Medicine and Biology Society, vol. 3, pp. 2273–2276, Cancun, Mexico, September 2003.

19. X.-S. Zhang, R. J. Roy, and E. W. Jensen, "EEG complexity as a measure of depth of anesthesia for patients," IEEE Transacions on Biomedical Engineering, vol. 48, no. 12, pp. 1424–1433, 2001.

20. S. Mund, "Ziv-Lempel complexity for periodic sequences and its cryptographic application," in Advances in Cryptology— EUROCRYPT '91, pp. 114–126, Brighton, UK, April 1991.

21. K.Q. Wang, L.S. Xu, L. Wang, Z. G. Li, and Y. Z. Li, "Pulse baseline wander removal using wavelet approximation," in Proceedings of the 30th Annual Conference of Computers in Cardiology (CinC '03), pp. 605–608, Thessaloniki, Chalkidiki, Greece, September 2003.

22. M. A. Navakatikyan, C. J. Barrett, G. A. Head, J. H. Ricketts, and S. C. Malpas, "A real-time algorithm for the quantification of blood pressure waveforms," IEEE Transactions on Biomedical Engineering, vol. 49, no. 7, pp. 662–670, 2002.

23. G. Gratze, J. Fortin, A. Holler, et al., "A software package for non-invasive, real-time beat-to-beat monitoring of stroke volume, blood pressure, total peripheral resistance and for assessment of autonomic function, " Computers in Biology and Medicine, vol. 28, no. 2, pp. 121–142, 1998.

24. K. G. Belani, J. J. Buckley, and M. O. Poliac, "Accuracy of radial artery blood pressure determination with the Vasotrac, " Canadian Journal of Anesthesia, vol. 46, no. 5, pp. 488–496, 1999.

25. L.-S. Xu, D. Zhang, and K.-Q. Wang, "Wavelet-based cascaded adaptive filter for removing baseline drift in pulse waveforms, " IEEE Transactions on Biomedical Engineering, vol. 52, no. 11, pp. 1973–1975, 2005.

26. D. Gusfield and J. Stoye, "Linear time algorithms for finding and representing all the tandem repeats in a string, " Journal of Computer and System Sciences, vol. 69, no. 4, pp. 525–546, 2004.

Chapter 8
Spatial and Spectrum Feature Extraction

Abstract In this chapter, we present a study on computational pulse diagnosis based on blood flow velocity signal. First, the blood flow velocity signal is collected using Doppler ultrasound device and preprocessed. Then, by locating the fiducial points, we extract the spatial features of blood flow velocity signal and further present a Hilbert-Huang transform-based method for spectrum feature extraction. Finally, support vector machine is applied for computation pulse diagnosis. Experiment results show that the proposed method is effective and promising in distinguishing healthy people from patients with cholecystitis or nephritis.

8.1 Introduction

Pulse diagnosis, one of the most important diagnostic methods in traditional Chinese medicine (TCM), has been used in disease examination and in guiding medicine selection for thousands of years [1]. In traditional Chinese pulse diagnosis (TCPD) theory [1], the wrist radial pulse signals, which are caused by the fluctuation of blood flow in radial artery, contain rich and critical information which can reflect the state of human viscus, i.e., gallbladder, kidneys, stomach, lungs, and so on [2]. That is, the pathologic change of these internal organs can be reflected from the variations of rhythm, velocity, and strength of radial pulse by which an experienced practitioner can tell a person's healthy condition. Moreover, TCPD is noninvasive and convenient for effective diagnosis. The diagnostic results of TCPD, however, sincerely depend on the practitioner's subjective analysis and sometimes may be unreliable and inconsistent. Therefore, it is necessary to develop computational pulse signal analysis techniques to make TCPD standard and objective. In recent years, techniques developed for measuring, processing, and analyzing the physiological signals [3–5] are considered in computational pulse signal research [6–8]. A series of pulse signal acquisition systems [9, 10] have recently been developed, and a number of methods have been proposed to analyze the digitized pulse signals [11–15].

By far, considerable achievements have been obtained in the development of computational pulse diagnosis based on the analysis of pulse signal acquired by pressure [9] or photoelectric sensors [10]. Since the information utilized in TCPD is

© Springer Nature Singapore Pte Ltd. 2018
D. Zhang et al., *Computational Pulse Signal Analysis*,
https://doi.org/10.1007/978-981-10-4044-3_8

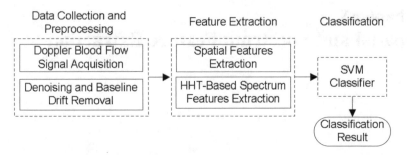

Fig. 8.1 Schematic diagram of the proposed computational pulse diagnosis method

comprehensive and complicated, photoelectric or pressure sensors cannot acquire all the necessary information for pulse diagnosis. Thus it is necessary to develop new types of sensors, to develop appropriate feature extraction methods, and to test the feasibility of other types of pulse signal.

Doppler ultrasonic blood flow inspection and measurement [16] is widely used as a noninvasive clinical check technique to evaluate the dynamic characteristics of peripheral artery. Thus, the effectiveness of Doppler ultrasonic blood flow signal for computational pulse diagnosis has been recognized and preliminarily investigated [17–19]. In this chapter, we systematically investigate the acquisition, preprocessing, feature extraction, and classification of Doppler ultrasonic blood flow signal and propose to use both spatial and spectrum features for computational pulse diagnosis.

Generally speaking, as shown in Fig. 8.1, the proposed scheme involves three major modules: data collection and preprocessing, feature extraction, and classification. In the first module, blood flow signal of the wrist radial artery is first collected by Doppler ultrasound device and then denoised using empirical mode decomposition (EMD)-based method [18]. In the feature extraction module, spatial features are first extracted, and then a Hilbert-Huang transform (HHT)-based method is adopted to extract the spectrum features. Finally, in the classification module, the support vector machine (SVM) classifier is used to distinguish healthy person from patients with two typical visceral diseases, cholecystitis and nephritis.

The remainder of this chapter is organized as follows. Section 8.2 describes the procedure of data acquisition and preprocessing. In Sect. 8.3, we first extract the spatial features of blood flow signal, and then a HHT-based method is proposed to effectively extract the spectrum features. The classification results are described in Sect. 8.4. Finally, Sect. 8.5 concludes this chapter.

8.2   Data Acquisition and Preprocessing

In our scheme, blood flow signals of the wrist radial artery are collected by a Doppler ultrasonic acquisition device. At the beginning of the signal acquisition, the operator uses his/her finger to feel the fluctuation of pulse at the patient's styloid process of radius to figure out a rough area where the ultrasound probe is then put on and moved around carefully until the most significant signal is detected. Then, a stable signal segment with 30 s is recorded and stored. The raw data acquired is represented in the form of Doppler spectrogram (see Fig. 8.2a), of which the up envelope corresponds to the blood flow velocity signal.

In the preprocessing, the blood flow velocity signal is first extracted and is then further processed to remove the noise and the baseline drift. An EMD-based method described in our former work [18] is adopted for denoising. To address the baseline drift problem, the wavelet-based cascade adaptive filter method [20] is adopted. As an example, Fig. 8.2b shows an extracted blood flow velocity signal, and Fig. 8.2c shows the result of blood flow velocity signal after denoising and baseline drift removal.

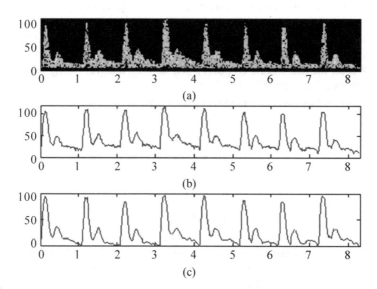

Fig. 8.2 An illustration of the preprocessing of wrist blood flow signal, where: (**a**) is a typical Doppler spectrogram of blood flow signal; (**b**) is the blood flow velocity signal extracted from Doppler spectrogram; (**c**) is the blood flow signal after denoising and baseline drift removal

8.3 Feature Extraction

This section describes the feature extraction methods used in our scheme. First, the spatial features of blood flow velocity signals are extracted. Then we discuss how to utilize the Hilbert-Huang transform (HHT), which includes empirical mode decomposition (EMD) and Hilbert transform, for spectrum feature extraction.

8.3.1 Spatial Feature Extraction of Blood Flow Velocity Signal

Blood flow velocity signal is a semi-periodic signal where each period signal is constructed by a primary wave, a secondary wave, and a dicrotic notch (see Fig. 1.6). Spatial feature is mainly means the fiducial points based feature introduced in Chap. 1.

The procedure of detecting fiducial point location is described as follows:

Step 1. Find the onsets of each period using the method described in [20], and then locate the points a and a_1, and their corresponding time labels are t_a and t_{a1}.

Step 2. Detect the peak point b of the primary wave in $[t_a, t_a + (t_{a1} - t_a)/3]$, and obtain the time label t_b and the amplitude h_b corresponding to b.

Step 3. Detect the subsequent peak point d within the time interval $[t_b, t_b + (t_{a1} - t_b)/2]$, and obtain its corresponding time label t_d and amplitude h_d.

Step 4. Detect the dicrotic notch point c within time interval $[t_b, t_d]$, and obtain its time labels t_c and amplitude h_c.

Step 5. Calculate the parameters in this period by:

$$\left. \begin{array}{l} T = t_{a_1} - t_a \\ T_{ba} = t_b - t_a \\ T_{cb} = t_c - t_b \\ T_{dc} = t_d - t_c \\ T_{a_1 b} = t_{a_1} - t_b \end{array} \right\}, \tag{8.1}$$

Step 6. Repeat Step 1–Step 5 until all the fiducial points of blood flow velocity signal are detected. After all the fiducial points are detected, we adopt the mean of relative ratios between different fiducial point information as spatial features because they are more stable.

8.3.2 EMD-Based Spectrum Feature Extraction

In this section, we first introduce the Hilbert-Huang transform (HHT) and then discuss how to utilize HHT for spectrum feature extraction of blood flow velocity signals.

8.3.2.1 Hilbert-Huang Transform

Hilbert-Huang transform (HHT) [21] is an adaptive signal processing method for analyzing nonlinear and nonstationary signals. In HHT, Hilbert spectrum, a time-frequency-energy spectrum of a signal, is generated for signal analysis. The cores of HHT are empirical mode decomposition and Hilbert transform.

Empirical Mode Decomposition Empirical mode decomposition (EMD) is a successful method used to generate a decomposition of signal into several individual components, intrinsic mode functions (IMFs) [21]. An IMF must satisfy the following two criteria: (1) the numbers of extrema and the number of zero-crossings of an IMF are equal or differ at most by one; (2) at any point, the mean value of the envelope defined by the local maxima and the envelope defined by the local minima is zero.

With EMD, a signal $S(t)$ is decomposed into a series of $\text{IMF}_n(t)$ and a residue $r(t)$. For expression convenience, the residue $r(t)$ is treated as the last IMF. Consequently, the original signal $S(t)$ can be reconstructed by IMFs:

$$S(t) = \sum_{n=1}^{N} \text{IMF}_n(t), \tag{8.2}$$

where N is the numbers of IMFs.

Hilbert Transform Hilbert transform of $\text{IMF}_n(t)$ is defined as:

$$Y_n(t) = \frac{1}{\pi} P \int_{-\infty}^{\infty} \frac{\text{IMF}_n(\tau)}{1 - \tau} d\tau, \tag{8.3}$$

where P denotes the Cauchy principal value [21].

With Hilbert transform, an analytic signal $Z_n(t)$ can be generated using $\text{IMF}_n(t)$ and the corresponding $Y_n(t)$, forming a complex conjugate pair defined as:

$$Z_n(t) = \text{IMF}_n(t) + iY_n(t) = a_n(t) e^{j\phi_n(t)}, \tag{8.4}$$

where $a_n(t)$ and $\varphi_n(t)$ are instantaneous amplitude and phase defined as:

$$a_n(t) = \sqrt{\left(\text{IMF}_n(t)\right)^2 + \left(Y_n(t)\right)^2}. \tag{8.5}$$

and

$$\phi_n(t) = \arctan\left(Y_n(t)\Big/\text{IMF}_n(t)\right), \tag{8.6}$$

respectively. Furthermore, the frequency of $Z_n(t)$ could be calculated as:

$$f_n(t) = \frac{1}{2\pi} \frac{d\phi_n(t)}{dt}. \tag{8.7}$$

8.3.2.2   Feature Extraction by Hilbert-Huang Transform

The procedure to use HHT for blood flow velocity signal feature extraction is described as follows:

For each blood velocity signal $S(t)$, EMD is applied to decompose it into a series of IMFs which satisfy:

$$S(t) = \sum_{n=1}^{N} \text{IMF}_n(t) \qquad t = 1, 2, \ldots m, \tag{8.8}$$

where N is the number of IMFs and m is the length of $S(t)$.

For each $\text{IMF}_n(t)$, we extract $a_n(t)$ and $f_n(t)$ using Eqs. (8.5) and (8.7) and then define the average amplitude h the average frequency of each $\text{IMF}_n(t)$ as μ:

$$\bar{h}_n = \sum_{t=1}^{m} a_n(t) / m, \tag{8.9}$$

$$\bar{\omega}_n = \sum_{t=1}^{m} a_n(t) f_n(t) / \sum_{t=1}^{m} a_n(t). \tag{8.10}$$

We define the energy P_n of $\text{IMF}_n(t)$ as:

$$P_n = \frac{\sum_{t=1}^{m} \left|\text{IMF}_n(t)\right|^2}{\sqrt{\sum_{n=1}^{N} \sum_{t=1}^{m} \left|\text{IMF}_n(t)\right|^2}}. \tag{8.11}$$

Using Eqs. (8.9, 8.10, and 8.11), for each blood flow velocity signal $S(t)$, we extract $3 \times N$ parameters $\left\{\bar{h}_n,, \bar{\omega}_n,, P_n\right\}$, which form a vector to be used for blood flow velocity signal classification.

8.4   Experimental Result and Discussion

In this section, the extracted features by methods described in Section 8.3 are tested on our blood flow velocity dataset. The dataset includes 33 healthy persons, 25 nephritis patients, and 25 cholecystitis patients. All of the data were collected at Harbin 211 Hospital using our Doppler ultrasonic analyzer. Before the classification, all the blood flow velocity signals are segmented to have the same length with the result that each has 2060 points.

For the HHT-based feature extraction method, all the 2060 points of data are used. Figures 8.3 and 8.4 show the EMD of a healthy person and a nephritis patient. EMD is an adaptive signal processing method. For different signals the numbers of

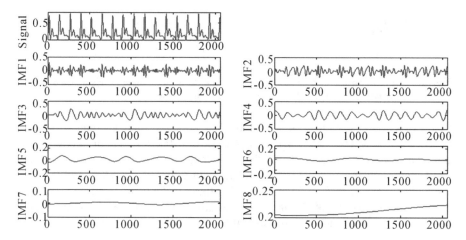

Fig. 8.3 EMD of blood flow velocity signal of a healthy person

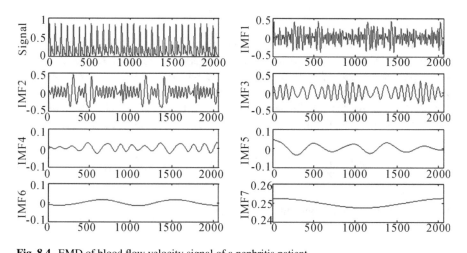

Fig. 8.4 EMD of blood flow velocity signal of a nephritis patient

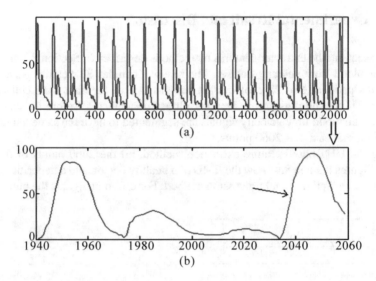

Fig. 8.5 Data processing for spatial feature extraction: (**a**) is an example of segmented data with the incomplete last span of data; (**b**) is partial enlarged view of (**a**)

their IMFs may not be the same. For blood flow velocity signal, the typical numbers of IMFs are between 7 and 9. Since the number of IMFs differs in different signals, the feature vectors extracted from different signal are not guaranteed to have the same feature dimension. For each blood velocity signal, there is less oscillation in the higher order of IMFs, which means that these IMFs contain the direct current component of the original signal. So, we discard the higher-order IMFs and use the first five lower-order IMFs (IMF1 to IMF5) for feature extraction. Then a fifteen-dimensional vector is extracted as:

$$E = \left\{ \overline{h}_n,, |\overline{\omega}_n,, |P_n,, |n \in [1,,\cdots,,5] \right\}. \tag{8.12}$$

For the spatial feature extraction method, since we have fixed the length of blood flow velocity signal and the periods of different signals are not the same, there may be a span at the end of each segmented data which could not cover a complete period, and some spatial feature could not be extracted in that span of signal (see Fig. 8.5). Thus, we discard that span and only use the remained part for spatial feature extraction. Using the method described in Sect 8.3.1, we form a vector:

$$S = \left\{ \frac{\overline{T}_{ba}}{\overline{T}},,,,,, \frac{\overline{T}_{cb}}{\overline{T}},,,,,, \frac{\overline{T}_{dc}}{\overline{T}},,,,,, \frac{\overline{T}_{a'b}}{\overline{T}_{ba}},,,,,, \frac{\overline{h}_c}{h_b},,,,,, \frac{\overline{h}_d}{h_b},,,,,, \right\}, \tag{8.13}$$

where "–" denotes the mean value of parameters.

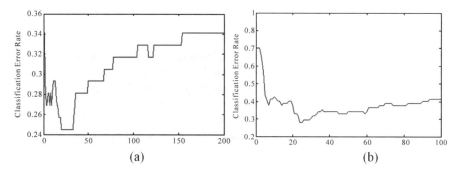

Fig. 8.6 The influence of C and α on the classification error rate: (**a**) α is fixed to 10 and C varies from 0.5 to 200; (**b**) C is fixed to 10 and α varies from 0.5 to 100

Table 8.1 Classification result using SVM

Sample class	Samples	Classification result	Accuracy	Average accuracy
Cholecystitis patients	25	14	56%	
Nephritis patients	25	23	92%	75%
Healthy people	33	26	79%	

Using both spatial and spectrum feature extraction, we extract two vectors E and S for each blood flow velocity signal and formulize them into a new vector $T = \{E, S\}$ for effective pulse classification.

In our experiments, we adopt support vector machine (SVM) [22] with Gaussian RBF kernel for that it has good generalization on small dataset. Our experiments were done under the MATLAB environment by using the SVM-KM toolbox [23]. In SVM, we should determine the values of two hyper-parameters, C and α. Figure 8.6 shows the influence of the two parameters on the classification error rate. According to the result shows in Fig. 8.6, we choose $C = 20$ and $\alpha = 25$. In order to reduce the bias, we adopt ten runs of a three-folder cross validation, and the classification results are listed in Table 8.1.

Table 8.1 shows that the proposed method achieves the highest accuracy, 92%, in the classification of the nephritis patients' group, and the lowest accuracy, 56%, in the cholecystitis patients' group. For all the three groups, the experiment achieves an acceptable accuracy of 75.9% in average.

The similar work of adopting pulse signals to classify healthy people from patient with nephritis and cholecystitis was reported in [24], where the pulse signals were acquired by a typical pressure sensor. The size of dataset used in [24] is comparable with that of this chapter. Compared with the results of [24], our works get a promotion in discriminating nephritis patients from the other two classes where the accuracy was equal to 92%. This result shows that the Doppler spectrogram is superior to pressure sensor in nephritis diagnosis and thus may contain valuable complementary information for pulse diagnosis.

8.5 Summary

The wrist pulse signal of a person contains important information about the pathologic changes of the person's body condition. In this chapter, we establish a systematic approach for computational pulse diagnosis by studying the quantitative features of blood flow velocity signal of radial artery. First, the spatial features were extracted by locating several fiducial points of the blood flow velocity signal. Then, a HHT-based feature extraction method was proposed and a series of spectrum features were extracted. Experimental results show that blood flow velocity signal carries important information for computational pulse diagnosis, and the proposed method achieves an accuracy of over 75% in classifying the healthy person from the patients with cholecystitis and nephritis. In the future, we will build large-scale dataset with more kinds of diseases to further verify this new computational pulse diagnosis approach and analyze the heterogeneity and complementarities of blood flow velocity signal and other types of pulse signal.

References

1. Li, S.Z. Pulse diagnosis. Hoc Ku Huyuh and G Seifert, Sydney, 1985.
2. Bob, F. The secret of Chinese pulse diagnosis. Blue Poppy Press, Boulder,1995.
3. Mahesh, V., Kandaswamy, A., Vimal, C. and Sathish, B. "ECG arrhythmia classification based on logistic model tree," Journal of Biomedical Science and Engi-neering, 2, 405–411,2009.
4. Dickhaus, H. and Heinrich, H. "Classifying biosignals with wavelet networks: A method for noninvasive diagnosis," IEEE Engineering in Medicine and Biology Magazine, 15, 103–111, 1996.
5. McGuirk, S.P., Ewert, D., Barron, D.J. and Coote, J.H. "Electrocardiographic interference and conductance volume measurements," Journal of Biomedical Science and Engineering, 2, 491–498, 2009.
6. Fei, Z.F. "Contemporary sphygmology in traditional Chinese medicine," People's Medical Publishing House, Beijing, 2003.
7. Wang, H. and Cheng, Y. "A quantitative system for pulse diagnosis in traditional Chinese medicine," Proceedings of the 27th Annual Conference on Engineering in Medicine and Biology Society, 6, 5676–5679, 2005.
8. Fu, S.E. and Lai, S.P. "A system for pulse measurement and analysis of Chinese medicine," Proceedings of the 11th Annual International Conference on Engineering in Medicine and Biology Society, 5, 1695–1696, 1989.
9. Tyan, C.C., Liu, S.H., Chen, J.Y., Chen, J.J. and Liang, W.M. "A novel noninvasive measurement technique for analyzing the pressure pulse waveform of the radial artery," IEEE Transactions on Biomedical Engineering, 55, 288–297, 2008.
10. Hertzman, A.B. "The blood supply of various skin areas as estimated by the photoelectric plethysmograph," American Journal Physiology, 124, 328–340, 1938.
11. Chun, T.L. and Ling, Y.W. "Spectrum analysis of human pulse," IEEE Transactions on Biomedical Engineering, 30, 348–352, 1983.
12. Lu, W.A., Lin Wang, Y.Y. and Wang, W.K. "Pulse analysis of patients with severe liver problems: Studying pulse spectrums to determine the effects on other organs," IEEE Engineering in Medicine and Biology Magazine, 18, 73–75, 1999.

13. Zhu, L., Yan, J., Tang, Q. and Li, Q. "Recent progress in computerization of TCM," Journal of Communication and Computer, 3, 78–81, 2006.
14. Chen, C.Y., Wang, W.K., Kao, T., Yu, B.C. and Chiang, B.C. "Spectral analysis of radial pulse in patients with acute uncomplicated myocardial infarction," Japanese Heart Journal, 34, 131–143, 1993.
15. Yu, G.L., Lin Wang, Y. Y. and Wang, W.K. "Resonance in the kidney system of rats," American Journal Physiology Heart and Circulatory Physiology, 267, 1544–1548, 1994.
16. Sigel, B. A brief history of Doppler ultrasound in the diagnosis of peripheral vascular disease," Ultrasound in Medicine and Biology, 24, 169–176, 1998.
17. Zhang, D.Y., Zhang, L., Zhang, D. and Zheng, Y. "Wavelet based analysis of Doppler ultrasonic wrist pulse signals," Proceedings of the IEEE International Conference on Biomedical Engineering and Informatics, 2, 539–543, 2008.
18. Zhang, D.Y., Wang, K.X., Wu, X.Q., Huang, B. and Li, N.M. "Hilbert-Huang transform based Doppler blood flow signals analysis," Proceedings of the IEEE International Conference on Biomedical Engineering and Informatics, 1-5, 2009.
19. Lee, Y.J., Lee, J. and Kim, J.Y. "A study on characteristics of radial arteries through ultrasonic waves," Proceedings of the 30th Annual International Conference on Engineering in Medicine and Biology Society, 2008, 2453–2456, 2008.
20. Xu, L.S., Zhang, D. and Wang, K.Q. "Wavelet-based cascaded adaptive filter for removing baseline drift in pulse waveforms," IEEE Transactions on Biomedical Engineering, 52, 1973–1975, 2005.
21. Huang, N.E., Shen, Z., Long, S.R., Tung, C.C. and Liu, H.H. "The empirical mode decomposition and the Hilbert spectrum for nonlinear and non-stationary time series analysis," Proceedings of the Royal Society, 454, 903–995, 1998.
22. Burges, C.J.C. (1998) "A tutorial on support vector machines for pattern recognition," Data Mining and Knowledge Discovery, 2, 121–167, 1998.
23. Canu, S., Grandvalet, Y., Guigue, V. and Rakotomamonjy, A. "SVM and Kernel methods Matlab toolbox," perception systèmes et information, INSA de Rouen, Rouen, France. http://asi.insa-rouen.fr/enseignants/~arak otom/toolbox/index.html
24. Guo, Q.L., Wang, K.Q., Zhang, D.Y. and Li, N.M."A wavelet packet based pulse waveform analysis for cholecystitis and nephrotic syndrome diagnosis," Proceedings of the 2008 International Conference on Wavelet Analysis and Pattern Recognition, 2, 513–517, 2008.

Chapter 9
Generalized Feature Extraction for Wrist Pulse Analysis: From 1-D Time Series to 2-D Matrix

Abstract Though many literatures on pulse feature extraction have been published, they just handle the pulse signals as simple 1-D time series and ignore the information within the class. This chapter presents a generalized method of pulse feature extraction, extending the feature dimension from 1-D time series to 2-D matrix. The conventional wrist pulse features correspond to a particular case of the generalized models. The proposed method is validated through pattern classification on actual pulse records. Both quantitative and qualitative results relative to the 1-D pulse features are given through diabetes diagnosis. The experimental results show that the generalized 2-D matrix feature is effective in extracting both the periodic and nonperiodic information. And it is practical for wrist pulse analysis.

9.1 Introduction

Radial arterial pulse is an important physiological signal which contains vital information of the health status. It has been extensively used as one of the four diagnostic methods in Traditional Chinese medicine (TCM) since ancient times [1, 2]. The Chinese medicine practitioners used to judge the health status of patients by feeling the pulsations at the wrist with fingers. However, it takes at least 5 years of experiences for a practitioner to master the pulse diagnosis skill. And inconsistent diagnostic results may be obtained among different practitioners. As a result, it is regarded as an empirical science which prevents the progress of the pulse diagnosis. A scientific way of studying the pulse should be to acquire the digital wrist pulse waveforms and to analyze the correlations between the pulse patterns and the diseases by using the computational methods [3].

Modern clinical studies have demonstrated that the loss of arterial elasticity and endothelial function is correlated with certain diseases such as hypertension, hypercholesterolemia, and diabetes [4]. These diseases eventually decrease the flexibility of vasculature and increase the stress to the blood circulatory system. As a result, the health conditions of the internal organs such as coronary heart disease [5], diabetes [6], arteriosclerosis [7], and ventricular tachycardia [8] are able to manifest in the pulsations.

© Springer Nature Singapore Pte Ltd. 2018
D. Zhang et al., *Computational Pulse Signal Analysis*,
https://doi.org/10.1007/978-981-10-4044-3_9

Generally speaking, the computational pulse diagnosis needs the techniques of signal processing and pattern recognition. The whole procedure consists of three stages, data collection and preprocessing, feature extraction, and pattern classification. At the first stage, a pulse acquisition platform is introduced to obtain the digital wrist pulse waveforms [9]. And then the pulse denoising and baseline wandering adjustment are performed to remove the artifacts in the coarse pulse datasets [10].

In the feature extraction module, two categories of methods have been proposed to analyze the digital wrist pulse signals. The first category is regarded as the expert system and studied in the early ages. Murthy et al. [11] proposed digital models for efficient representation of arterial pressure pulse and respiratory volume waveforms. The pole angers of the model were selected as the features and a Bayes classifier was applied to separate the abnormal signals from the normal ones in respiration pathways. Shu and Sun [4] used collective Gamma density functions to fit the wrist pulse waveforms via multidimensional variable analysis. And four classification indices, wavelength, the relative phase difference, rate parameter, and peak ratio, were extracted from the model to interpret the pulse waveform patterns objectively. Xu et al. [12] extracted a feature vector of 17 pulse shape parameters and chose fuzzy neural network for classification based on expert knowledge. However, these feature extraction methods were proposed to distinguish the pulse patterns defined based on their experiences. And the correlation relationships between pulse patterns and certain diseases were not researched.

In order to analyze the pulse waveforms more objectively, many methods using the biochemical criterions are proposed for pulse diagnosis and form the second category, statistical system. The pulse patterns are determined by the biochemical criterions, but not the expert knowledge [3]. Liu et al. [13] used multiscale sample entropy algorithm to compare the healthy pulse patterns and the disease samples and achieved a classification accuracy of 76.3%. Chen et al. [14–16] proposed AR model and Gaussian model to fit the wrist pulse curves. These features are time domain features. Zhang et al. [17] presented the spatial features and Hilbert-Huang transform-based spectrum feature to classify the healthy subjects from patients with cholecystitis or nephritis. Guo et al. [18] used the wavelet transform to extract diagnostic parameters related with cholecystitis and nephrotic syndrome. Liu et al. [19] combined multiple heterogeneous pulse features to enhance the classification and obtained encouraging results. Although the feature extraction methods in these researches are heterogeneous in nature, the pulse waveforms are regarded as having strict periodicity. And this assumption is invalid for actual pulse waveforms. Since the wrist pulse waveform is not a determinate periodical signal and the single-period changes a lot from cycle to cycle, which are verified in our experiments.

This chapter aims to propose a systematic approach with focus on the wrist pulse feature extraction. The conventional pulse feature extraction methods from time domain and frequency domain, including pulse shape, pulse width, improved Gaussian models, pulse energies, and pulse frequency components, are first introduced. Then, we extend the pulse dimension from 1-D time series to 2-D matrix description. And periodic decomposition is introduced to explain the essence of the pulse waveforms. The wrist pulse is considered as a combination of periodic stationary time series and nonperiodic distribution. The previous methods are mainly focused on the periodic components and turn out to be a subspace of the generalized 2-D pulse matrix description. The nonperiodic subspace within the class is also important for the pulse diagnosis. Based on the generalized pulse model, we combine the conventional features from periodic space and the 2-D matrix features from nonperiodic space. After the feature extraction, PCA and LDA are applied to reduce the feature dimension and select the disease-sensitive features, respectively. These selected features are then taken as the inputs to the support vector machine (SVM) classifier for pulse pattern classification. In this chapter, we construct a pulse dataset collected from 125 healthy persons and 125 diabetes patients to compare the proposed 2-D matrix features with the previous methods. In addition, a pulse database composed of 100 healthy women and 100 pregnant women is also established to validate the effectiveness of the proposed approach.

The remainder of this chapter is organized as follows. In Sect. 9.2, we describe the wrist pulse acquisition platform and the related preprocessing methods. In Sect. 9.3, the traditional pulse features from both time domain and frequency domain are introduced. In Sect. 9.4, the motivation and the method of 2-D pulse matrix feature extraction are presented. And the feature fusion and selection are then explained. The experiment comparisons between traditional 1-D pulse features and the 2-D matrix features are discussed in Sect. 9.5. Finally, a conclusion is given in Sect. 9.6.

9.2   Wrist Pulse Acquisition and Preprocessing Methods

9.2.1   Wrist Pulse Acquisition Platform

The Chinese medicine practitioners used to feel the wrist pulse of patients at Cun, Guan, and Chi three positions. In this chapter, the pulse acquisition platform with multichannel and fusion sensor arrays proposed in Ref. [9] is used to collect the wrist pulse signals at the three positions (see Fig. 6.2). Velcro strap is applied to fasten the pulse transducer owning to the convenience in clinical practice. The pressure sensors transfer the physical pulsations to quantitative voltage outputs, and the photoelectric sensor arrays detect the changes of blood flow. Then these electric signals are processed by amplification and filtering module, analog to digital conversion and micro digital signal processing (DSP) in order. Finally, the digital pulse waveforms are stored in Microsoft Database (MDB) through a universal serial bus (USB) interface for further processing and analysis.

The pulse data collection includes three steps. First, the rough positions of "Cun," "Guan," and "Chi" are manually searched by fingertips. Once the positions are ensured, the transducer is put on the wrist to the right place by aligning each channel with the corresponding position. Then, the intervals and centers of the three channels are subtly adjusted by the setting knobs to obtain more stable pulse signals with higher amplitudes. The third step is to apply proper pressures to the sensors by step

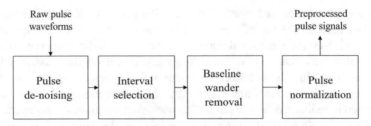

Fig. 9.1 The flowchart of the pulse preprocessing method

motors and to record the acquired pulse waveforms. Therefore, pulse beatings at the wrist are collected by the sensor arrays straight at the three body parts of "Cun," "Guan," and "Chi." And the sampling time is controlled to last 1 min. Several samples of each subject are collected following the three steps to reduce the measurement errors. Compared with the single-point pulse systems, capturing pulse signals from three channels is more accurate by considering the spatial information [9]. In addition, sensor arrays can provide pulse location, which is not available by using the single-point sensor.

9.2.2   Wrist Pulse Preprocessing

The pulse signal, known as a weak physiological signal, is easily corrupted by the artifacts. Talking, slight body movement and skin vibration all contribute to the signal noise. Besides, the baselines of the pulses often drift owing to the respirations. To remove these artifacts is necessary for more accurate wrist pulse feature extraction.

In this chapter, the pulse preprocessing consists of four stages (see Fig. 9.1). The coarse pulse waveforms are first denoised by a cascade filter based on wavelet decomposition [10]. Then, the interval selection is performed to remove the distortions. Next, the wrist pulse baseline drift is adjusted by using the curve fitting methods. Finally, the pulse normalization is developed before feature extraction.

9.3   Conventional Pulse Feature

Since the wrist pulse waveforms are typical 1-D time series, the traditional 1-D digital signal processing methods are first taken into consideration. In this section, the conventional pulse features extracted from time domain and frequency domain are presented. The time domain feature is composed of pulse shape information, pulse width, the model fitting parameters, and pulse energy. And the frequency domain feature includes pulse cycle intervals, frequency components, and wavelet coefficients.

9.3.1 Time Domain Feature

The duration of pulse acquiring for each subject is controlled to last at least 1 min. Figure 9.2 presents a typical wrist pulse waveform collected by our pulse acquisition platform. It reveals that wrist pulse is a classical periodical signal similar to other physiological signals such as ECG. In each cycle, the pulse signal could be divided into an ascending limb and a descending limb. The ascending limb is a monotone increasing section without any characteristic points. While at the descending limb, there exists several important extreme points which makes the pulse waveforms various and different. The wrist pulse at the latter half is usually regarded as the superimposition of two waves, a tidal wave with higher amplitude and a dicrotic wave with lower amplitude.

The distinctive characteristic of the pulse is caused by the rhythmic contraction and relaxation of the heart [20]. The ascending limb before percussion wave, the wave with highest amplitudes, reflects the heart systole. It is generated when the left ventricle of the heart is in contraction forcing blood into the aorta. The descending limb after the percussion wave reflects the diastole. And the tidal wave and the dicrotic wave are generated by the phenomenon of wave reflection. Meanwhile, peripheral resistance and artery compliance have an effect on the descending limb.

The amplitude of percussion wave is affected by the cardiac contractility and ejection fraction. Consequently, the percussion wave mainly contains the heart and rhythmic states. And the descending limb contains information of the periphery of the arterial system and plays a major role in determining the wrist pulse patterns [16]. Therefore, in the time domain, our focus is which is crucial for pulse diagnosis. And the feature illustrated in Tables 1.1 and 1.2 was adopted in this chapter as the time domain features.

In spatial dimension, the radial arterials vary in width from individual to individual. It is an important physiological symbol for judging the fullness or tension of pulse patterns in TCM. As the pulse width is produced by the fluid content of blood

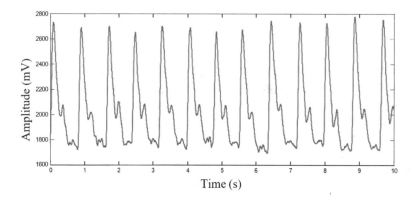

Fig. 9.2 Typical wrist pulse waveform obtained by our system

Fig. 9.3 Fitting surface of the pulse array waveforms

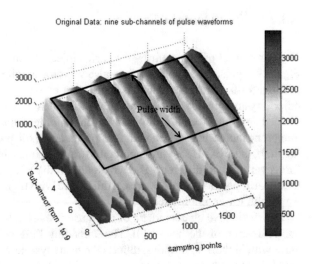

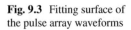

vessels and correlated with the conditions of vessel [21], the change of vessel form usually indicates the change of healthy states. Thus, the sensor array design is used in our pulse acquisition platform to obtain the pulse width information. The sensor array is placed in the vertical direction over the radial artery to cover the vessel lateral section. And the surface fitting algorithm is employed to simulate the spatial blood flow of radial artery under the skin. Figure 9.3 shows the fitting curves by using spline interpolation and the amplitudes of pulse signals in the array decrease from the artery center. There is a reference frame, in which X-axis is the time value, Y-axis is the fitting of nine channels, and Z-axis is the amplitudes of the pulse waveforms. The pulse width is extracted from the fitting surface by calculating the intervals with pulse amplitudes above the threshold in Y-axis direction.

Model fitting is widely used for matching the time series data. Pulse features extracted from the Gaussian model is also studied by Chen et al. [16]. They thought the single-period pulse signals should be expressed by a two-term Gaussian function with an offset as below:

$$f\left(x|,A_1|,\tau_1|,\sigma_1|,A_2|,\tau_2|,\sigma_2|,d\right) = A_1{}^* e^{-\left((x-\tau_1)/\sigma_1\right)^2} + A_2{}^* e^{-\left((x-\tau_2)/\sigma_2\right)^2} + d. \quad (9.1)$$

The percussion wave and the secondary wave are represented by $A_1{}^* e^{-\left((x-\tau_1)/\sigma_1\right)^2}$ and $A_2{}^* e^{-\left((x-\tau_2)/\sigma_2\right)^2}$, respectively, where A_1 and A_2 stand for the amplitude of the two waves, d is the baseline, τ_1 and τ_2 are the centers of the two waves, and σ_1 and σ_2 denote the wave width. These seven coefficients represent the amplitude, phase and shape of the two waves and are extracted as the fitting features.

However, the wrist pulse is composed of "percussion wave," "tidal wave," and "dicrotic wave" in each cycle [20]. It could not be segmented into a two-wave form accurately. Therefore, the two-term Gaussian model is insufficient for matching the three-wave time series, which will result in the pulse information loss. Moreover, the optimization of the Gaussian model fitting is also required to obtain more accurate representation.

In this chapter, we introduce the mixed Gaussian model without a constant term in the fitting equations as below:

$$f\left(x|A_i,\tau_i,\sigma_i\right)=\sum_{i=1}^{n}A_i^{*}e^{-\left((x-\tau_i)/\sigma_i\right)^2}.$$ (9.2)

The constant term is not selected due to the nonlinearity of the baseline. These coefficients are obtained by using the nonlinear least squares formulation to fit the Gaussian model to the wrist pulse signal by using the toolbox in Matlab.

Figure 9.4 shows the comparisons of the mixed Gaussian models from two-term to five-term for pulse fitting. From above, it can be seen that the wrist pulse waveform can be well matched by a four-term Gaussian model with the lease error of all. And three parameters, including sum square error (SSE), R-square, and root mean square error (RMSE), are introduced to evaluate the performance.

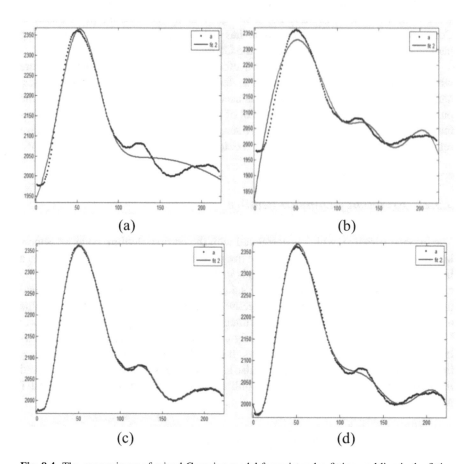

(a)

(b)

(c)

(d)

Fig. 9.4 The comparisons of mixed Gaussian model for wrist pulse fitting; red line is the fitting curve: (**a**) two-term Gaussian model, (**b**) three-term Gaussian model, (**c**) four-term Gaussian model, and (**d**) five-term Gaussian model

Table 9.1 Comparisons of the Gaussian model

Gaussian model	Two-term	Three-term	Four-term
SSE (10^4)	8.296	12.51	0.1438
R-square	0.9731	0.9595	0.9995
RSME	19.64	24.29	2.623

The evaluation of the Gaussian model is given in Table 9.1. It can be seen that the pulse wave represented by a four Gaussian model has the least SSE and RSME, and the R-square which measures how successful the fit is in explaining the variation of the data indicates a better fit with a value closer to 1. Why is the four-term Gaussian model a better fit for pulse waveform? The reason is that the pulse wave is proved to have three waves in each cycle, and each wave corresponds to a Gaussian peak in the fitting. As the constant term is not included in the fitting equations, an extra Gaussian peak is needed to fit the baseline. In the four-term Gaussian model, a large value of σ_i means a wave more like a straight line and denotes the pulse baseline. Consequently, the four-term Gaussian has the best performance, and the fitting parameters $\{A_i, \tau_i, \sigma_i\}$ are extracted as the Gaussian model feature.

In TCM, the power of the pulse waveform denotes the static contact pressure when feeling one's pulsations. And this feature is divided into three categories, named "Fu," "Zhong," and "Chen." It is used by TCM practitioners for judging the pulse depth and accounted as the symbol of physical weakness. In this chapter, this feature is captured by using the pressure sensors. The baseline of the pressure pulse reflects the static contact pressure and is extracted as the pulse energy feature.

9.3.2   Frequency Domain Feature

The interval variance, which is correlated with the cardiac rhythm, plays an important role in heart disease diagnosis. The irregular cardiac rhythm usually indicates a heart disease. Thus, the abnormal periods in the wrist pulse waveform are found by using the variance analysis [22]. Figure 9.5 displays the normal pulse waveform and the pulse with abnormal periods, respectively. In our experiments, the mean value and the variance of the periods are calculated as the period frequency information.

The Fourier transform (FT) is a widely used signal processing method for viewing the frequency spectrum components. It provides the complementary frequency information within the single-period pulse signals besides the interval variance. And the frequency components within the pulse period are calculated by using the FT method below:

$$X_k = \sum_{n=0}^{N-1} x_n e^{-2\pi k i \frac{n}{N}}, k = 0, \cdots, N-1, \tag{9.3}$$

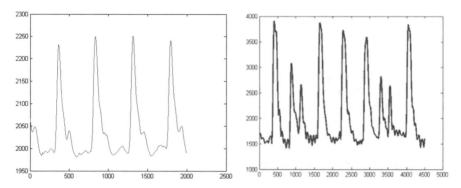

Fig. 9.5 Pulse periods with normal periods and abnormal periods

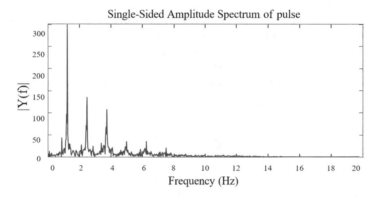

Fig. 9.6 The pulse frequency spectrum within single-period

where x_n is the pulse time series and N denotes the pulse length. Figure 9.6 shows the single-sided amplitude spectrum of the pulse signal. As the periods of the wrist pulse belong to the range from 30/min to 120/min, the first spectrum peak which denotes the period frequency lies in the band from 0.5 Hz to 2 Hz. The latter spectrum peaks describe the higher frequency information within the periods. The first three spectrum peaks and the corresponding amplitudes are extracted as the frequency feature.

Wavelet transform is applied to extract the wavelet features of each band in the pulse waveforms. By using the eight-level "db6" wavelet transform, we decompose pulse signals into eight bands, one coarse band, and seven detailed bands. The wavelet energy features of each band are calculated as below:

$$E_{cD_i} = \sum_{k=1}^{l\_cD_i} cD_i\left(k\right)^2, i = 1,\cdots,8, \tag{9.4}$$

$$E_{cA_8} = \sum_{k=1}^{l\_cA} cA_8 (k)^2 . \tag{9.5}$$

In wavelet analysis, the approximations cA_8 are the high-scale, low-frequency components of the wrist pulse signals. And the details cD_i are the low-scale and high-frequency components.

9.4   2–D Pulse Feature Extraction

9.4.1   Motivation

The wrist pulse is usually regarded as a quasiperiodic signal by former researches. In that case, if anyone knows one period of the pulse signal, the entire signal is also determined. As a result, they all attempt to analyze the wrist pulse signals under the assumptions that the wrist pulse signal is a repetitive process with high autocorrelations and can be accurately predicted by the values from previous periods. Thus, the autoregression (AR) model [15] has been used for the wrist pulse representation as below:

$$f(t) = \sum_{i=1}^{n} a_i f(t-i) + \varepsilon_f (t), \tag{9.6}$$

where a_i is the ith AR coefficient and $\varepsilon_f (t)$ is the modeling error. The coefficients are obtained by using the least square method. The identified model $\{a_i\}$ is then used to fit the input pulse waveforms. They assume that the AR model which is trained from healthy persons will accurately predict the signal from a healthy subject and will not well predict the pulse signal from a patient [15].

However, the wrist pulse is not a determinate process that can be accurately expressed by a mathematic function. Although the rough framework of each period seems to be similar, and the length meets the periodical requirements. The detail varies in local extreme points, amplitudes, and slope factors. Therefore, these characteristics make the wrist pulse various in each single period. Figure 9.6 shows the segments of original pulse waveforms from a healthy person and a patient, respectively. The pulse in the upper panel is collected from a diabetic patient and the lower panel shows a healthy pulse. We can find that the pulse shape of the two signals is different as a whole. But if we take a local view point, the single-period signals change a lot from cycle to cycle, especially in the patient's pulse. Even the forth single-period pulse signal of the diabetes is very close to the forth one of the healthy person. In this situation, one may fail to distinguish the diabetes from the healthy sample if the pulse is regarded as a determinate periodical signal.

The previous pulse feature extraction algorithms via selecting one single-period or the average single-period pulse both ignore the shape various among the periods.

In this chapter, we define the degrees of single-period disparities as the pulse intra-class distance. It gives an evaluation criterion of the wrist pulse signal how it is consistent or various within each periods. Moreover, the pulse information from the entire signal should be extracted to avoid the overgeneralizations. Just choosing one period of pulse will lead to the false-positive classification.

9.4.2 Matrix Description for Pulse Waveforms

In order to completely extract the pulse features from the entire signal, we extend the pulse feature dimension from 1-D time series to 2-D matrix. The conventional wrist pulse features mainly focus on the local details of a single-period segment or the global statistical characteristics. The wrist pulse waveforms are just considered as cycle stationary time series. In this chapter, we redefine the wrist pulse as a combination of periodic stationary time series and nonperiodic distribution. Thus, the wrist pulse signal is decomposed into two-dimensional independent components. It is given by the formula below:

$$x(t) = f(t) + \varepsilon(t), \tag{9.7}$$

where $x(t)$ represents the original entire pulse signal of a subject, $f(t)$ is the periodic components of the wrist pulse and satisfies the autocorrelation, and T is the period:

$$f(t) = f(t+T), \forall t. \tag{9.8}$$

The residual term $\varepsilon(t)$ denotes the nonperiodic components. Thus, the wrist pulse signal is composed of two-dimensional information. One dimension is the periodic component, and the conventional pulse features are extracted in this space. The second dimension is the nonperiodic component containing the pulse intra-class distance information. If $\varepsilon(t) = 0$, the conventional pulse model is the special case of the generalized pulse signal representation.

Since the first dimension of the generalized model is a periodic term, we take the pulse cycle as the basic length. Thus, the pulse period segmentation is applied to obtain the basic signals. We treat the valleys as the partitioned points. The valley detection algorithm is introduced as follows:

Step 1. Perform the Fourier transform to find out the basic frequency, and the basic period T is calculated as $T = 1/f$.

Step 2. Detect the peak and valley of the pulse signal within initial window $[0,T]$. The obtained peak point is the maximum point P_1 of the first period, while valley is the minimum point V_1. And their corresponding positions at timing axis are t_1, respectively.

Step 3. After t_1 and t_2 are determined, then we slide the window step by step to update P_1, V_1 and find out the second peak and valley point P_2, V_2 in time interval $\lfloor t_1 + T/2, t_1 + 3\,T/2 \rfloor$.

Step 4.   Once the peak and valley points P_i, V_i are detected, the wrist pulse is segmented into single-period pulse signals between two consecutive valleys
V_i and V_{i+1} .

The wrist pulse waveform of each subject is considered as a space expanded by
the segmented single-period signals. Thus, the data structure of wrist pulse waveform is transformed from time series $x(t) \in R^L$ into a set X':

$$x(t) \mapsto X' = \bigcup_{i=1}^{N} s_i'. \tag{9.9}$$

The single-period waveforms s_i' of each sample are regarded as the basic elements of the set X'. The single-period pulses with unequal sampling points caused
by irregular heart rhythm and measurement errors are resampled to the same length
by using the linear interpolation method. The algorithm is given by the formula
below:

$$t_i = \left[1 + \frac{(n-1)(m_i'-1)}{m-1} \right], \tag{9.10}$$

$$w_i = 1 + \frac{(n-1)(m_i'-1)}{m-1} - t_i, \tag{9.11}$$

$$s_i(n) = (1-w_i)s_i'(t_i) + w_i s_i'(t_i+1), n = 1, 2, \cdots, m, \tag{9.12}$$

where s_i' denotes the coarse segmented pulse signals with m_i' sampling points. s_i is
the resampled pulse with m points; in this chapter m is set to 100 based on the experiences. "[ ]" is the integer conversion.

Then, the data structure of the wrist pulse waveform for each sample is transformed from the time series set X' into matrix description $X \in R^{m \times N}$:

$$X' = \bigcup_{i=1}^{N} s_i' \mapsto X = [s_1, s_2, \cdots, s_n]. \tag{9.13}$$

And each column $s_i = [s_i(1), \ldots, s_i(m)]^T$ is a complete cycle segmented from the
original signal. The periodic component should be contained in every segmented
signal s_i as the single-period pulses are without self-similarity. Therefore, we can
also acquire the matrix description $F \in R^{m \times N}$ and $D \in R^{m \times N}$ for the periodic component and nonperiodic component of the segmented wrist pulse, respectively:

$$f(t) = \bigcup_{i=1}^{N} f_i' \mapsto F = [f_1, f_2, \cdots f_n], \tag{9.14}$$

$$\varepsilon(t) = \bigcup_{i=1}^{N} \varepsilon_i' \mapsto D = [\varepsilon_1, \varepsilon_2, \cdots, \varepsilon_n]. \tag{9.15}$$

Due to the periodicity theorem, $f_i = f$, $\forall i$ always exists. The single-period pulse signal of the set is then expressed by the formula below:

$$s_i = f + \varepsilon_i$$
$$X = [f + \varepsilon_1, f + \varepsilon_2, \cdots, f + \varepsilon_n] = F + D^{\cdot} \tag{9.16}$$

In this chapter, F is named as the periodic space and D is the nonperiodic space. And f is the periodic component of the entire signal. We extract this periodic component by averaging the elements in the matrix as below:

$$f = \frac{1}{N} \sum_{i=1}^{N} s_i. \tag{9.17}$$

The periodic component f stands for the global averaging pulse waveform in each segmented single-period pulse signals. The relationship between the segmented single-period pulse signals is shown by the formula below:

$$s_i - s_j = \varepsilon_i - \varepsilon_j. \tag{9.18}$$

The nonperiodic component ε_i measures the signal difference from the averaging and denotes the specificity of each cycle. It is various in each vector s_i and the set of $\{\varepsilon_i\}$ presents a distribution of the nonperiodic space. The previous researches are all developed on the pulse periodic space. And our focus is on extracting the intra-class distribution in the nonperiodic space plus the conventional periodic space.

Figure 9.7 presents the novel thoughts of wrist pulse analysis. The pulses are considered as bringing distinguishing information caused by individual differences. Bao et al. [23] have applied the physiological signals of subjects for authentication. We intend to reduce the disturbances from individual differences and focus on the

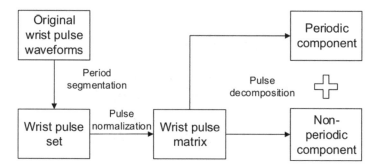

Fig. 9.7 A framework of the 2-D pulse features

characteristics of the disease influences. A reasonable assumption is that wrist pulse has two-dimensional independent information. One dimension is the conventional pulse features that is regarded as the individual-dependent space, and the second dimension is the disease-sensitive pulse space which is superimposed on the individual-dependent space.

In general, we assume that the intra-class distribution in the nonperiodic space has several orthogonal directions μ_j. The segmented single-period pulse is then expressed by the formula below:

$$s_i = \frac{1}{N} \sum_{m=1}^{N} s_m + \sum_{j=1}^{P} a_{ij} \mu_j, \tag{9.19}$$

$$u_i^T u_j = \begin{cases} 0, i \neq j \\ 1, i = j \end{cases}. \tag{9.20}$$

And we intend to find the principal directions in which most of the nonperiodic component energies are concentrated:

$$\widetilde{S}_i = \frac{1}{N} \sum_{m=1}^{N} s_m + \sum_{j=1}^{P} a_{ij} \mu_j, d < p. \tag{9.21}$$

The energies of the residual term are then given by the formula below:

$$\xi = \sum_{i=1}^{N} \left(s_i - \widetilde{s}_i \right)^T \left(s_i - \widetilde{s}_i \right) = \sum_{i=1}^{N} \left(\sum_{j=d+1}^{P} a_{ij} \mu^T, \sum_{j=d+1}^{P} a_{ij} \mu_j \right) = \sum_{i=1}^{N} \sum_{j=d+1}^{P} a_{ij}^2. \tag{9.22}$$

where we can obtain the coefficients a_{ij} from Eq. (9.19):

$$a_{ij} = \mu_j^T \left(s_i - \frac{1}{N} \sum_{m=1}^{N} s_m \right). \tag{9.23}$$

Then,

$$\begin{aligned} \xi &= \sum_{i=1}^{N} \sum_{j=d+1}^{P} a_{ij}^2 = \sum_{j=d+1}^{P} \sum_{i=1}^{N} a_{ij}^2 \\ &= \sum_{j=d+1}^{P} \sum_{i=1}^{N} \mu_j^T \left(s_i - \frac{1}{N} \sum_{m=1}^{N} s_m \right) \left(s_i - \frac{1}{N} \sum_{m=1}^{N} s_m \right)^T \mu_j \\ &= \sum_{j=d+1}^{P} \mu_j^T \sum_{i=1}^{N} \left(s_i - \frac{1}{N} \sum_{m=1}^{N} s_m \right) \left(s_i - \frac{1}{N} \sum_{m=1}^{N} s_m \right)^T \mu_j. \end{aligned} \tag{9.24}$$

Since the nonperiodic space is defined as $D = X - F$, thus,

$$\sum_{i=1}^{N}\left(s_i - \frac{1}{N}\sum_{m=1}^{N}s_m\right)\left(s_i - \frac{1}{N}\sum_{m=1}^{N}s_m\right)^T = DD^T, \qquad (9.25)$$

$$\xi = \sum_{j=d+1}^{p} \mu_j^T DD^T \mu_j. \qquad (9.26)$$

To minimize the residual energies ξ, the Lagrangian multiplier method is applied as below:

$$f\left(\mu_i\right) = \sum_{j=d+1}^{p} \mu_j^T DD^T \mu_j - \sum_{j=d+1}^{p} \lambda_j \left(\mu_j^T \mu_j - 1\right), \qquad (9.27)$$

where $\dfrac{\partial f}{\partial \mu_j} = DD^T \mu_j - \lambda_j \mu_j = 0$, therefore, μ_j is the eigenvectors of the matrix DD^T

and the residual energies is then transformed into the formula below:

$$\xi = \sum_{j=d+1}^{p} \mu_j^T \lambda_j^T \mu_j = \sum_{j=d+1}^{p} \lambda_j. \qquad (9.28)$$

We sort the eigenvectors by the corresponding eigenvalues and choose the first five directions and the energies as the intra-class distribution in the experiment as follows:

$$f\left(D\right) = \left[\mu_1^T, \cdots, \mu_5^T, \lambda_1, \cdots, \lambda_5\right]. \qquad (9.29)$$

The nonperiodic space of the wrist pulse is mainly expanded by the selected five directions, and the errors of the residual energies ξ are the least under this feature extraction. The selected vectors denote the main intra-class distribution directions; the eigenvalues show the intra-class distance in these directions. While the periodic space is simply expanded by the single component $f\left(F\right) = \left[\sum_{m=1}^{N} s_m / N\right]^T$, the two-dimensional wrist pulse features, intra-class distributions and conventional pulse features, are combined as the fusion feature of the 2-D pulse matrix and given by $f(X) = [f(F), f(D)]$. Figure 9.8 shows the feature extension process.

Figure 9.9 presents the proposed feature extraction procedure. For each pulse sample in our database, the preprocessed wrist pulse signals collected from the sensor array are first analyzed to obtain the spatial information of pulse width. The wrist pulse from the sensor array shows high similarities, and the array signal analysis attempts to choose the most valuable information and exclude the redundant characteristics. On the basis of array selection, period analysis, Fourier transform, and wavelet transform are developed to extract the pulse features in frequency domain. In time domain, local extreme values are first detected as the conventional pulse shape features. And then, the pulse amplitudes and fitting

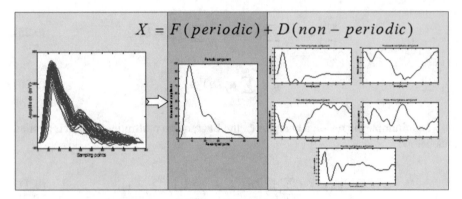

Fig. 9.8 Segmented single-period pulse signals and the nonperiodic space

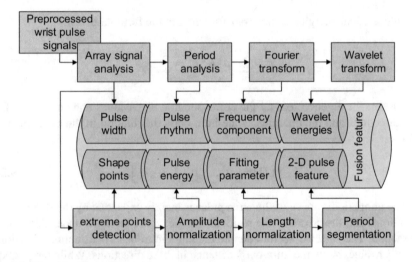

Fig. 9.9 The pulse feature extraction procedure

parameters are extracted. At last, the period segmentation is developed to obtain the 2-D pulse features.

Thus, we have extracted a pulse fusion feature vector for a subject. However, the shape points are associated with the frequency components and the fitting parameters. Some closely correlated parameters exist in the feature vector and these correlated parameters should be eliminated. When we get the feature matrix for all the subjects, PCA is then developed to reduce the feature redundancy and the dimension. So far a no tightly correlated feature vector has been obtained. However, the reduced features are still subject to further feature selection. Since the individual differences are included in the pulse features, the disease-sensitive features are required for the disease diagnosis. Consequently, we propose a linear discriminant analysis (LDA)-based approach to select the disease-sensitive features. Assuming that a training pulse dataset is available with N_1 wrist pulse signals from the healthy subjects and N_2 pulse signals from the patients, the reduced fusion features are denoted as $f = \left[f_{h,1}, \cdots f_{h,N_1}, f_{p,1}, \cdots f_{p,2} \right]^T$. The statistical feature difference between these two groups can be calculated as:

$$S_{f^i} = \frac{\left(f_h^i - f_p^i \right)^2}{p(w_1) S_{w_1} + p(w_2) S_{w_2}}, \tag{9.30}$$

where f_h^i and f_p^i are the means of i-th feature of the feature vector $f_{h,i}$ and $f_{p,j}$, respectively. And the within-class scatter matrix is defined as:

$$S_w = p(w_1) S_{w_1} + p(w_2) S_{w_2} = \frac{N_1 S_1^2 + N_2 S_2^2}{N_1 + N_2}, \tag{9.31}$$

where S_1^2 and S_2^2 are the variances i-th feature of the feature vector $f_{h,i}$ and $f_{p,j}$, respectively. For each feature in the feature vector, the statistical linear discriminant ability between the healthy persons and patients reflects the sensitivity of this feature to the disease. A large value of S_{f^i} usually means a good indicator for disease classification. Consequently, the features that have large statistical differences should be selected and the features with small differences between the two patterns should not be used for classification.

9.5 Experiments

Related experiments are conducted to verify the performance of the proposed pulse features in disease diagnosis. Our pulse dataset consists of 1554 wrist pulse samples which are gathered from Guangdong Hospital of Traditional Chinese Medicine. The database is composed of 148 healthy persons, 872 subhealthy persons, and 534 persons with certain diseases such as diabetes, nephritis, and cardiopathy. The patients with a healthy or subhealthy status are judged by the recent healthy check, and the wrist pulses of subjects with certain diseases are collected from the corresponding ward in the hospital. And the final labels are checked by the doctors through the patients' medical record.

The original wrist pulse signals are preprocessed by the denoising, baseline drift removal, array selection, and period segmentation stages sequentially. The proposed fusion pulse features are then extracted after the pulse preprocessing. The methods of PCA and LDA are developed to reduce the feature dimension and select the disease-sensitive features, respectively. Last, the support vector machine (SVM) with radial basis function (RBF) kernel is selected as the classifiers to separate the pulse patterns.

9.5.1 Diabetes Diagnosis

In the first experiment, we use the wrist pulse samples to distinguish healthy subjects and patients known to be afflicted with diabetes. The diabetes were confirmed by comparing patients' levels with standard clinical blood markers. The pulse dataset contains 148 healthy persons and 534 persons with certain diseases. And the diabetic in the disease group occupied a large part. Thus, we randomly choose 125 healthy samples and 125 diabetes samples from the dataset.

We adopt the fivefold cross-validation procedure to reduce the influence caused by the sample partition. The pulse samples from healthy subject and diabetic are randomly divided into five equal folds, respectively. Each fold contains 25 healthy samples and 25 diabetes pulse samples. Each time we select four of them to form the training set and leave one fold as the testing set for verification. The pulse features including the pulse shape, pulse width, pulse energy, pulse frequency, Gaussian models, wavelet coefficients, and matrix pulse features are all extracted for classification. And the fusion pulse features are also obtained by combining the feature vectors together in serial strategy for comparison. After the original feature dimension reduced by projecting the samples onto the PCA subspace, the diabetes sensitive features are selected. Then, the classifier of KNN and RBF-SVM are introduced to construct a proper classification hyper plane by using these features and to predict the pattern of test samples, respectively. The specification parameters of the RBF kernel are determined by using the grid searching technique. The average classification accuracy of the fivefold cross validation is finally calculated as indicators of the system performance.

Table 9.2 shows the experiment results of the classification. The accuracy is not satisfied if only a single type of pulse features is selected for diabetes diagnosis. And the best performance is obtained by using the Gaussian fitting models, reaching an accuracy of 65%. And the experiment also demonstrates that the RBF-SVM is superior to the KNN in diabetes diagnosis, since the RBF-SVM is a nonlinear classifier and the pulse signals are produced by a nonlinear system.

The classification rate is increased to 71.2% by using the fusion of the 1-D conventional pulse features, including shape, width, energy, frequency, Gaussian fitting

Table 9.2 Classification results

Features	Accuracy	
	KNN	RBF-SVM
Shape feature	55.2	64.2
Pulse width	55.6	59
Pulse energy	55	58
Pulse frequency	52	61.2
Gaussian models	57.4	65
Wavelet coefficient	55	60
1-D Fusion features	65	71.2
Matrix features	68	85.6
2-D Fusion features	71.6	91.6

Table 9.3 Diabetes diagnosis comparison

Features	Sensitivity (%)	Specificity (%)	Accuracy (%)
Heterogeneous features [19]	75.8	88.9	79.4
WPT [14]	88.9	77.1	85.4
ARPE [14]	91.7	80.0	88.0
2-D fusion features	94.6	88.6	91.6

parameters, and wavelet coefficients. And the proposed matrix pulse features performance better than the conventional fusion features. The classification accuracy is increased by 14.4%, up to 85.6% on diabetes diagnosis. In this experiment, the best performance is obtained by combining the conventional pulse features with the matrix features which contain the two-dimensional information of the wrist pulse. An accuracy of 91.6% is finally achieved with a ratio of 20.4% increase compared with the best performance of conventional pulse features.

In addition, we also compare the proposed 2-D fusion pulse feature extraction method with the other researches on diabetes diagnosis. Table 9.3 presents the comparison result. Liu et al. [19] introduce a combination of heterogeneous features for wrist pulse diagnosis through multiple kernel learning classifiers. And the classification accuracy reaches 79.4%. Chen et al. [14] propose two pulse feature extraction methods, wavelet package transform (WPT) and auto-regressive prediction error (ARPE), for pulse diagnosis. And the classification rate for diabetes diagnosis is 85.4% and 88.0%, respectively. From Table 9.2, it can be seen that the proposed 2-D fusion feature method is superior to these conventional pulse extraction methods.

9.5.2 Pregnancy Diagnosis

In the second experiments, we intend to classify the pregnant woman from the healthy subject by using the 2-D pulse fusion features. As in TCM, the Chinese medicine practitioners were able to judge whether a woman was pregnant or not just by feeling the pulsations.

By collaborating with the fourth affiliated hospital of Harbin medical university (Harbin, Heilongjiang Province, China), we collected an experimental pulse database, including 100 wrist pulse samples of pregnant women for testing. The pregnant pulse samples were collected from the patients at the obstetrics gynecological ward. And the pregnancy durations of the patients are from 4 weeks to 36 weeks. Besides, we construct a dataset of nonpregnant women for classification. In order to reduce the influences caused by ages and health conditions, the nonpregnant samples are collected from healthy women at the ages from 20 to 35, the same as the pregnant women. And the labels of healthy status are determined according to the recent health check at the hospital. In this study, the fivefold cross-validation procedure is also developed with each fold containing 20 nonpregnant women and 20

Table 9.4 Pregnancy diagnosis result

Methods	Sensitivity (%)	Specificity (%)	Accuracy (%)
1-D fusion features	70.4	66.0	68.2
2-D fusion features	82.4	77.2	79.8

pregnant women. Table 9.4 summarizes the accuracy of the pregnancy diagnosis via the proposed pulse feature extraction method. We can see that the conventional 1-D fusion feature method just achieves the classification accuracy of 68.2%. And the accuracy is increased to 79.8% by using the proposed 2-D fusion features method. The result demonstrates that the nonperiodic feature space of the pulse contains discriminatory information between the pregnant women and the nonpregnant women. And it is a significant supplement to the conventional pulse features in pregnancy diagnosis.

9.6   Summary

The pulse feature extraction is an important stage in pulse diagnosis. As a large amount of redundant information and interferences are included in the pulses, several methodologies for extracting the useful pulse information from the database are proposed. From the time domain, the pulse characteristic points, pulse width, energies, and Gaussian models are calculated. From the frequency domain, the pulse rhythm and frequency features are extracted. Besides the conventional pulse feature extraction, we propose a 2-D matrix description for pulse signals. The pulse signal is considered as bringing two-dimensional information, periodic component and nonperiodic component. The periodic component contains the conventional pulse features and is the special case of the generalized 2-D pulse features. An experiment has been developed to test the effectiveness of the proposed 2-D pulse features. The experimental results testify that the proposed algorithm outperforms the previous conventional pulse features in diabetes diagnosis.

References

1. G. Maciocia, S. Foster, W. H. Hylton, R. Weiss, M. Tierra, H. Santillo, et al., "The foundations of Chinese medicine: A comprehensive text," London, UK: Churchill Livingstone, 2005.
2. G. Maciocia, Diagnosis in Chinese medicine: a comprehensive guide: Elsevier Health Sciences, 2013.
3. S. Lukman, Y. He, and S.-C. Hui, "Computational methods for Traditional Chinese Medicine: A survey," Computer Methods and Programs in Biomedicine, vol. 88, pp. 283–294, 12.2007.
4. J.-J. Shu and Y. Sun, "Developing classification indices for Chinese pulse diagnosis," Complementary Therapies in Medicine, vol. 15, pp. 190–198, 9, 2007.

5. S. S. Franklin, S. A. Khan, N. D. Wong, M. G. Larson, and D. Levy, "Is pulse pressure useful in predicting risk for coronary heart disease? The Framingham Heart Study," Circulation, vol. 100, pp. 354–360, 1999.
6. Y. Chen, L. Zhang, D. Zhang, and D. Zhang, "Wrist pulse signal diagnosis using modified Gaussian models and Fuzzy C-Means classification," Medical engineering & physics, vol. 31, pp. 1283–1289, 2009.
7. S. A. CARTER, "Indirect systolic pressures and pulse waves in arterial occlusive disease of the lower extremities," Circulation, vol. 37, pp. 624–637, 1968.
8. H. M. Haqqani, J. B. Morton, and J. M. Kalman, "Using the 12-Lead ECG to Localize the Origin of Atrial and Ventricular Tachycardias: Part 2—Ventricular Tachycardia," Journal of cardiovascular electrophysiology, vol. 20, pp. 825–832, 2009.
9. D. Wang, D. Zhang, and G. Lu, "A Novel Multichannel Wrist Pulse System With Different Sensor Arrays," Instrumentation and Measurement, IEEE Transactions on, vol. PP, pp. 1–1, 2015. doi: https://doi.org/10.1109/TIM.2014.2357599
10. D. Wang and D. Zhang, "Analysis of pulse waveforms preprocessing," in Computerized Healthcare (ICCH), 2012 International Conference on, 2012, pp. 175–180.
11. I. S. N. Murthy and G. Sita, "Digital models for arterial pressure and respiratory waveforms," Biomedical Engineering, IEEE Transactions on, vol. 40, pp. 717–726, 1993.
12. L. Xu, M. Q.-H. Meng, K. Wang, W. Lu, and N. Li, "Pulse images recognition using fuzzy neural network," Expert systems with applications, vol. 36, pp. 3805–3811, 2009.
13. L. Liu, N. Li, W. Zuo, D. Zhang, and H. Zhang, "Multiscale sample entropy analysis of wrist pulse blood flow signal for disease diagnosis," in Intelligent Science and Intelligent Data Engineering, Springer, 2013, pp. 475–482.
14. Y. Chen, D. Zhang, and Z. Dongyu, "Pattern Classification for Doppler Ultrasonic Wrist Pulse Signals," in Bioinformatics and Biomedical Engineering , 2009. ICBBE 2009. 3rd International Conference on, 2009, pp. 1–4.
15. Y. Chen, L. Zhang, D. Zhang, and D. Zhang, "Computerized wrist pulse signal diagnosis using modified auto-regressive models," Journal of Medical Systems, vol. 35, pp. 321–328, 2011.
16. D. Wang, D. Zhang, and G. Lu. "A robust signal preprocessing framework for wrist pulse analysis." Biomedical Signal Processing and Control, vol. 23, pp. 62–75, 2016.
17. D.-Y. Zhang, W.-M. Zuo, D. Zhang, H.-Z. Zhang, and N.-M. Li, "Wrist blood flow signal-based computerized pulse diagnosis using spatial and spectrum features," Journal of Biomedical Science and Engineering, vol. 3, p. 361, 2010.
18. Q.-L. Guo, K.-Q. Wang, D.-Y. Zhang, and N.-M. Li, "A wavelet packet based pulse waveform analysis for cholecystitis and nephrotic syndrome diagnosis," in Wavelet Analysis and Pattern Recognition, 2008. ICWAPR'08. International Conference on, 2008, pp. 513–517.
19. L. Liu, W. Zuo, D. Zhang, N. Li, and H. Zhang, "Combination of heterogeneous features for wrist pulse blood flow signal diagnosis via multiple kernel learning," Information Technology in Biomedicine, IEEE Transactions on, vol. 16, pp. 598–606, 2012.
20. L. Xu, M. Q.-H. Meng, C. Shi, K. Wang, and N. Li, "Quantitative analyses of pulse images in Traditional Chinese Medicine," Medical Acupuncture, vol. 20, pp. 175–189, 2008.
21. Y.-F. Chung, C.-S. Hu, C.-C. Yeh, and C.-H. Luo, "How to standardize the pulse-taking method of traditional Chinese medicine pulse diagnosis," Computers in Biology and Medicine, vol. 43, pp. 342–349, 5/1/ 2013.
22. L. Xu, M. Q.-H. Meng, X. Qi, and K. Wang, "Morphology variability analysis of wrist pulse waveform for assessment of arteriosclerosis status," Journal of medical systems, vol. 34, pp. 331–339, 2010.
23. S.-D. Bao, Y.-T. Zhang, and L.-F. Shen, "Physiological signal based entity authentication for body area sensor networks and mobile healthcare systems," in Engineering in Medicine and Biology Society, 2005. IEEE-EMBS 2005. 27th Annual International Conference of the, 2005, pp. 2455–2458.

Chapter 10
Characterization of Inter-Cycle Variations for Wrist Pulse Diagnosis

Abstract Although pulse signal is quasiperiodic, most feature extraction methods usually consider it as a whole or only use a single cycle, neglecting the variations between pulse cycles. To characterize both the inter- and intra-cycle variations, in this chapter we propose three feature extraction methods, i.e., simple combination, multi-scale entropy, and complex network. The simple combination method is a direct extension of conventional single-cycle feature extraction method by concatenating features from multiple cycles. The multi-scale entropy method measures the inter- and intra-cycle variations using entropies of different scales. The complex network method transforms the pulse signal from time domain to network domain and measures the inter-cycle variations using the statistical properties on complex network. Experimental results show that the presented features are effective in characterizing both inter- and intra-cycle variations and can obtain better performance in pulse diagnosis.

10.1 Introduction

Diagnosis has played an important role in oriental medicine for thousands of years [1–3]. Generally, wrist pulse signal is produced by cardiac contraction, but also affected by the characteristics of blood and the vessel, making it effective in analyzing both cardiac and non-cardiac diseases [1]. However, traditional pulse diagnosis is a subjective skill which needs years of training and practice to master and the diagnosis result relies on the personal experience of the practitioner [4]. For different practitioners, the diagnosis results may be inconsistent. To overcome these limitations, computational pulse diagnosis has recently been studied to make pulse diagnosis objective and quantitative, and researchers have verified the connections of pulse signal with several certain diseases, e.g., pancreatitis, diabetes, appendicitis, duodenal bulb ulcer, cholecystitis, and nephritis [5–14].

Computational pulse diagnosis usually involves four modules, i.e., acquisition, preprocessing, feature extraction, and classification. The acquisition module is used to collect pulse samples. A lot of systems have been proposed to collect the pulse signal from the patient's wrist, where pressure, photoelectric, and Doppler ultrasound

© Springer Nature Singapore Pte Ltd. 2018
D. Zhang et al., *Computational Pulse Signal Analysis*,
https://doi.org/10.1007/978-981-10-4044-3_10

sensors are the most common sensors used in these systems [14–16]. The aim of the preprocessing module is to remove some artifact in the collected sample such as noise and baseline drift, increasing the accuracy and stability of subsequent feature extraction and classification [17–19]. Sometimes the segmentation is also included in the preprocessing module [20, 21]. The feature extraction module extracts discriminative feature from the pulse signal [5, 22]. The classification module generates a model to classify the pulse signal into different health conditions [9–11].

Among the four modules of computational pulse diagnosis, feature extraction plays a critical role and has received increasing research interests. By far, a number of feature extraction methods have been proposed, which can be roughly grouped into two subcategories: single cycle-based and whole signal-based ones. Single cycle-based methods [8, 10–13, 23–27] extract the features from each single cycle, while whole signal-based methods [5, 6, 22, 28–38] extract the features directly from the whole signal.

Typical single cycle-based method aims to characterize the properties of single cycle in pulse signal. It usually needs the segmentation step in preprocess to get each pulse cycle. To extend it for feature representation of the whole pulse signal, one natural strategy is to use the average over different cycles [39]. Fiducial point-based features [11, 13, 23–25, 27], model fitting features [10, 26], and elastic distance features [8, 40] are three popular single cycle-based features. Fiducial point-based features were inspired by traditional Chinese medicine which measures the position of some key points within a pulse cycle like the peaks and valleys, their amplitude ratios, the period, the area under the cycle, and so on. Model fitting features were extracted using some model, e.g., Gaussian mixture model, to fit the single pulse cycle and extract the fitting parameters as features. Elastic distances were also applied on single pulse cycle, such as dynamic time warping and time warping edit distance.

Whole signal-based feature extraction methods usually do not need the segmentation and extract the features to characterize the property of the whole signal. The most popular whole signal-based feature extraction methods are those transform-based methods which transform the pulse signal to the transform domain such as frequency domain or wavelet domain and extract the coefficients or other statistics, e.g., Fourier frequency spectrum features, Hilbert-Huang transform features, wavelet features, and wavelet packet features [6, 28–33]. Besides the transform-based methods, the entropy features, auto-regressive features, Lyapunov exponents features, PCA features, ICA features, and some other features were also usually applied on the whole pulse signal [5, 34–38]. It should be noted that most whole signal-based methods can also be used for feature extraction from single cycle, e.g., the entropy feature in [34], and some single cycle-based methods can also be applied to the whole signal, e.g., the elastic distance-based method in [12].

Note that pulse signal is quasiperiodic. However, both single cycle-based and whole signal-based methods are limited in characterizing the inter-cycle variations of pulse signal. The single cycle-based features usually are capable of characterizing the variations within the pulse cycle. The variations between different pulse cycles cannot be characterized. The whole signal-based features can characterize the overall property of the pulse signal, thus can both characterize the intra-cycle variations and inter-cycle variations to some extent, but we cannot distinguish the intra-cycle features from inter-cycle features. The inter-cycle variations play more crucial role in the diagnosis of some diseases like arrhythmia, while intra-cycle variations play more crucial role in the diagnosis of some diseases like diabetes. Thus, separation of inter- and intra-cycle variations would allow us design disease-specific classification methods, resulting in improved diagnosis accuracy.

In traditional Chinese medicine (TCM), pulse signal was analyzed from different aspects such as the rate, rhythm, depth, length, width, arterial tension, pulse force, pulse occlusion, and pulse contour [1], where some of them are appropriate to be characterized using the intra-cycle variations, while the others should be attributed to the inter-cycle variations. Thus, it is important to develop novel methods to extract the features for characterizing both intra- and inter-cycle variations of pulse signal.

In this chapter we focus on the characterization of the intra- and inter-cycle variations of pulse signal. Three inter-cycle variations sensitive methods are introduced in this work, i.e., the simple combination method, the multi-scale entropy method, and the complex network method. The simple combination method uses single cycle-based method to extract intra-cycle features and simply concatenates features from multiple cycles to describe the inter-cycle variations. The multi-scale entropy method measures the intra-cycle variations and inter-cycle variations from the entropies with series of scales. Complex network method transforms the pulse signal from time domain to network domain and measures the inter-cycle variations via the organization of the network. Moreover, in the complex network method, fiducial point features are also adopted to characterize the intra-cycle variations. With these studies, we intend to introduce some new features for inter-cycle feature extraction and to validate the importance of the inter-cycle variations for pulse diagnosis.

The remainder of the chapter is organized as follows. Section 10.2 introduces the quasi-property of the pulse signal. Section 10.3 provides the detailed description of the three inter-cycle variation sensitive feature extraction methods. Section 10.4 provides the experimental results to demonstrate the effectiveness of these features in pulse diagnosis. Finally, Sect. 10.5 gives several concluding remarks.

10.2   The Quasiperiodic Pulse Signals

As a quasiperiodic signal, pulse signal is composed of multiple pulse cycles, but the pulse cycles are not completely the same. Figure 10.1 shows an example of two pulse signals. One can see that each pulse signals contains a set of pulse cycles. For clarity we mark these pulse cycles as C_1, C_2, C_3, etc. Figure 10.1a is a healthy person; these pulse cycles are similar but different to each other, e.g., the position of C_9's main peak is relatively higher than those of the other cycles and the secondary peak of C_1 is higher than those of the other cycles. For person with disease such as arrhythmias,

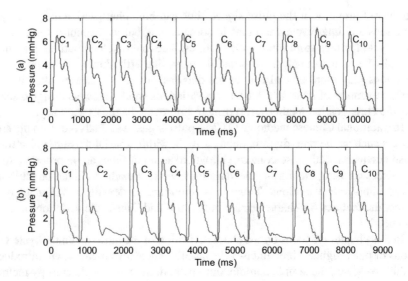

Fig. 10.1 Quasiperiodic pulse signals. (**a**) Healthy person. (**b**) Arrhythmia patient

the difference will be even obvious, as shown in Fig. 10.1b. One can see the periods of C_2 and C_7 in Fig. 10.1b are clearly longer than those of the other circles.

The quasiperiodic property of pulse signal should be attributed to two major reasons. First, the pulse signal is generated by cardiac contraction and relaxation. The heart rhythm is not completely periodic, and some diseases, e.g., arrhythmias, may further increase the nonperiodic property of heartbeat. Second, the arterial system is a complex nonlinear anisotropic and viscoelastic system including tapered, curved, and branching tubes, which can further decrease the periodic property of pulse signal.

10.3   Characterization of Inter-Cycle Variations

In this section we provide three methods to characterize the inter-cycle variations of pulse signal, i.e., the simple combination method, the multi-scale entropy method, and the complex network method. First, we introduce the preprocessing method and the single cycle-based feature extraction. Then, we describe the three feature extraction methods.

10.3.1   Preprocessing

The sampled pulse signal usually contains high-frequency noise and suffers from baseline drift caused by breathing and body movement. Moreover, for the segmentation-dependent feature extraction, segmentation of pulse cycles usually is

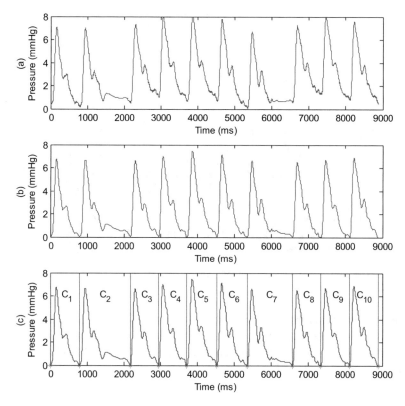

Fig. 10.2 Preprocessing of pulse signal. (**a**) Signal before preprocessing, (**b**) signal after preprocessing, and (**c**) segmentation of pulse cycles

required. In the following, we introduce the preprocessing method for denoising, baseline drift removal, and segmentation.

We use wavelet denoising to remove the high-frequency noise and use CAF [41] to remove the baseline drift. Then, we segment the pulse signal into pulse cycles according to the local maximum and the local minimum of the pulse signal. Figure 10.2 shows the preprocessing result of a pulse signal. Figure 10.2a shows the original sampled pulse signal which contains noise and baseline drift. After denoising and baseline drift removal, the quality of the pulse signal can be improved, as shown in Fig. 10.2b. Figure 10.2c shows the segmented pulse signal, where the red star denotes the start point of each cycle.

10.3.2   The Simple Combination Method

In this subsection we introduce the simple combination method to enhance the capacity of single-cycle feature extraction method in characterizing inter-cycle variations. Here we use fiducial point-based method as an example and extend it to the simple combination method.

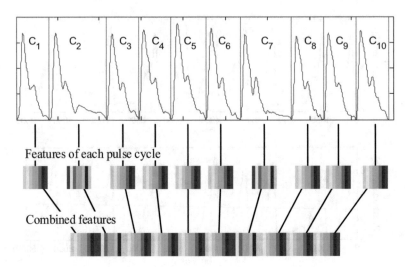

Fig. 10.3 The simple combination method: combination of features according to the original sequence

Features extracted from single pulse cycle such as fiducial point-based features only reflect the intra-cycle properties but fail to describe the inter-cycle variations. One natural solution is to extract single-cycle features from each cycle and concatenate all these features to form a feature vector, as shown in Fig. 10.3. The combined feature vector contains information from every pulse cycle and thus can describe the inter-cycle variations.

When using the simple combination method, the combination sequence may affect the diagnosis performance. The combination according to the original sequence may not be the optimal choice for disease diagnosis. Figure 10.4 shows three pulse signals: signal in Fig. 10.4a follows the pattern "ABB," signal in Fig. 10.4b is time shift of signal in Fig. 10.4a, and signal in Fig. 10.4c follows the pattern "AAB." Obviously the distance between signals in Fig. 10.4a, b should be smaller than signals in Fig. 10.4a, c. However, if we combine the fiducial point features according to their original sequence, assuming that the distance between feature vector of cycle A and cycle B is 1, the Euclidean distance between signals in Fig. 10.4a, b is $\sqrt{7}$, while the Euclidean distance between signals in Fig. 10.4a, c is $\sqrt{3}$. One can see that the distance between signals in Fig. 10.4a, c is smaller than that between signal in Fig. 10.4a and its time shift. Thus, the combination according to the original sequence is not robust against the time shift.

To avoid this, one can use the average of features over different cycles to form a feature vector. However, the average feature vector loses too much information about the distribution of the features and usually cannot outperform the single cycle-based method.

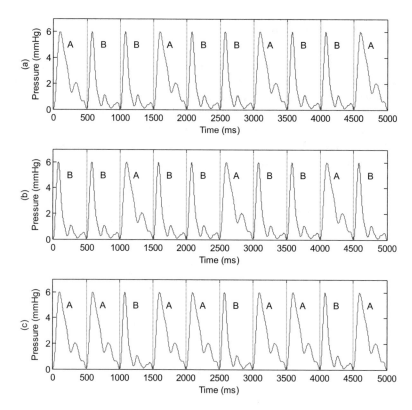

Fig. 10.4 The sequence problem. (**a**) A pulse signal that follows the "ABB" pattern, (**b**) time shift of signal (**a**), and (**c**) a pulse signal that follows the "AAB" pattern

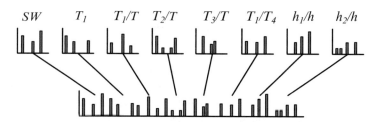

Fig. 10.5 The simple combination method: combination of histograms

To preserve the feature distribution information and to reduce the influence of the sequence, we combine the histogram of each feature instead of directly combining features from each pulse cycle. For example, for the eight fiducial point-based features, we calculate the histogram of each feature and combine the eight histograms to form the final features, as shown in Fig. 10.5.

10.3.3   Multi-scale Entropy

In this subsection we introduce the multi-scale entropy method to characterize both inter-cycle variations and intra-cycle variations. Sample entropy is a whole signal-based feature which reflects the overall unpredictability of the pulse signal, and by extracting the sample entropy from multiple scales, we further distinguish the intra-cycle features from inter-cycle features to some extent.

For a pulse signal $X = [x_1, x_2, \ldots x_N]$and a fixed window size m, we can form a sequence of vectors $X_m(1)$, $X_m(2)$,..., $X_m(N-m + 1)$, where $X_m(i) = [x_i, x_{i + 1}, \ldots, x_{i + m-1}]$. We define:

$$B_i^m(r) = \frac{\text{num}\left(d\left[X_m(i), X_m(j)\right] < r\right)}{N - m + 1} \quad j = 1, 2 \ldots N - m, j \neq i, \qquad (10.1)$$

$$B^m(r) = \frac{1}{N - m} \sum_{i=1}^{N-m} \ln\left(B_i^m(r)\right), \qquad (10.2)$$

$$A_i^m(r) = \frac{\text{num}\left(d\left[X_{m+1}(i), X_{m+1}(j)\right] < r\right)}{N - m + 1} \quad j = 1, 2 \ldots N - m, j \neq i, \qquad (10.3)$$

$$A^m(r) = \frac{1}{N - m} \sum_{i=1}^{N-m} \ln\left(A_i^m(r)\right), \qquad (10.4)$$

where r is the threshold and is the Chebyshev distance of $X(i)$ and $X(j)$. Sample entropy is defined as [42]:

$$\text{SampEn}(m,,r,,N) = -\log \frac{A^m(r)}{B^m(r)}. \qquad (10.5)$$

In most articles, the values of the parameters used to calculate sample entropy or approximate entropy are $m = 2$ and r is 0.15 times standard derivation of the signal [42, 43], and then the sample entropy will not depend on the variance of the amplitude of the pulse signal. In this work m is also set to 2, and since the pulse signal was normalized before the calculation of sample entropy, r is set to 0.15 directly.

Sample entropy measures the complexity and regularity of time series data and is reported effective in the study of experimental clinical cardiovascular and other biological time series [35, 42, 44]. However, from the definition of entropy, one can see that it is hard to distinguish the intra-cycle features from inter-cycle features using sample entropy. For example, the sample entropy of signal in Fig. 10.6a, b is almost the same; however it is obvious that both intra- and inter-cycle differences exist between Fig. 10.6a, b.

To alleviate this limitation, one can use multi-scale entropy to reveal unpredictability with long-range correlations on multiple spatial and temporal scales [45, 46].

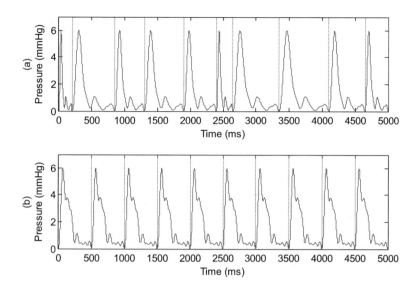

Fig. 10.6 Pulse signal with similar sample entropy

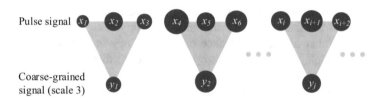

Fig. 10.7 Coarse-graining process

In multi-scale entropy method, multiple pulse signals in different scales were generated from one pulse signal by "coarse-graining" process using a series of scale factors. For a scale factor k, the pulse signal was divided into N/k non-overlapping groups, and each group contains k samples. The coarse-graining process averaged the data points within these groups and formed a coarse-grained signal with scale factor k. The element of the coarse-grained time series is calculated as [47]:

$$y_j(k) = \frac{1}{k} \sum_{i=k(j-1)+1}^{jk} x_i. \qquad (10.6)$$

Figure 10.7 is an example of coarse-graining process with scale factor $k = 3$ and $y_j(3) = \frac{x_i + x_{i+1} + x_{i+2}}{3}$, where $i = 3j-2$.

By applying the coarse-graining process using a series of scale factors, multiple pulse signals in different scales were generated from the pulse signal, and then we can extract the entropy feature in different scales. The entropy of this pulse signal in

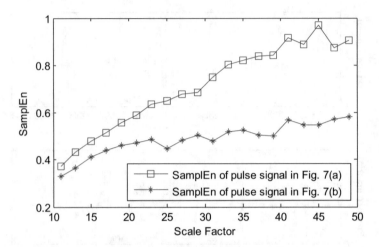

Fig. 10.8 Multi-scale entropy of pulse signals in Fig. 10.6

different scales can reveal the unpredictability with different spatial and temporal scales.

Figure 10.8 is the multi-scale sample entropy of signal in Fig. 10.6. One can see that when the scale factor is small, the sample entropy of signal in Fig. 10.6a, b is close to each other and the difference of their entropy increases with the scale. Therefore, multiple scale sample entropy is helpful to distinguish the intra-cycle features from inter-cycle features.

In the experiment of pulse signal analysis, we noted that the SampEn can reveal the unpredictability from both intra- and inter-cycle variations of pulse signal; what's more SampEn with smaller scales reflected more the intra-cycle variations, and with the increase of scale, the fraction of the inter-cycle variations will increase. Figure 10.9 shows three pulse signals, signals in Fig. 10.9a, b have almost the same pulse cycles except the cycle length, and thus signals in Fig. 10.9a, b only have inter-cycle difference. Signals in Fig. 10.9a, c are both periodic signal, and thus signals in Fig. 10.9a, c don't have inter-cycle differences, and they only have intra-cycle differences.

Figure 10.10 shows the multi-scale sample entropy of signals in Fig. 10.9. One can see that the entropy of signals in Fig. 10.9a, b is similar in small scales and the difference of their entropy increases with the scale. Since signals in Fig. 10.9a, b only have inter-cycle difference, the difference of their sample entropy with large scale is because of the inter-cycle difference. They have similar entropy with small scale because they have similar pulse cycles. Therefore, we believe that the sample entropy with small scale reflected more about the intra-cycle variations and the sample entropy with large scale is helpful in describing the inter-cycle variations of pulse signals. For the multi-scale entropy of Fig. 10.9a, c, one can see that with the small scale the difference of their entropy is relatively large and with the growth of the scale the difference of their entropy diminished, which also demonstrate the same conclusion because Fig. 10.9a, c doesn't have inter-cycle variations, but they are different in intra-cycles.

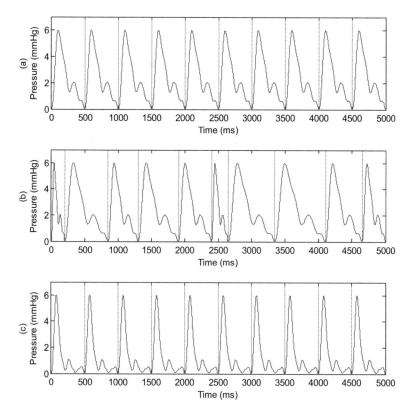

Fig. 10.9 Pulse signals with only intra-cycle variations or intra-cycle variations

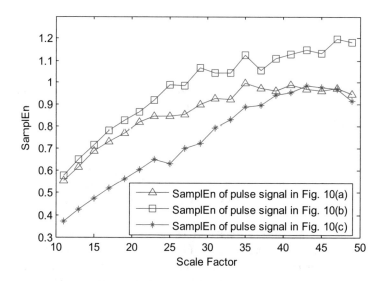

Fig. 10.10 Multi-scale entropy of pulse signals in Fig. 10.9

10.3.4   The Complex Network Method

In this subsection we introduce the complex network method to characterize inter-cycle variations directly. By transforming the pulse signal from time domain to network domain, we analyze the pulse signal via the structure of the network.

Complex networks describe a wide range of systems in nature and society such as cells and the Internet. In the earlier research, Zhang and Small [48] proposed a method to explore the dynamics of quasiperiodic time series via complex network. Representing the time series through the corresponding complex network can transform time series from the time domain to the network domain, which allows the dynamics of the time series to be studied via structure of the network. The property of network structure can be quantified by a number of topological statistics, and these statistics can provide new information about the phase space geometry of pulse cycles within a long pulse signal. Thus it would be an effective way to describe the relationship between different pulse cycles.

Construction of the Complex Network A network is composed by vertexes and edges. We hope the network should describe the connections between different pulse cycles; therefore we use the pulse cycles as vertexes of the network. To add the connections between vertexes (edges), we use a metric which can measure the similarity between pulse cycles to decide whether there is an edge. Considering the continuity and smoothness of pulse cycles, two similar pulse cycles should be close in phase space, and thus we can use phase space distance as the distance between two pulse cycles. We denote D_{ij} as the distance of two pulse cycles C_i and C_j in time domain, and D_{ij} can be calculated using their phase space distance:

$$D_{ij} = \min_{l=0,1,...\#l_j - l\#} \frac{1}{\min\left(l_j, l_i\right)} \sum_{k=1}^{\min\left(l_j, l_i\right)} X_k - Y_{k+l}, \tag{10.7}$$

where X_k and Y_k is the kth point of C_i and C_j and l_i and l_j are the lengths of C_i and C_j.

The correlation coefficient is another metric of the similarity between pulse cycle C_i and C_j. The larger the coefficient, the higher level of similarity, and thus we can also use the correlation coefficient as the distance between pulse cycle C_i and C_j in time domain, where D_{ij} can be calculated by:

$$D_{ij} = \max_{l=0,1,...,l_j - l_i} \frac{\text{cov}\left[C_i\left(1:l_i\right), C_j\left(1+l:l_i+l\right)\right]}{\sqrt{V\left[C_i\left(1:l_i\right)\right]}\sqrt{V\left[C_j\left(1+l:l_i+l\right)\right]}}. \tag{10.8}$$

Both the phase space distance and correlation coefficient can be used to measure the similarity between two pulse cycles [49]. In this work we use the correlation coefficient as the metric of the distance because it is more robust to noise. After we have the vertexes and the distance metric, we can construct the network. The network can either be constructed to a weighted network or a binary network. To get a weighted network, we can apply a fully connected network on these vertexes, and then use the distance as the weight of the edges. To get a binary network, we first get a weighted network, and then we set a threshold on these weights. If the weights are smaller (or larger if we use phase space distance) than the threshold, we remove the corresponding edges from the fully connected network to get a binary network.

For simplicity we use the binary network. Figure 10.11 shows networks constructed from the example pulse signal in Fig. 10.2 with different thresholds. From Fig. 10.11 one can see that the threshold is a very important parameter when constructing binary network. It will greatly change the shape of the network. The larger the threshold, the network will have fewer edges because larger threshold removes

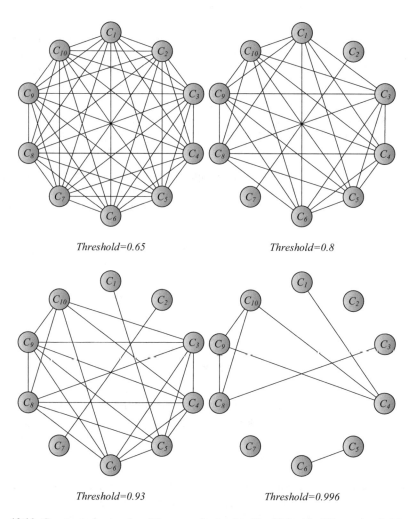

Fig. 10.11 Constructed networks of the example signal in Fig. 10.2 with different threshold

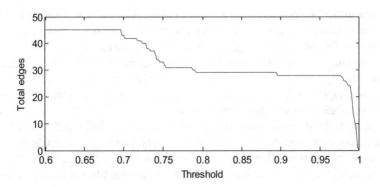

Fig. 10.12 Total edges variance with threshold

more edges from the fully connected networks. For the signal in Fig. 10.2, if the threshold is smaller than 0.69, the network will be a fully connected network (45 edges). If the threshold increases to 0.996, the network will only have eight edges. If the threshold is one, no edges will appear in the constructed network. Figure 10.12 shows the edge numbers of networks obtained with different thresholds. The choice of threshold would also affect the diagnosis performance. In this work a number of thresholds were tested, and the threshold with best diagnosis performance was used. One can also use some optimization algorithm to find the optimal threshold.

The Statistics of the Network After constructing the complex network, some basic statistical properties [50] of the network were investigated to characterize the connection between pulse cycles, including the degree of each node, the average path length, and the clustering coefficient.

The degree of a pulse cycle is the number of edges incident to the vertex. For any vertex i, its degree deg_i describes the similarity of the pulse cycle with the other ones.

The average path length is the average shortest distance between all pairs of pulse cycles. The average path length is defined as:

$$L = \frac{1}{\frac{1}{2}N(N-1)}\sum_{i>j}d_{ij},$$
(10.9)

where N is the number of pulse cycles and d_{ij} is the shortest distance between pulse cycle C_i and C_j in the network domain (different with D_{ij} which is the distance in time domain). For binary network the distance d_{ij} is equal to the minimum number of edges necessary to connect C_i and C_j. It is a measure of the efficiency of the network.

The clustering coefficient is the fraction of edges between the topological neighbors of a vertex with respect to the maximum possible edges. Suppose a vertex i has k_i neighbors, then at most $k_i(k_i-1)/2$ edges can exist between them when every neighbors are connected with each other. Let E_i denote the edges really exist, and the clustering coefficient is defined as:

$$C_i = \frac{2E_i}{k_i(k_i - 1)}. \tag{10.10}$$

The clustering coefficient is a measure of degree to which pulse cycles in a pulse signal tend to cluster together.

The Sequence Problem Except the average path length, the other two kinds of features are connected with the vertexes. Similar to the simple combination method, the sequence of the vertexes used to construct the feature vector may influence the disease diagnosis performance. Actually it is a common problem when using multiple segmentation-dependent features to characterize the inter-cycle variations.

We can use the similar strategy as we do in the simple combination method, i.e., using the averaged statistics or using the histogram method.

If we use the averaged statistics, we can use the averaged degree and the global clustering coefficient. The global clustering coefficient C is the average of C_i over all pulse cycle i. It can also be calculated in a more graphic formulation [51]:

$$C = \frac{3 \times \text{number of triangles}}{\text{number of connected triples}}, \tag{10.11}$$

where triangles are trios of vertexes in which each vertex is connected to both of the others, and connected triples are trios in which at least one is connected to both others, the factor 3 accounting for the fact that each triangle contributes to three connected triples.

We can also use histogram which can preserve the distribution information of these statics features. For the degree of the vertexes, we use a series of sorted degree intervals (bins) to form a degree histogram, and for the clustering coefficient, we can also form a clustering coefficient histogram. Moreover, for the average path length, we can also extend it to distance histogram to describe the distribution of the shortest distance between vertexes. Then, the degree histogram, clustering coefficient histogram, and distance histogram are used as the complex network features.

Including Single-Cycle Features to the Complex Network Method Besides the correlation coefficient and the phase space distance, we can also use the Euclidian distance of some single-cycle features as the distance between pulse cycles. For example, we can use Euclidian distance of fiducial point features as the distance between different pulse cycles and extend fiducial point feature into network domain by creating a fiducial point network. The fiducial point network can characterize the variations of these key points between pulse cycles. Using complex network method, we can extend some single-cycle features to network domain. Similar to the simple combination method, the complex network method is another way to extend the single-cycle features' capacity to characterize the inter-cycle variations.

Joint Features The simple combination method and multi-scale entropy can be used to describe both the intra-cycle features and inter-cycle features. The simple combination method contains the feature from each pulse cycle; therefore it can describe the intra-cycle features. The multi-scale entropy contains the entropy of small scale which can also describe the intra-cycle information. While the complex network method is mainly designed for the measure of the inter-cycle variations, it is limited in measuring the intra-cycle information. Thus we should add some intra-cycle features when using the network method to obtain higher diagnosis performance. In this chapter we use the fiducial point features of an averaged cycle together with the network method to enhance the capability of describing the intra-cycle features.

10.4   Experimental Results

In this section, using two diseases, i.e., arrhythmia and diabetes, we present case studies to evaluate the diagnosis performance of the presented feature extraction methods.

The definition of arrhythmia is any of a group of conditions in which the electrical activity of the heart is irregular, faster or slower than normal [52]. In this chapter, arrhythmia only refers to irregular heartbeat because it closely tied to inter-cycle variations. Thus the inter-cycle features are expected to be effective in arrhythmia diagnosis problem.

Except arrhythmia, we also consider another disease, i.e., diabetes, whose connection with inter-cycle variations is less direct. We use diabetes diagnosis problem to validate if the inter-cycle variations have contributions to the diagnosis performance of disease without obvious connection with inter-cycle variations.

10.4.1   Datasets

By collaborating with Hong Kong Yao Chung Kit Diabetes Assessment Centre and Harbin Binghua Hospital, we construct a dataset of 475 volunteers, including 71 volunteers with arrhythmia, 200 healthy volunteers, and 205 volunteers with diabetes. To avoid the imbalance of the dataset, we randomly select a subset from healthy dataset and diabetes dataset in the arrhythmia disease diagnosis experiment. To avoid the potential influence of biological factors, we also ensure that the distributions of gender and age of volunteers with diabetes or arrhythmia are similar with those of healthy volunteers. Table 10.1 lists a summary of the dataset used in arrhythmia and diabetes diagnosis experiment.

Table 10.1 Summary of datasets

		Age distribution				Gender distribution	
		1~40	40~50	50~60	>60	Male	Female
H/A	H	10	34	21	15	40	40
	A	9	29	19	14	33	38
H/D	H	10	40	71	79	128	72
	D	5	36	68	96	134	71
H/A/D	H	10	34	21	15	40	40
	A	9	29	19	14	33	38
	D	5	36	23	16	41	39

10.4.2 Experiments and Results

In the experiment the simple combination method, multi-scale entropy, and the complex network method are tested on the dataset. Moreover, we also compare these three methods with other feature extraction methods, i.e., Hilbert-Huang transform (HHT), wavelet transform, and fiducial point-based method.

The wavelet method, HHT method, and multi-scale entropy method are whole signal-based feature extraction methods and do not need segmentation. The fiducial point method, the simple combination method, and the complex network method need segmentation before feature extraction.

For the simple combination method, we use fiducial point features as an example and extend it to simple combination framework. For the complex network method, we use network statistics features together with fiducial point features of the average pulse cycle. Moreover, we also extend fiducial point method to the complex network method in the experiment.

Figure 10.13 shows three typical signals with different healthy conditions in the dataset. Figure 10.13a is a typical healthy pulse signal, Fig. 10.13b is a typical arrhythmia pulse signal, and Fig. 10.13c is a typical diabetes pulse signal. In Fig. 10.13, the first column is the signal, the second column is their corresponding complex network under threshold 0.93, and the last column is their average cycle.

One can see that the network is effective in describing the inter-cycle variations and the network structure of the arrhythmia sample is clearly different to the others. The adding of the averaged cycle-based features can further enhance the capability of describing the intra-cycle variations between healthy sample and diabetes sample.

Based on these features, we use the support vector machine (SVM) for classification [53]. The results of arrhythmia experiment using different features are shown in the first column of Table 10.2. For the complex network method, a series of threshold was tested, and the threshold with best classification accuracy was used as the final threshold. Figure 10.14 shows the classification accuracy and the corresponding threshold tested in the arrhythmia experiment. One can see that at first the accuracy increases with the growth of the threshold, and when the threshold is close to

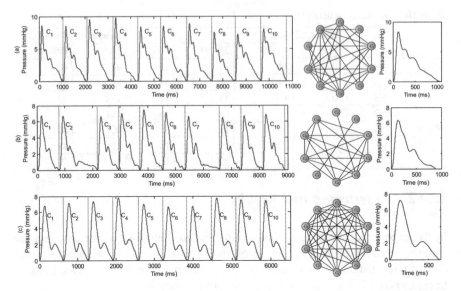

Fig. 10.13 Typical signals of different healthy conditions, their mean cycle and complex network under threshold 0.93. (**a**) Typical healthy signal. (**b**) Typical arrhythmia signal. (**c**) Typical diabetes signal

Table 10.2 Arrhythmia and diabetics diagnosis performance

	H/A	H/D	H/A/D
Wavelet	70.9%	71.6%	51.5%
HHT	77.5%	75.3%	56.3%
Fiducial point	51.7%	69.6%	41.1%
Fiducial point[a]	86.8%	76.7%	62.3%
Fiducial point[b]	85.4%	76.0%	64.5%
Multi-scale entropy	88.7%	84.0%	71.9%
Complex network	92.1%	84.4%	72.3%

Fiducial point[a] Fiducial point method extended to simple combination method
Fiducial point[b] Fiducial point method extended to complex network method
H healthy, *A* arrhythmia, *D* diabetes

1, the accuracy drops dramatically. In the arrhythmia experiment, we chose the 0.865 as the final threshold, and the best accuracy is 92.1%.

Note that the threshold would greatly change the shape of the network. Using a small threshold will get a network with more edges and using a large threshold will get a network with less edges. The accuracy with threshold below 0.6 is very low because when the threshold is very small, nearly all of the pulse signal was transformed to a fully connected network, and thus this network is very similar to each other. With the growth of the threshold, some edges were removed from this network, and the network of pulse signal sampled from different volunteers becomes different in organization. Gradually, the network can characterize the inter-cycle

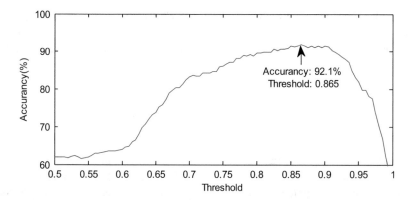

Fig. 10.14 Performance with different threshold in diabetes experiment

variations of the pulse signal, and the accuracy grows up. When the threshold becomes too large, more and more edges were removed, only a few edges were left in the network, the network no longer has the capability to characterize inter-cycle variations of pulse signals, and the classification performance starts falling.

In arrhythmia diagnosis experiment, the multi-scale entropy features, complex network features, and two extensions of point features get better performance than other features. This may be because irregular heartbeats result in the variations between pulse cycles; therefore features which may describe the inter-cycle variations can reveal this change and achieve relatively higher performance. The fiducial point method applied on single pulse cycle has the lowest performance which may result in single-cycle feature extraction methods that are not capable of describing the inter-cycle variations. After extending the fiducial point feature to the simple combination method and the complex network method, the increased diagnosis performance can be obtained.

Wavelet and HHT can obtain higher classification rates than fiducial point feature in arrhythmia diagnosis. These methods were not designed to describe the difference between pulse cycles, but these methods use the long pulse signal as a whole, and the inter-cycle variations may also result in some changes in the whole pulse signal; thus these methods can be characterized by the inter-cycle variations to some extent.

The diagnosis performance of diabetes is shown in the second column of Table 10.2. From the result one can see that the multi-scale entropy feature and complex network feature also get better performance than other features. For the fiducial point feature after extending it to simple combination method and complex network method, increased performance was obtained which means in the diabetes experiment, the inter-cycle variations also have contributions to the diagnosis performance. Since the diabetes is not closely connected with inter-cycle variations as arrhythmia, the performance improvement of the two extensions of fiducial point feature in diabetes diagnosis is not as much as that in arrhythmia diagnosis experiment.

We also give the multi-class diagnosis performance in the third column of Table 10.2. One can see that in the multi-class experiment, features which can characterize both the intra- and inter-cycle variations also achieve higher accuracy than the others.

10.5 Summary

In this chapter, we propose three feature extraction methods to utilize the inter-cycle variations of pulse signal for disease diagnosis, i.e., the simple combination method, the multi-scale entropy method, and the complex network method. The simple combination method extends the fiducial point-based method and combines the histograms from individual single-cycle features to characterize the inter-cycle variations. The multi-scale entropy method measures the inter- and intra-cycle variations by measuring the unpredictability of the pulse signal in different scale, and we pointed out that sample entropy with small scale reflected more about the intra-cycle variations and the sample entropy with large scale reflected more about the inter-cycle variations of pulse signals. The complex network method transforms the pulse signal from time domain to network domain and analyzes the inter-cycle variations based on the statistics of the network structure.

By taking both inter- and intra-cycle variations into account, the proposed methods achieve higher classification accuracy than the competing methods, and among the three proposed methods, complex network is more effective. The experimental results show that the inclusion of inter-cycle features can not only significantly improve some diseases closely related with heart rhythm, e.g., arrhythmia, but also can benefit the diagnosis of some diseases without obvious connections with inter-cycle variations, e.g., diabetes.

References

1. S. Walsh and E. King, Pulse Diagnosis: A Clinical Guide. Sydney Australia: Elsevier, 2008.
2. V. D. Lad, Secrets of the Pulse. Albuquerque, New Mexico: The Ayurvedic Press, 1996.
3. E. Hsu, Pulse Diagnosis in Early Chinese Medicine. New York, American: Cambridge University Press, 2010.
4. R. Amber and B. Brooke, Pulse Diagnosis Detailed Interpretations For Eastern & Western Holistic Treatments. Santa Fe, New Mexico: Aurora Press, 1993.
5. Y. Chen, L. Zhang, D. Zhang, and D. Zhang, "Computerized wrist pulse signal diagnosis using modified auto-regressive models," Journal of Medical Systems, vol. 35, pp. 321–328, Jun 2011.
6. Q. Guo, K. Wang, D. Zhang, and N. Li, "A wavelet packet based pulse waveform analysis for cholecystitis and nephrotic syndrome diagnosis," in IEEE International Conference on Wavelet Analysis and Pattern Recognition, Hong Kong, China, 2008, pp. 513–517.

7. S. Charbonnier, S. Galichet, G. Mauris, and J. P. Siche, "Statistical and fuzzy models of ambulatory systolic blood pressure for hypertension diagnosis," IEEE Transactions on Instrumentation and Measurement, vol. 49, pp. 998–1003, 2000.

8. D. Zhang, W. Zuo, D. Zhang, H. Zhang, and N. Li, "Classification of pulse waveforms using edit distance with real penalty," EURASIP Journal on Advances in Signal Processing, vol. 2010, p. 28, 2010.

9. L. Liu, W. Zuo, D. Zhang, and D. Zhang, "Learning with multiple Gaussian distance kernels for time series classification " in IEEE International Conference on Advanced Computer Control, Harbin,China, 2011, pp. pp.624–628.

10. Y. Chen, L. Zhang, D. Zhang, and D. Zhang, "Wrist pulse signal diagnosis using modified Gaussian Models and Fuzzy C-Means classification," Medical Engineering & Physics, vol. 31, pp. 1283–1289, Dec 2009.

11. L. Liu, W. Zuo, D. Zhang, N. Li, and H. Zhang, "Combination of heterogeneous features for wrist pulse blood flow signal diagnosis via multiple kernel learning," IEEE Transactions on Information Technology in Biomedicine, vol. 16, pp. 599–607, Jul 2012.

12. L. Liu, W. Zuo, D. Zhang, N. Li, and H. Zhang, "Classification of wrist pulse blood flow signal using time warp edit distance," Medical Biometrics, vol. 6165, pp. 137–144, 2010.

13. D. Zhang, W. Zuo, D. Zhang, H. Zhang, and N. Li, "Wrist blood flow signal-based computerized pulse diagnosis using spatial and spectrum features," Journal of Biomedical Science and Engineering, vol. 3, pp. 361–366, 2010.

14. H.-T. Wu, C.-H. Lee, C.-K. Sun, J.-T. Hsu, R.-M. Huang, and C.-J. Tang, "Arterial Waveforms Measured at the Wrist as Indicators of Diabetic Endothelial Dysfunction in the Elderly," IEEE Transactions on Instrumentation and Measurement, vol. 61, pp. 162–169, 2012.

15. C. C. Tyan, S. H. Liu, J. Y. Chen, J. J. Chen, and W. M. Liang, "A novel noninvasive measurement technique for analyzing the pressure pulse waveform of the radial artery," IEEE Transactions on Biomedical Engineering, vol. 55, pp. 288–297, Jan 2008.

16. P. Wang, W. Zuo, and D. Zhang, "A Compound Pressure Signal Acquisition System for Multichannel Wrist Pulse Signal Analysis," Instrumentation and Measurement, IEEE Transactions on, vol. PP, pp. 1–1, 2014.

17. L. Xu, D. Zhang, and K.Wang, "Wavelet-based cascaded adaptive filter for removing baseline drift in pulse waveforms," Biomedical Engineering, IEEE Transactions on, vol. 52, pp. 1973–1975, 2005.

18. D. Wang and D. Zhang, "Analysis of pulse waveforms preprocessing," in Computerized Healthcare (ICCH), 2012 International Conference on, 2012, pp. 175–180.

19. H. Wang, X. Wang, J. R. Deller, and J. Fu, "A Shape-Preserving Preprocessing for Human Pulse Signals Based on Adaptive Parameter Determination," IEEE Transactions on Biomedical Circuits and Systems, vol. PP, pp. 1–1, 2013.

20. C. Xia, Y. Li, J. Yan, et al., "A Practical Approach to Wrist Pulse Segmentation and Single-period Average Waveform Estimation," in IEEE International Conference on BioMedical Engineering and Informatics 2008, pp. 334–338.

21. W. Karlen, J. M. Ansermino, and G. Dumont, "Adaptive pulse segmentation and artifact detection in photoplethysmography for mobile applications," in IEEE International Conference of the Engineering in Medicine and Biology Society, 2012, pp. 3131–3134.

22. D. Zhang, D. Zhang, L. Zhang, and Y. Zheng, "Wavelet Based Analysis of Doppler Ultrasonic Wrist-pulse Signals," in International Conference on BioMedical Engineering and Informatics, Sanya, China, 2008, pp. 539–543.

23. L. Xu, M. Q. H. Meng, R. Liu, and K. Wang, "Robust peak detection of pulse waveform using height ratio," in International Conference of the IEEE Engineering in Medicine and Biology Society, Vancouver, BC, Canada, 2008, pp. 3856–3859.

24. L. Xu, M. Q. H. Meng, K. Wang, W. Lu, and N. Li, "Pulse images recognition using fuzzy neural network," Expert systems with applications, vol. 36, pp. 3805–3811, 2009.

25. Y. Wang, X. Wu, B. Liu, Y. Yi, and W. Wang, "Definition and application of indices in Doppler ultrasound sonogram," Shanghai Journal of Biomedical Engineering, vol. 18, pp. 26–29, Aug 1997.
26. J.-J. Shu and Y. Sun, "Developing classification indices for Chinese pulse diagnosis," Complementary therapies in medicine, vol. 15, pp. 190–198, 2007.
27. C. Xia, Y. Li, J. Yan, Y. Wang, H. Yan, R. Guo, et al., "Wrist Pulse Waveform Feature Extraction and Dimension Reduction with Feature Variability Analysis," in International Conference on Bioinformatics and Biomedical Engineering, Shanghai, China, 2008, pp. 2048–2051.
28. C. T. Lee and L. Y. Wei, "Spectrum analysis of human pulse," IEEE Transactions on Biomedical Engineering, vol. BME-30, pp. 348–352, Jun 1983.
29. D. Zhang, K. Wang, X. Wu, B. Huang, and N. Li, "Hilbert-Huang transform based doppler blood flow signals analysis," in 2009 2nd International Conference on Biomedical Engineering and Informatics, BMEI 2009, October 17, 2009–October 19, 2009, Tianjin, China, 2009, p. IEEE Engineering in Medicine and Biology Society.
30. D. Zhang, L. Zhang, D. Zhang, and Y. Zheng, "Wavelet based analysis of doppler ultrasonic wrist-pulse signals," in IEEE International Conference on BioMedical Engineering and Informatics, Sanya, Hainan, China, 2008, pp. 539–543.
31. Q. Wu, "Power Spectral Analysis of Wrist Pulse Signal in Evaluating Adult Age," in International Symposium on Intelligence Information Processing and Trusted Computing, 2010, pp. 48–50.
32. G. Guo and Y. Wang, "Research on the pulse-signal detection methods using the HHT methods," in International Conference on Electric Information and Control Engineering, Wuhan, China, 2011, pp. 4430–4433.
33. B. Thakker, A. L. Vyas, O. Farooq, D. Mulvaney, and S. Datta, "Wrist pulse signal classification for health diagnosis," in International Conference on Biomedical Engineering and Informatics, Shanghai, China 2011, pp. 1799–1805.
34. N. Arunkumar and K. M. M. Sirajudeen, "Approximate entropy based ayurvedic pulse diagnosis for diabetics - a case study," in IEEE International Conference on Trendz in Information Sciences and Computing, Chennai,India, 2011, pp. 133–135.
35. N. Arunkumar, S. Jayalalitha, S. Dinesh, A. Venugopal, and D. Sekar, "Sample entropy based ayurvedic pulse diagnosis for diabetics," in International Conference on Advances in Engineering, Science and Management Nagapattinam , India, 2012, pp. 61–62.
36. J. M. Irvine, S. A. Israel, W. Todd Scruggs, and W. J. Worek, "eigenPulse: Robust human identification from cardiovascular function," Pattern Recognition, vol. 41, pp. 3427–3435, 2008.
37. W. Yang, L. Zhang, and D. Zhang, "Wrist-Pulse Signal Diagnosis Using ICPulse," in International Conference on Bioinformatics and Biomedical Engineering, Wuhan, China, 2009, pp. 1–4.
38. J. Yan, C. Xia, H. Wang, et al., "Nonlinear Dynamic Analysis of Wrist Pulse with Lyapunov Exponents," in International Conference on Bioinformatics and Biomedical Engineering Shanghai, China, 2008, pp. 2177–2180.
39. C. Xia, Y. Li, J. Yan, Y. Wang, H. Yan, R. Guo, et al., "A practical approach to wrist pulse segmentation and single-period average waveform estimation," in International Conference on BioMedical Engineering and Informatics, Sanya, China, 2008, pp. 334–338.
40. L.Wang, K.Wang, and L.Xu, "Recognizing wrist pulse waveforms with improved dynamic time warping algorithm," in IEEE International Conference on Machine Learning and Cybernetics, 2004, pp. 3644–3649 vol.6.
41. L. Xu, D. Zhang, and K. Wang, "Wavelet-based cascaded adaptive filter for removing baseline drift in pulse waveforms," IEEE Transactions on Biomedical Engineering, vol. 52, pp. 1973–1975, Nov 2005.
42. J. S. Richman and J. R. Moorman, "Physiological time-series analysis using approximate entropy and sample entropy," American Journal of Physiology-Heart and Circulatory Physiology, vol. 278, pp. H2039-H2049, 2000.

43. S. M. Pincus, "Approximate entropy as a measure of system-complexity," Proceedings of the National Academy of Sciences, vol. 88, pp. 2297–2301, Mar 1991.
44. D. E. Lake, J. S. Richman, M. P. Griffin, and J. R. Moorman, "Sample entropy analysis of neonatal heart rate variability," American Journal of Physiology-Regulatory, Integrative and Comparative Physiology, vol. 283, pp. R789-R797, 2002.
45. M. Costa, A. L. Goldberger, and C. K. Peng, "Multiscale entropy analysis of biological signals," Physical Review E, vol. 71, pp. 1–18, Feb 2005.
46. M. Costa, A. L. Goldberger, and C. K. Peng, "Multiscale entropy analysis of complex physiologic time series," Physical Review Letters, vol. 89, pp. 1–4, Aug 5 2002.
47. M. Costa, A. L. Goldberger, and C. K. Peng, "Multiscale entropy analysis of complex physiologic time series," Physical Review Letters, vol. 89, pp. 068102/1-068102/4, 2002.
48. J. Zhang and M. Small, "Complex network from pseudoperiodic time series: Topology versus dynamics," Physical Review Letters, vol. 96, pp. 1–4, 2006.
49. J. Zhang, X. Luo, and M. Small, "Detecting chaos in pseudoperiodic time series without embedding," Physical Review E, vol. 73, pp. 1–5, 2006.
50. R. Albert and A.-L. Barabási, "Statistical mechanics of complex networks," Reviews of modern physics, vol. 74, pp. 47–97, 2002.
51. M. E. Newman, S. H. Strogatz, and D. J. Watts, "Random graphs with arbitrary degree distributions and their applications", Physical Review E, vol. 64, p. 026118, 2001.
52. W. J. Mandel, Cardiac arrhythmias: their mechanisms, diagnosis and management. Mishawaka, USA: Lippincott Williams & Wilkins, 1995.
53. C. J. C. Burges, "A tutorial on support vector machines for pattern recognition," Data Mining and Knowledge Discovery, vol. 2, pp. 121–167, Jun 1998.

Part V
Pulse Analysis and Diagnosis

Chapter 11
Edit Distance for Pulse Diagnosis

Abstract In this chapter, by referring to the edit distance with real penalty (ERP) and the recent progress in k-nearest neighbors (KNN) classifiers, we propose two novel ERP-based KNN classifiers. Taking advantage of the metric property of ERP, we first develop an ERP-induced inner product and a Gaussian ERP kernel, then embed them into difference-weighted KNN classifiers, and finally develop two novel classifiers for pulse waveform classification. The experimental results show that the proposed classifiers are effective for accurate classification of pulse waveform.

11.1 Introduction

Traditional Chinese pulse diagnosis (TCPD) is a convenient, noninvasive, and effective diagnostic method that is widely used in traditional Chinese medicine (TCM) [1]. In TCPD, practitioners feel for the fluctuations in the radial pulse at the styloid processes of the wrist and classify them into the distinct patterns which are related to various syndromes and diseases in TCM. This is a skill which requires considerable training and experience and may produce significant variation in diagnosis results for different practitioners. So in recent years, techniques developed for measuring, processing, and analyzing the physiological signals [2, 3] have been considered in quantitative TCPD research as a way to improve the reliability and consistency of diagnoses [4–6]. Since then, much progress has been received: a range of pulse signal acquisition systems have been developed for various pulse analysis tasks [7–9]; a number of signal preprocessing and analysis methods have been developed in pulse signal denoising, baseline rectification [10], and segmentation [11]; many pulse feature extraction approaches have been proposed by using various time-frequency analysis techniques [12–14]; many classification methods have been studied for pulse diagnosis [15, 16] and pulse waveform classification [17–19].

Pulse waveform classification aims to assign a traditional pulse pattern to a pulse waveform according to its shape, regularity, force, and rhythm [1]. However, because of the complicated intra-class variation in pulse patterns and the inevitable

© Springer Nature Singapore Pte Ltd. 2018
D. Zhang et al., *Computational Pulse Signal Analysis*,
https://doi.org/10.1007/978-981-10-4044-3_11

influence of local time shifting in pulse waveforms, it has remained a difficult problem for automatic pulse waveform classification. Although researchers have developed several pulse waveform classification methods such as artificial neural network [18, 21, 22], decision tree [20], and wavelet network [23], most of them are only tested on small datasets and usually cannot achieve satisfactory classification accuracy.

Recently, various time series matching methods, e.g., dynamical time warping (DTW) [24] and edit distance with real penalty (ERP) [25], have been applied for time series classification. Motivated by the success of time series matching techniques, we suggest utilizing time series classification approaches for addressing the intra-class variation and the local time shifting problems in pulse waveform classification. In this chapter, we first develop an ERP-induced inner product and a Gaussian ERP (GERP) kernel function. Then, with the difference-weighted KNN (DFWKNN) framework [26], we further present two novel ERP-based classifiers: the ERP-based difference-weighted KNN classifier (EDKC) and the kernel difference-weighted KNN with Gaussian ERP kernel classifier (GEKC). Finally, we evaluate the proposed methods on a pulse waveform dataset of five common pulse patterns, moderate, smooth, taut, unsmooth, and hollow. This dataset includes 2470 pulse waveforms, which is the largest dataset used for pulse waveform classification to the best of our knowledge. Experimental results show that the proposed methods achieve an average classification rate of 91.74%, which is higher than those of several state-of-the-art approaches.

The remainder of this chapter is organized as follows. Section 11.2 introduces the main modules in pulse waveform classification. Section 11.3 first presents a brief survey on ERP and DFWKNN and then proposes two novel ERP-based classifiers. Section 11.4 provides the experimental results. Finally, Sect. 11.5 concludes this chapter.

11.2   The Pulse Waveform Classification Modules

Pulse waveform classification usually involves three modules: a pulse waveform acquisition module, a preprocessing module, and a feature extraction and classification module. The pulse waveform acquisition module is used to acquire pulse waveforms with satisfactory quality for further processing. The preprocessing module is used to remove the distortions of the pulse waveforms caused by noise and baseline drift. Finally, using the feature extraction and classification module, pulse waveforms are classified into different patterns (Fig. 11.1).

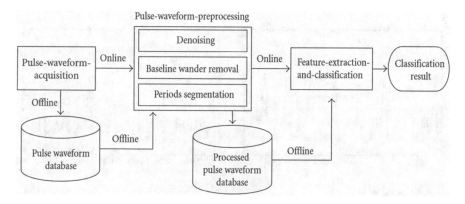

Fig. 11.1 Schematic diagram of the pulse waveform classification modules

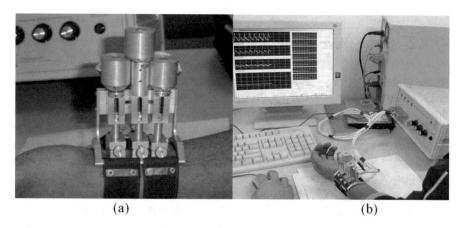

Fig. 11.2 The pulse waveform acquisition system: (**a**) the motor-embedded pressure sensor and (**b**) the whole pulse waveform acquisition system

11.2.1   Pulse Waveform Acquisition

Our pulse waveform acquisition system is jointly developed by the Harbin Institute of Technology and the Hong Kong Polytechnic University. The system uses a motor-embedded pressure sensor, an amplifier, a USB interface, and a computer to acquire pulse waveforms. During the pulse waveform acquisition, the sensor (Fig. 11.2a) is attached to the wrist and contact pressure is applied by the computer-controlled automatic rotation of motors and mechanical screws. Pulse waveforms acquired by the pressure sensors are transmitted to the computer through the USB interface. Figure 11.2b shows an image of the scene of the pulse waveform collection.

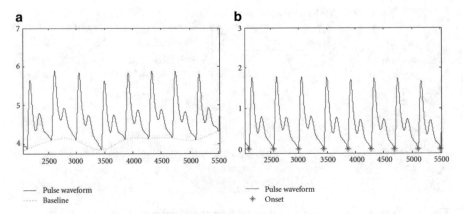

Fig. 11.3 Pulse waveform baseline drift correction: (**a**) pulse waveform distorted by baseline drift and (**b**) pulse waveform after baseline drift correction

11.2.2   Pulse Waveform Preprocessing

In the pulse waveform preprocessing, it is necessary to first remove the random noise and power line interference. Moreover, as shown in Fig. 11.3a, the baseline drift caused by factors such as respiration would also greatly distort the pulse signal. We use a *Daubechies* 4 wavelet transform to remove the noise by empirically comparing the performance of several wavelet functions and correct the baseline drift using a wavelet-based cascaded adaptive filter previously developed by our group [10].

Pulse waveforms are quasiperiodic signals where one or a few periods are sufficient to classify a pulse shape. So we adopt an automatic method to locate the position of the onsets, split each multiperiod pulse waveform into several single periods, and select one of these periods as a sample of our pulse waveform dataset. Figure 11.3b shows the result of the baseline drift correction and the locations of the onsets of a pulse waveform.

11.2.3   Feature Extraction and Classification

TCPD recognizes more than 20 kinds of pulse patterns which are defined according to criteria such as shape, position, regularity, force, and rhythm. Several of these are not settled issues in the TCPD field, but we can say that there is general agreement that, according to the shape, there are five pulse patterns, namely, moderate, smooth, taut, hollow, and unsmooth. Figure 11.4 shows the typical waveforms of these five pulse patterns acquired by our pulse waveform acquisition system. All of these pulses can be defined according to the presence, absence, or strength of three types of waves or peaks: percussion (primary wave), tidal (secondary wave), and dicrotic (triplex wave), which are denoted by P, T, and D, respectively, in Fig. 11.4. A

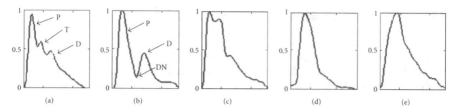

Fig. 11.4 Five typical pulse patterns classified by shape: (**a**) moderate, (**b**) smooth, (**c**) taut, (**d**) hollow, and (**e**) unsmooth pulse patterns

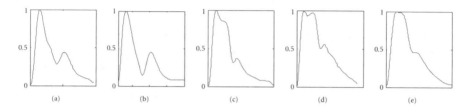

Fig. 11.5 Inter- and intra-class variations of pulse patterns: (**a**) a moderate pulse with unnoticeable tidal wave is similar to (**b**) a smooth pulse; taut pulse patterns may exhibit different shapes, for example, (**c**) typical taut pulse, (**d**) taut pulse with high tidal wave, and (**e**) taut pulse with tidal wave merged with percussion wave

moderate pulse usually has all three types of peaks in one period, a smooth pulse has low dicrotic notch (DN) and unnoticeable tidal wave, a taut pulse frequently exhibits a high-tidal peak, an unsmooth pulse exhibits unnoticeable tidal or dicrotic wave, and a hollow pulse has rapid descending part in percussion wave and unnoticeable dicrotic wave.

However, pulse waveform classification may suffer from the problems of small interclass and large intra-class variation. As shown in Fig. 11.5, moderate pulse with unnoticeable tidal wave is similar to smooth pulse. For taut pulse, the tidal wave sometimes becomes very high or even merges with the percussion wave. Moreover, the factors such as local time axis distortion would make the classification problem more complicated.

So far, a number of pulse waveform classification approaches have been proposed, which can be grouped into two categories: the representation-based and the similarity measure-based methods. The representation-based methods first extract representative features of pulse waveforms using techniques such as spatiotemporal analysis [14], fast Fourier transform (FFT) [12], and wavelet transform [13]. Then the classification is performed in the feature space by using various classifiers, for example, decision tree [22] and neural network [18, 20, 21].

For the similarity measure-based methods, classification is performed in the original data space by using certain distance functions to measure the similarity of different pulse waveforms. Our pulse waveform classification approaches belong to the similarity measure-based method, where we first propose an ERP-induced inner product and a Gaussian ERP kernel and then embed them into the DFWKNN and KDFWKNN classifiers [26, 27]. In the following section, we will introduce the proposed methods in detail.

11.3   The EDCK and GEKC Classifiers

In this section, we first provide a brief survey on related work, that is, ERP, DFWKNN, and KDFWKNN. Then we explain the basic ideas and implementations of the ERP-based DFWKNN classifier (EDKC) and the KDFWKNN with Gaussian ERP kernel classifier (GEKC).

11.3.1   Edit Distance with Real Penalty

The ERP distance is a state-of-the-art elastic distance measure for time series match-ing [25]. During the calculation of the ERP distance, two time series, $a = [a_1, \ldots, a_m]$ with m elements and $b = [b_1, \ldots, b_n]$ with n elements, are aligned to the same length by adding some symbols (also called gaps) to them. Then each element in a time series is either matched to a gap or an element in the other time series. Finally the ERP distance between a and b, $d_{erp}(a,b)$, is recursively defined as:

$$
d_{\mathrm{erp}}(\mathbf{a},\mathbf{b}) = \begin{cases} \sum_{i=1}^{m} |a_i - g|, & \text{if } n = 0 \\[2mm] \sum_{i=1}^{n} |b_i - g|, & \text{if } m = 0 \\[2mm] \min \begin{cases} d_{\mathrm{erp}}\left(\mathrm{Rest}(\mathbf{a}), \mathrm{Rest}(\mathbf{b})\right) + |a_1 - b_1|, \\ d_{\mathrm{erp}}\left(\mathrm{Rest}(\mathbf{a}), \mathbf{b}\right) + |a_1 - g|, \\ d_{\mathrm{erp}}\left(\mathbf{a}, \mathrm{Rest}(\mathbf{b})\right) + |b_1 - g| \end{cases}, & \text{otherwise} \end{cases}
\quad , (11.1)
$$

where $\mathrm{Rest}(\mathbf{a}) = [a_2, \ldots, a_m]$ and $\mathrm{Rest}(\mathbf{b}) = [b_2, \ldots, b_n]$, $|\cdot|$ denote the l_1-norm and g is a constant with a default value $g = 0$ [25]. From (Eq. 11.1), one can see that the distance $d_{erp}(\mathbf{a},\mathbf{b})$ can be derived by recursively calculating the ERP distance of their subsequences until the length of one subsequence is zero. By incorporating gaps in aligning time series of different lengths, the ERP distance is very effective in han-dling the local time shifting problem in time series matching. Besides, the ERP distance satisfies the triangle inequality and is a metric [25].

11.3.2   DFWKNN and KDFKNN

DFWKNN and KDFWKNN are two recently developed KNN classifiers with clas-sification performance comparable with or better than several state-of-the-art clas-sification methods [26]. Let X be a dataset of n samples $\{\mathbf{x}_1, \ldots, \mathbf{x}_n\}$ and the corresponding class labels are $\{y_1, \ldots, y_n\}$ with each element from $\{\omega_j | j \in [1, \ldots, c]\}$, where c denotes the number of classes. For a test sample $\mathbf{x}$, its k-nearest neighbors from X are found using the Euclidean distance to form a matrix $\mathbf{X}^{nn} = \left[\mathbf{x}_1^{nn}, \ldots, \mathbf{x}_k^{nn}\right]$. In DFWKNN, the weights of the k-nearest neighbors are defined as a vector $w = [w_1, \ldots, w_k]^T$, which can be obtained by solving the following constrained optimization problem:

$$\mathbf{w} = \arg \min_{\mathbf{w}} \left\|\frac{1}{2}\mathbf{x} - \mathbf{X}^{nn}\mathbf{w}\right\|^2.$$

$$\text{subject to } \sum_{i=1}^{k} w_i = 1 \tag{11.2}$$

By defining the Gram matrix as:

$$\mathbf{G} = \left[\mathbf{x} - \mathbf{x}_1^{nn}, \ldots, \mathbf{x} - \mathbf{x}_k^{nn}\right]^T \left[\mathbf{x} - \mathbf{x}_1^{nn}, \ldots, \mathbf{x} - \mathbf{x}_k^{nn}\right], \tag{11.3}$$

the weight vector w can be obtained by solving $Gw = 1_k$, where 1_k is a $k \times 1$ vector with all elements equal to 1. If the matrix G is singular, there is no inverse of G, and the solution of w would be not unique. To avoid this case, a regularization method is adopted by adding the multiplication of a small value with the identity matrix, and the weight vector w can be obtained by solving the system of linear equations:

$$\left[\mathbf{G} + \eta \mathbf{I}_k \text{tr}(\mathbf{G}) / k\right]\mathbf{w} = \mathbf{1}_k, \tag{11.4}$$

where tr($\mathbf{G}$) is the trace of G, $\eta \in [10^{-3} \sim 10^0]$ is the regularization parameter, k is the number of nearest neighbors of x, and $\mathbf{I}_k$ is a $k \times k$ identity matrix. Finally, using the weighted KNN rule, the class label $\omega_{j\max} = \arg\max_{\omega j} \left(\sum_{y^{nn} = \omega j} w_i\right)$ is assigned to the sample x. By defining the kernel Gram matrix, DFWKNN can be extended to KDFWKNN. Using the feature mapping F: $x \rightarrow \phi(x)$ and the kernel function $\kappa(x, x') = \langle \phi(x), \phi(x')\rangle$, the kernel Gram matrix G^κ is defined as:

$$\mathbf{G}^\kappa = \left[\phi(\mathbf{x}) - \phi(\mathbf{x}_1^{nn}), \ldots, \phi(\mathbf{x}) - \phi(\mathbf{x}_k^{nn})\right]^T$$
$$\left[\phi(\mathbf{x}) - \phi(\mathbf{x}_1^{nn}), \ldots, \phi(\mathbf{x}) - \psi(\mathbf{x}_k^{nn})\right] \tag{11.5}$$

In KDFWKNN, the weight vector w is obtained by solving:

$$\left[\mathbf{G}^\kappa + \eta \mathbf{I}_k \text{tr}(\mathbf{G}^\kappa) / k\right]\mathbf{w} = \mathbf{1}_k. \tag{11.6}$$

For a detailed description of KDFWKNN, please refer to [26].

11.3.3   The EDKC Classifier

Current similarity measure-based methods usually adopt the simple nearest neighbor classifier. The combination of similarity measure with advanced KNN classifiers is expected to be more promising. So, by using DFWKNN, we intend to develop a more effective classifier, the ERP-based DFWKNN classifier (EDKC), for pulse waveform classification. Utilizing the metric property of the ERP distance, we first develop an ERP-induced inner product and then embed this novel inner product into DFWKNN to develop the EDKC classifier. Let $\langle\cdot,\cdot\rangle_{erp}$ denote the ERP-induced inner product. Since ERP is a metric. We can get the following heuristic deduction:

$$d_{erp}^2\left(\mathbf{x},\mathbf{x}'\right) = \mathbf{x}-\mathbf{x}',\mathbf{x}-\mathbf{x}'_{erp} = \mathbf{x},\mathbf{x}_{erp}+\mathbf{x}',\mathbf{x}'_{erp}-2\mathbf{x},\mathbf{x}'_{erp},$$
$$\Rightarrow d_{erp}^2\left(\mathbf{x},\mathbf{x}'\right) = d_{erp}^2\left(\mathbf{x},\mathbf{x}_0\right)+d_{erp}^2\left(\mathbf{x}',\mathbf{x}_0\right)-2\mathbf{x},\mathbf{x}'_{erp}, \tag{11.7}$$

where $d_{erp}(\mathbf{x},\mathbf{x}')$ is the ERP distance between $\mathbf{x}$ and $\mathbf{x}'$, and the vector x_0 represents a zero-length time series. Then the ERP-induced inner product of x and x' can be defined as follows:

$$\mathbf{x},\mathbf{x}'_{erp} = \frac{1}{2}\left(d_{erp}^2\left(\mathbf{x},\mathbf{x}_0\right)+d_{erp}^2\left(\mathbf{x}',\mathbf{x}_0\right)-d_{erp}^2\left(\mathbf{x},\mathbf{x}'\right)\right). \tag{11.8}$$

In (11.3), the element at the ith row and the jth column of the Gram matrix G is defined as $G_{ij} = x-x_i^{nn},x-x_j^{nn}$ where $\langle\cdot,\cdot\rangle$ denotes the regular inner product. In EDKC, we replace the regular inner product with the ERP-induced inner product to calculate the Gram matrix G_{erp}, which can be rewritten as follows:

$$\mathbf{G}_{erp} = \mathbf{K}_{erp}+\mathbf{x},\mathbf{x}_{erp}\mathbf{1}_{kk}-\mathbf{1}_k\mathbf{k}_{erp}^T-\mathbf{k}_{erp}\mathbf{1}_k^T, \tag{11.9}$$

where $\mathbf{k}_{erp}$ is a $k \times k$ matrix with the element at ith row and jth column $\mathbf{K}_{erp}(i,j) = \mathbf{x}_i^{nn},\mathbf{x}_j^{nn}{}_{erp}$, $\mathbf{k}_{erp}$ is a $k \times 1$ vector with the ith element $\mathbf{k}_{erp}(i) = \mathbf{x},\mathbf{x}_i^{nn}{}_{erp}$, and $\mathbf{1}_{kk}$ is a $k \times k$ matrix of which each element equals 1. Once we obtain the Gram matrix G_{erp}, we can directly use DFWKNN for pulse waveform classification by solving the linear system of equations defined in (Eq. 11.4). The detailed algorithm of EDKC is shown as Algorithm 11.1 (Table 11.1).

Table 11.1   The average classification rates (%) of different methods

Pulse waveform	1NN-Euclidean	1NN-DTW	1NN-ERP	Wavelet network [23]	IDTW [19]	EDKC	GEKC
Moderate	86.11	82.44	88.31	87.23	87.31	89.94	91.25
Smooth	85.02	81.16	86.31	85.36	80.38	86.00	87.09
Taut	95.76	87.95	95.10	89.63	93.15	95.50	96.88
Hollow	86.75	82.44	87.56	85.63	80.44	86.88	89.38
Unsmooth	84.06	70.81	84.75	80.63	89.50	85.00	86.88
Average	87.36	83.19	89.79	87.08	88.90	90.36	91.74

Algorithm 11.1 ERP-Based DFWKNN Classifier (EDKC)

Input: The unclassified sample x, the training samples $X = \{x_1,\ldots,x_n\}$ with the corresponding class labels $\{y_1,\ldots, y_n\}$, the regularization parameter η, and the number of nearest neighbors k

    Output: The predicted class label ω_{jmax} of the sample $\mathbf{x}$

1. Use the ERP distance to obtain the k-nearest neighbors $\mathbf{X}^{nn} = \left[\mathbf{x}_1^{nn},\cdots,\mathbf{x}_k^{nn} \right]$ of the sample x and their corresponding class labels $\left[y_1^{nn},\ldots,y_k^{nn} \right]$

2. Calculate the GERP-induced inner product between samples x and each of its   nearest   neighbors
$$\mathbf{k}_{\mathrm{erp}}\left(i\right) = \left\langle \mathbf{x},\mathbf{x}_i^{nn} \right\rangle_{\mathrm{erp}} = \left(d_{\mathrm{erp}}^2\left(\mathbf{x},\mathbf{x}_0\right) + d_{\mathrm{erp}}^2\left(\mathbf{x}_i^{nn},\mathbf{x}_0\right) - d_{\mathrm{erp}}^2\left(\mathbf{x},\mathbf{x}_i^{nn}\right) \right)/2$$

3. Calculate the ERP-induced inner product of the k-nearest neighbors of sample x,
$$\mathbf{K}_{\mathrm{erp}}\left(i,j\right) = \left\langle \mathbf{x}_j^{nn},\mathbf{x}_i^{nn} \right\rangle_{\mathrm{erp}}$$

4. Calculate the self-inner product of the sample $\mathbf{x}$, $\langle \mathbf{x},\mathbf{x} \rangle_{\mathrm{erp}}$

5. Calculate $\mathbf{G}_{\mathrm{erp}} = \mathbf{K}_{\mathrm{erp}} + \langle \mathbf{x},\mathbf{x} \rangle_{\mathrm{erp}} \mathbf{1}_{kk} - \mathbf{1}_k \mathbf{k}_{\mathrm{erp}}^{\mathrm{T}} - \mathbf{k}_{\mathrm{erp}} \mathbf{1}_k^{\mathrm{T}}$

6. Calculate w by solving $[\mathbf{G}_{\mathrm{erp}} + \eta \mathbf{I}_k \mathrm{tr}(\mathbf{G}_{\mathrm{erp}})/k]\mathbf{w} = \mathbf{1}_k$

7. Assign the class label $\omega_{j\max} = \arg\max_{\omega j}(\sum_{y_i^{nn}=\omega_j} w_i)$ to the sample x

11.3.4   The GEKC Classifier

The Gaussian RBF kernel [28] is one of the most common kernel functions used in kernel methods. Given two time series x and x' with the same length n, the Gaussian RBF kernel is defined as:

$$K_{\mathrm{RBF}}\left(\mathbf{x},\mathbf{x}'\right) = \exp\left(-\frac{\|\mathbf{x}-\mathbf{x}'\|_2^2}{2\sigma^2} \right), \tag{11.10}$$

where σ is the standard deviation. The Gaussian RBF kernel requires that the time series should have the same length, and it cannot handle the problem of time axis distortion. If the length of two time series is different, resampling usually is required to normalize them to the same length before further processing. Thus Gaussian RBF kernel usually is not suitable for the classification of time series data. Actually Gaussian RBF kernel can be regarded as an embedding of Euclidean distance in the form of Gaussian function. Motivated by the effectiveness of ERP, it is interesting to embed the ERP distance into the form of Gaussian function to derive a novel kernel function, the Gaussian ERP (GERP) kernel. By this way, we expect that the GERP kernel would be effective in addressing the local time shifting problem and be more suitable for time series classification in kernel machines. Given two time series x and x', we define the Gaussian ERP kernel function on X as:

$$K_{\text{erp}}\left(\mathbf{x},\mathbf{x}'\right) = \exp\left(-\frac{d_{\text{erp}}^2\left(\mathbf{x},\mathbf{x}'\right)}{2\sigma^2}\right), \tag{11.11}$$

where σ is the standard deviation of the Gaussian function. We embed the GERP kernel into KDFWKNN by constructing the kernel Gram matrix $G\kappa_{\text{erp}}$ defined as:

$$\mathbf{G}_{\text{erp}}^{\kappa} = \mathbf{K}_{\text{erp}}^{\kappa} + \mathbf{1}_{kk} - \mathbf{1}_k\left(\mathbf{k}_{\text{erp}}^{\kappa}\right)^{\text{T}} - \mathbf{k}_{\text{erp}}^{\kappa}\mathbf{1}_k^{\text{T}}, \tag{11.12}$$

where $\mathbf{K}_{\text{erp}}^{\kappa}$ is a $k \times k$ matrix with its element at ith row and jth column,

$$\mathbf{K}_{\text{erp}}^{\kappa}\left(i,j\right) = K_{\text{erp}}\left(\mathbf{x}_j^{nn},\mathbf{x}_i^{nn}\right), \tag{11.13}$$

and $\mathbf{k}_{\text{erp}}^{\kappa}$ is a $k \times 1$ vector with its ith element,

$$\mathbf{k}_{\text{erp}}^{\kappa}\left(i\right) = K_{\text{erp}}\left(\mathbf{x},\mathbf{x}_i^{nn}\right). \tag{11.14}$$

Once we have obtained the kernel Gram matrix $\mathbf{G}_{\text{erp}}^{\kappa}$, we can use KDFWKNN for pulse waveform classification by solving the linear system of equations defined in (Eq. 11.6). The details of the GEKC algorithm are shown as Algorithm 11.2.

11.4   Experimental Results

In order to evaluate the classification performance of EDKC and GEKC, by using the device described in Sect. 11.2.1, we construct a dataset which consists of 2470 pulse waveforms of five pulse patterns, including moderate (M), smooth (S), taut (T), hollow (H), and unsmooth (U). All of the data are acquired at the Harbin Binghua Hospital under the supervision of the TCPD experts. All subjects are patients in the hospital between 20 and 60 years old. Clinical data, for example, biomedical data and medical history, are also obtained for reference. For each subject, only the pulse signal of the left hand is acquired, and three experts are asked to determine the pulse pattern according to their pulse signal and the clinical data. If the diagnosis results of the experts are the same, the sample is kept in the dataset; else it is abandoned. Table 11.2 lists the number of pulse waveforms of each pulse pattern. To the best of our knowledge, this dataset is the largest one used for pulse waveform classification.

Table 11.2 Dataset used in our experiments

Pulse	Moderate	Smooth	Taut	Hollow	Unsmooth	Total
Number	800	550	800	160	160	2470

Algorithm 11.2 Gaussian ERP Kernel Classifier (GEKC)

Input: The unclassified sample x, the training samples $X = \{x_1,\ldots,x_n\}$ with the corresponding class labels $\{y_1,\ldots,y_n\}$, the regularization parameter η, the kernel parameter σ, and the number of nearest neighbors k

    Output: The predicted class label $\omega_{j\max}$ of the sample **x**

1. Use the ERP distance to obtain the k-nearest neighbors $\mathbf{G}_{erp}^{\kappa}$ of the sample x and their corresponding class labels $\left[y_1^{nn},\ldots,y_k^{nn} \right]$

2. Calculate the GERP-induced inner product between samples x and each of its nearest neighbors $\mathbf{k}_{erp}^{\kappa}(i) = \exp\left(-d_{erp}^2\left(\mathbf{x},\mathbf{x}_i^{nn}\right)/2\sigma^2\right)$

3. Calculate the GERP-induced inner product of the k-nearest neighbors of x
$$\mathbf{K}_{erp}^{\kappa}(i,j) = \exp\left(-d_{erp}^2\left(\mathbf{x}_j^{nn},\mathbf{x}_i^{nn}\right)/2\sigma^2\right)$$

4. Calculate $\mathbf{G}_{erp}^{\kappa} = \mathbf{K}_{erp}^{\kappa} + \mathbf{1}_{kk} - \mathbf{1}_k\left(\mathbf{k}_{erp}^{\kappa}\right)^{\mathrm{T}} - \mathbf{k}_{erp}^{\kappa}\mathbf{1}_k^{\mathrm{T}}$

5. Calculate w by solving $\left[\mathbf{G}_{erp}^{\kappa} + \eta\mathbf{I}_k\,\mathrm{tr}\left(\mathbf{G}_{erp}^{\kappa}\right)/k \right]\mathbf{w} = \mathbf{1}_k$

6. Assign the class label $\omega_{j\max} = \arg\max_{\omega_j}(\sum_{y_i^{nn}=\omega_j} w_i)$ to the sample x

Table 11.3 The confusion matrix of EDKC

Actual	Predicted	M	S	T	H	U
M		**720**	59	19	2	0
S		68	**473**	3	6	0
T		22	5	**764**	3	6
H		7	9	4	**139**	1
U		1	1	20	2	**136**

We make use of only one period from each pulse signal and normalize it to the length of 150 points. We randomly split the dataset into three parts of roughly equal size and use the threefold cross-validation method to assess the classification performance of each pulse waveform classification method. To reduce bias in classification performance, we adopt the average classification rate of the ten runs of the threefold cross validation. Using the stepwise selection strategy [26], we choose the optimal values of hyper-parameters k, η, and σ: $k = 4$ and $\eta = 0.01$ for EDKC and $k = 31$, $\eta = 0.01$, and $\sigma = 16$ for GEKC. The classification rates of the EDKC and GEKC classifiers are 90.36% and 91.74%, respectively. Tables 11.3 and 11.4 list the confusion matrices of EDKC and GEKC, respectively.

To provide a comprehensive performance evaluation of the proposed methods, we compare the classification rates of EDKC and GEKC with several achieved accuracies in the recent literature [19, 21–23]. Table 11.5 lists the sizes of the dataset, the number of pulse waveform classes, and the achieved classification rates of several recent pulse waveform classifiers, including improved dynamic time warping (IDTW) [19], decision tree (DT-M4) [22], artificial neural network [21], and

Table 11.4 The confusion matrix of GEKC

		Predicted				
Actual		M	S	T	H	U
	M	**730**	54	15	1	0
	S	61	**479**	4	6	0
	T	16	2	**775**	1	6
	H	7	7	2	**143**	1
	U	0	1	19	1	**139**

Table 11.5 Comparison of different methods for pulse waveforms classification with their accuracies achieved in recent literature

Category	Methods	Dataset		Accuracy
		Size	Classes	
Representation-based methods	DT-M4 [22]	372	3	92.2%
	Wavelet network [23]	600	6	83%
	Artificial neural network [21]	63	3	73%
		21	2	90%
Similarity measure-based methods	IDTW [19]	1000	5	92.3%
	EDKC	2470	5	90.36%
	GEKC	2470	5	91.74%

wavelet network [23]. From Table 11.5, one can see that GEKC achieves higher accuracy than wavelet network [23] and artificial neural network [21]. Moreover, although IDTW and DT-M4 reported somewhat higher classification rates than our methods, the size of the dataset used in our experiments is much larger than those used in these two methods, and DT-M4 is only tested on a three-class problem. In summary, compared with these approaches, EDKC and GEKC are very effective for pulse waveform classification.

To provide an objective comparison, we independently implement two pulse waveform classification methods listed in Table 11.5, that is, IDTW [19] and wavelet network [23], and evaluate their performance on our dataset. The average classification rates of these two methods are listed in Table 11.5. Besides, we also compare the proposed methods with several related classification methods, that is, nearest neighbor with Euclidean distance (1NN-Euclidean), nearest neighbor with dynamic time warping (1NN-DTW), and nearest neighbor with ERP distance (1NN-ERP). These results are also listed in Table 11.6. From Table 11.6, one can see that our methods outperform all the other methods in terms of the overall average classification accuracy.

Table 11.6 The average classification rates (%) of different methods

Pulse waveform	1NN-Euclidean	1NN-DTW	1NN-ERP	Wavelet network [23]	IDTW [19]	EDKC	GEKC
Moderate	86.11	82.44	88.31	87.23	87.31	89.94	91.25
Smooth	85.02	81.16	86.31	85.36	80.38	86.00	87.09
Taut	95.76	87.95	95.10	89.63	93.15	95.50	96.88
Hollow	86.75	82.44	87.56	85.63	80.44	86.88	89.38
Unsmooth	84.06	70.81	84.75	80.63	89.50	85.00	86.88
Average	87.36	83.19	89.79	87.08	88.90	90.36	91.74

11.5 Summary

By incorporating the state-of-the-art time series matching method with the advanced KNN classifiers, we develop two accurate pulse waveform classification methods, EDKC and GEKC, to address the intra-class variation and the local time shifting problems in pulse patterns. To evaluate their classification performance, we construct a dataset of 2470 pulse waveforms, which may be the largest dataset yet used in pulse waveform classification. The experimental results show that the proposed GEKC method achieves an average classification rate of 91.74%, which is higher than or comparable with those of other state-of-the-art pulse waveform classification methods. Another potential advantage of the proposed methods is to utilize the lower bounds and the metric property of ERP for fast pulse waveform classification and indexing [28].

References

1. S. Z. Li, Pulse Diagnosis, Paradigm Press, 1985.
2. H. Dickhaus and H. Heinrich, "Classifying biosignals with wavelet networks: a method for noninvasive diagnosis, " IEEE Engineering in Medicine and Biology Magazine, vol. 15, no. 5, pp. 103–111, 1996.
3. H. Adeli, S. Ghosh-Dastidar, and N. Dadmehr, "A wavelet- chaos methodology for analysis of EEGs and EEG subbands to detect seizure and epilepsy, " IEEE Transactions on Biomedical Engineering, vol. 54, no. 2, pp. 205–211, 2007.
4. H. Wang and Y. Cheng, "A quantitative system for pulse diagnosis in traditional Chinese medicine," in Proceedings of the 27th Annual International Conference of the Engineering in Medicine and Biology Society (EMBS '05), pp. 5676–5679, September 2005.
5. S. E. Fu and S. P. Lai, "A system for pulse measurement and analysis of Chinese medicine, " in Proceedings of the 11th Annual International Conference of the IEEE Engineering in Medicine and Biology Society, pp. 1695–1696, November 1989.
6. J. Lee, J. Kim, and M. Lee, "Design of digital hardware system for pulse signals, " Journal of Medical Systems, vol. 25, no. 6, pp. 385–394, 2001.
7. W. Ran, J. I. Jae, and H. P. Sung, "Estimation of central blood pressure using radial pulse waveform," in Proceedings of the International Symposium on Information Technology Convergence (ISITC '07), pp. 250–253, November 2007.
8. R. Leca and V. Groza, "Hypertension detection using standard pulse waveform processing," in Proceedings of IEEE Instrumentation and Measurement Technology Conference (IMTC '05), pp. 400–405, May 2005.

9. C.-C. Tyan, S.-H. Liu, J.-Y. Chen, J.-J. Chen, and W.-M. Liang, "A novel noninvasive measurement technique for analyzing the pressure pulse waveform of the radial artery," IEEE Transactions on Biomedical Engineering, vol. 55, no. 1, pp. 288–297, 2008.

10. L. Xu, D. Zhang, and K. Wang, "Wavelet-based cascaded adaptive filter for removing baseline drift in pulse waveforms," IEEE Transactions on Biomedical Engineering, vol. 52, no. 11, pp. 1973–1975, 2005.

11. C. Xia, Y. Li, J. Yan et al., "A practical approach to wrist pulse segmentation and single-period average waveform estimation," in Proceedings of the 1st International Conference on BioMedical Engineering and Informatics (BMEI '08), pp. 334–338, May 2008.

12. H. Yang, Q. Zhou, and J. Xiao, "Relationship between vascular elasticity and human pulse waveform based on FFT analysis of pulse waveform with different age," in Proceedings of the International Conference on Bioinformatics and Biomedical Engineering, pp. 1–4, 2009.

13. Q.-L. Guo, K.-Q. Wang, D.-Y. Zhang, and N.-M. Li, "A wavelet packet based pulse waveform analysis for cholecystitis and nephrotic syndrome diagnosis," in Proceedings of the International Conference on Wavelet Analysis and Pattern Recognition (ICWAPR '08), pp. 513–517, August 2008.

14. P.-Y. Zhang and H.-Y. Wang, "A framework for automatic time-domain characteristic parameters extraction of human pulse signals," EURASIP Journal on Advances in Signal Processing, vol. 2008, Article ID 468390, 9 pages, 2008.

15. L. Xu, D. Zhang, K. Wang, and L. Wang, "Arrhythmic pulses detection using Lempel-Ziv complexity analysis," EURASIP Journal on Applied Signal Processing, vol. 2006, Article ID 18268, 12 pages, 2006.

16. J.-J. Shu and Y. Sun, "Developing classification indices for Chinese pulse diagnosis," Complementary Therapies in Medicine, vol. 15, no. 3, pp. 190–198, 2007.

17. J. Allen and A. Murray, "Comparison of three arterial pulse waveform classification techniques," Journal of Medical Engineering and Technology, vol. 20, no. 3, pp. 109–114, 1996.

18. L. Xu, M. Q.-H. Meng, K. Wang, W. Lu, and N. Li, "Pulse images recognition using fuzzy neural network, " Expert Systems with Applications, vol. 36, no. 2, pp. 3805–3811, 2009.

19. L. Wang, K.-Q. Wang, and L.-S. Xu, "Recognizing wrist pulse waveforms with improved dynamic time warping algorithm, " in Proceedings of the International Conference on Machine Learning and Cybernetics, pp. 3644–3649, August 2004.

20. J. Lee, "The systematical analysis of oriental pulse waveform: a practical approach," Journal of Medical Systems, vol. 32, no. 1, pp. 9–15, 2008.

21. C. Chiu, B. Liau, S. Yeh, and C. Hsu, "Artificial neural networks classification of arterial pulse waveforms in cardiovascular diseases," in Proceedings of the 4th Kuala Lumpur International Conference on Biomedical Engineering, Springer, 2008.

22. H. Wang and P. Zhang, "A quantitative method for pulse strength classification based on decision tree," Journal of Software, vol. 4, no. 4, pp. 323–330, 2009.

23. L. S. Xu, K. Q. Wang, and L. Wang, "Pulse waveforms classification based on wavelet network," in Proceedings of the 27th Annual International Conference of the Engineering in Medicine and Biology Society (EMBS '05), pp. 4596–4599, September 2005.

24. B. Yi, H. V. Jagadish, and C. Faloutsos, "Efficient retrieval of similar time sequences under time warping," in Proceedings of the 14th International Conference on Data Engineering, pp. 201–208, February 1998.

25. L. Chen and R. Ng, "On the marriage of Lp-norms and edit distance," in Proceeding of the 30th Very Large Data Bases Conference, pp. 792–801, 2004.

26. W. Zuo, D. Zhang, and K. Wang, "On kernel difference weighted k-nearest neighbor classification," Pattern Analysis and Applications, vol. 11, no. 3–4, pp. 247–257, 2008.

27. M. R. Gupta, R. M. Gray, and R. A. Olshen, "Nonparametric supervised learning by linear interpolation with maximum entropy," IEEE Transactions on Pattern Analysis and Machine Intelligence, vol. 28, no. 5, pp. 766–781, 2006.

28. B. Schölkopf and A. J. Smola, Learning with Kernels, MIT Press, Cambridge, Mass, USA, 2002.

Chapter 12
Modified Gaussian Models and Fuzzy C-Means

Abstract In this chapter, a systematic approach is proposed to analyze the computation wrist pulse signals, with the focus placed on the feature extraction and pattern classification. The wrist pulse signals are first collected and preprocessed. Considering that a typical pulse signal is composed of periodically systolic and diastolic waves, a modified Gaussian model is adopted to fit the pulse signal and the modeling parameters are then taken as features. Consequently, a feature selection scheme is proposed to eliminate the tightly correlated features and select the disease-sensitive ones. Finally, the selected features are fed to a Fuzzy C-Means (FCM) classifier for pattern classification. The proposed approach is tested on a dataset which includes pulse signals from 100 healthy persons and 88 patients. The results demonstrate the effectiveness of the proposed approach in computation wrist pulse diagnosis.

12.1 Introduction

Pulse diagnosis has been successfully used for thousands of years in oriental medicine [1–6]. In traditional pulse diagnosis, practitioners use fingertips to feel the pulse beating at the measuring position of the radial artery. Since the wrist pulse signals contain vital information and can reflect the pathological changes of a person's body condition, the practitioners can then determine the person's health conditions. However, the accuracy of pulse diagnosis depends heavily on the practitioner's skills and experience. Different practitioners may not give identical results for the same patient [2, 3]. Therefore, it is necessary to develop computational pulse signal analysis techniques to standardize and objectify the pulse diagnosis method. The computational pulse signal analysis has shown promises to the modernization of traditional pulse diagnosis, such as the pulse pattern reorganization, the arterial wave analysis, and so on [7, 8]. Generally speaking, computational pulse signal diagnosis can be divided into three stages: data collection, feature extraction, and pattern classification. In the first stage of our work, the pulse signals are collected using a Doppler ultrasound device, and some preprocessing of the collected pulse signals has been performed. At the second stage, some diagnostic

© Springer Nature Singapore Pte Ltd. 2018
D. Zhang et al., *Computational Pulse Signal Analysis*,
https://doi.org/10.1007/978-981-10-4044-3_12

features that can reflect the characteristics of the measured pulse signals are extracted. These features can be time domain features (like Doppler parameters [9, 10]), frequency domain features extracted by the Fourier transform [7], or time-frequency features extracted by the wavelet transform [11–15]. By taking the extracted features as inputs, pattern classification can be carried out at the third stage to classify the signals into different groups, i.e., the healthy subjects or patients with particular types of diseases. The pattern classification methods adopted can be statistical methods, such as support vector machine (SVM) classifier [13, 16] and Bayesian classifier [5], or artificial neural network (ANN) methods [17]. Although some of the existing pulse signal diagnosis approaches have shown good results, the effectiveness of these methods needs further assessment due to the limited number of testing samples and the types of diseases.

This chapter aims to establish a systematic approach to the computational pulse signal diagnosis, with the focus placed on feature extraction and pattern classification. The collected wrist pulse signals are first denoised by the wavelet transform. To effectively and reliably extract the features of the pulse signals, a two-term Gaussian model is then adopted to fit the pulse signals. The reason of using this model is because each period of a typical pulse signal is composed of a systolic wave and a diastolic wave, both of which are bell-shaped. The obtained Gaussian models can provide reliable and distinctive features of the wrist pulse signal, such as the relative differences of the two waves with respect to amplitude, phase, and shape. Instead of directly using these features for pattern classification, a two-step feature selection scheme is performed. Firstly, the tightly correlated features are eliminated so that the pattern dimension is reduced to ensure the efficiency of computation. Secondly, the disease-sensitive features, which can best describe the symptoms and signs of disease, are selected by using the training datasets to improve the classification performance. These selected features are taken as the inputs to the fuzzy C-means (FCM) classifier for pattern classification. In this chapter, a pulse signal dataset, which contains pulse signals from 100 healthy persons and 88 patients, was established to validate the effectiveness of the proposed approach.

The remainder of this chapter is organized as follows. Section 12.2 describes the wrist pulse signal collection and preprocessing. A modified Gaussian model is proposed in Sect. 12.3 to model pulse signals and extract features. The feature selection scheme is also presented in this section. Section 12.4 presents the FCM clustering classification method to classify the pulse signals. Section 12.5 performs extensive experiments to validate the proposed method. Finally, the chapter is concluded in Sect. 12.6.

12.2   Wrist Pulse Signal Collection and Preprocessing

In our work, a USB-based Doppler ultrasonic blood analyzer (Edan Instruments, Inc.) is used to collect the wrist pulse signals (see Fig. 12.1). Through an USB interface, the collected signals are transmitted and stored in a PC for further processing

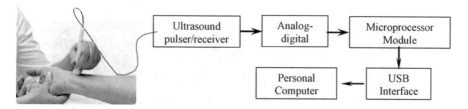

Fig. 12.1 Pulse signal collection using ultrasonic blood analyzer

and analysis. The signal collection process includes three steps. First is to find a rough location in the wrist. In traditional pulse diagnosis, the practitioners usually use three fingertips (index, middle, and ring fingers) to feel the pulse fluctuation on three positions, named "Cun," "Guan," and "Chi," in a patient's wrist [1, 3]. Since there is only one probe of the Doppler ultrasound device, we can only detect the pulse fluctuation at one position. Hence the pulse signal at the "Guan" position is detected because the fluctuation of pulse at this position is bigger than other positions. The second step is to get the most significant signal by moving the probe around the rough location while changing the angle of the probe against the skin; and finally, the wrist pulse signal can be recorded and saved in the form of Doppler spectrograms.

These three steps are repeated several times to collect several measurements of a subject so that the measurement error can be reduced. Compared with detecting pulse signal by using the pressure sensor, which is heavily interfered by the artery blood flowing in the wrist, capturing pulse signal through ultrasound scanning is more accurate by locating the probe directly on the styloid processes. In addition, ultrasound scanning can provide new information, which is not available by using the pressure sensor, because it can reflect the deep radial artery changes beneath the skin [18, 19].

Figure 12.2a shows the collected Doppler ultrasonic spectrogram of a typical wrist pulse signal. Before extracting features, the collected wrist pulse samples are preprocessed. First, the maximum velocity envelope of each spectrogram is extracted in order to reduce dimension of the signal (see Fig. 12.2b). Afterward, the low-frequency drift and high-frequency noise contained in the maximum velocity envelopes should be removed without the phase shift distortion. In this chapter, both the low-frequency drift and the high-frequency noise can be reduced simply by using a seven-level "db6" wavelet transform [20]. By subtracting the seventh level wavelet approximation coefficients, the low-frequency drift of the waveform is eliminated. Similarly, the high-frequency noise can be removed by subtracting the first level wavelet detail coefficients from the waveform. The result of drift and noise removal is shown in Fig. 12.2c.

It can be seen from Fig. 12.2 that the wrist pulse signal is not a random process but a cyclic wave with regularly occurring systolic and diastolic waves, which is confirmed in [21]. In this study, a sampled pulse signal is segmented into

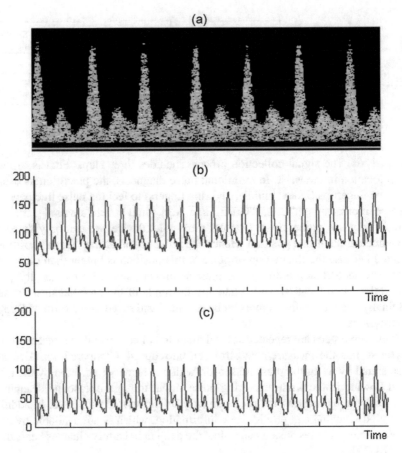

Fig. 12.2 (**a**) A typical wrist pulse Doppler spectrogram, (**b**) the maximum velocity envelope of this Doppler spectrogram, and (**c**) the wrist pulse signal after denoising and drift removal

single-period waveforms for further analysis. The procedures to extract each period are described as follows (illustrated in Fig. 12.3):

Step 1.   Perform the Fourier transform to find out the base frequency, denoted as f, of the signal. Then the base period T is calculated as $T = 1/f$.

Step 2.   Detect the peak point of the pulse signal within the time interval $[0, T]$. The obtained peak point, denoted as P_1, is the maximum point of the first period, and its corresponding time instant is t_1.

Step 3.   After t_1 is determined, we can find out the second peak point P_2 within the time interval $[t_1 + (T/2), t_1 + (3\ T/2)]$. Its corresponding time instant is denoted as t_2. The time interval between the two peak points P_1 and P_2 is calculated as $T' = t_2 - t_1$.

Step 4.   Similarly, the next peak point P_3 can be detected within the time interval $[t_2 + (T'/2), t_2 + (3\ T'/2)]$, and its corresponding time instant is t_3. It should

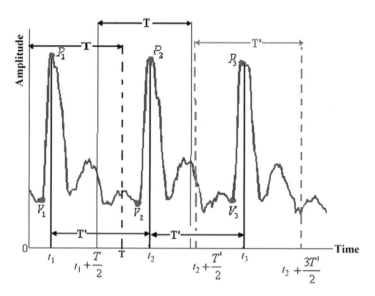

Fig. 12.3   Illustration of the wrist pulse signal segmentation process

be noted that T' is used here instead of T. The time interval between P_2 and P_3 is denoted as $T' = t_3 - t_2$.

Step 5.   Repeat step 4 until all the peak points for the pulse signal are detected. These peak points are denoted as P_i, $i = 1, \ldots, n$.

Step 6.   Once the peak points are detected, we can search for the start points on the left side of each peak point. On the left side of each P_i ($i = 2, \ldots, n$), find out the local minimum point (denoted as V_i) which is nearest to the Pi. The corresponding time instant of V_i is denoted as t_i'.

As a result, each start point Vi of the pulse signal can be detected. The pulse signal at each time interval $[t_i', t_{i+1}']$ ($i = 2, \ldots, n$) consists of two complete waves: a systolic wave and a diastolic wave. Thus the pulse signal can be partitioned into multiple cycles according to the start points (e.g., see Fig. 12.4).

12.3   Feature Extraction and Feature Selection

12.3.1   A Two-Term Gaussian Model

With the method described in Sect. 12.2, the wrist pulse signal can be partitioned into several single-period waveforms for further feature extraction. Figure 12.5a shows one typical period of a wrist pulse signal. A further examination of the waveform in Fig. 12.5a reveals that this single-period wrist pulse signal can be seen as the superimposition of two waves: a primary wave with higher amplitude and a

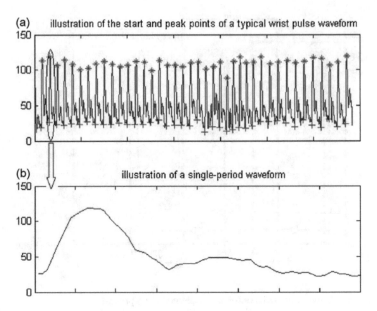

Fig. 12.4 (**a**) Illustration of the start and peak points for a typical wrist pulse signal; (**b**) a single-period waveform of the wrist pulse signal divided using the start point

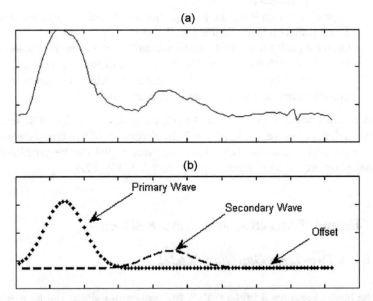

Fig. 12.5 Illustration of the decomposition of a single-period wrist pulse waveform. (**a**) A typical one-period wrist pulse waveform. (**b**) Two waves

secondary wave with lower amplitude and a phase shift. This distinctive characteristic is caused by the rhythmic contraction and relaxation of the heart [22]. The primary wave, also called as the systolic component, is generated when the left ventricle of the heart is in contraction forcing blood into the aorta. The secondary wave is due to the phenomenon of wave reflection, which is an echo of the primary wave and usually occurring when the left ventricle of the heart is in relaxation following systole. The primary wave mainly contains information of the heart itself while the secondary wave contains information of the reflection sites and the periphery of the arterial system [22]. Moreover, the secondary wave tends to increase the load to the heart and plays a major role in determining the wrist pulse waveform patterns [23]. Therefore, how to extract these two waves, particularly the secondary wave from the wrist pulse signal is crucial for diagnosis.

Since both of the two waves are "bell-shaped" curves with relative phase shift to each other, the pulse signal in Fig. 12.5a can be expressed by a two-term Gaussian function with an offset:

$$f(x\,|\,A_1,\tau_1,\sigma_1,A_2,\tau_2,\sigma_2,d) = A_1 * e^{-((x-\tau_1)/\sigma_1)^2} + A_2 * e^{-((x-\tau_2)/\sigma_2)^2} + d, \quad (12.1)$$

where the primary wave and the secondary wave are extracted as $A_1^* e^{-((x-\tau_1)/\sigma_1)^2} + d$ and $A_2^* e^{-((x-\tau_2)/\sigma_2)^2} + d$, respectively (refer to Fig. 12.5b). It can be seen from Eq. (12.1) that there exist seven coefficients in the Gaussian model: $A_1, A_2, r_1, r_2, a_1, a_2,$ and d. Among them, A_1 and A_2 determine the amplitudes of the two waves, d is the offset, r_1 and r_2 are the phases of the two waves, while σ_1 and σ_2 determine the width of two bell-shaped waves.

These coefficients are obtained by using the nonlinear least squares formulation to fit the Gaussian model to the wrist pulse signal. For simplicity, we assume that the Gaussian model for data fitting can be expressed as:

$$y = f(X,\beta) + \varepsilon, \quad (12.2)$$

where y is an n-by-1 wrist pulse signal, f is a function of β and X, β is a parameter vector including the seven coefficients in the Gaussian model, X is the n-by-m design matrix for the model, and ε is an n-by-1 vector of errors.

The fitting process can then be determined as follows:

Step 1.   Initial estimate of each parameter. Based on our experimental experience, some reasonable starting values of these parameters are made.

Step 2.   Produce the fitted curve for the current set of coefficients. The fitted response value $\hat{y}$ is given by $\hat{y} = f(X,\beta)$ and involves the calculation of the Jacobian of $f(X,\beta)$, which is defined as a matrix of partial derivatives taken with respect to the coefficients.

Step 3.   Adjust the coefficients and determine whether the fit improves. The direction and magnitude of the adjustment depend on the fitting algorithm. Some algorithms, such as trust-region [24], Levenberg-Marquardt [25], and Gauss-Newton [26], can be the options. In this study, trust-region

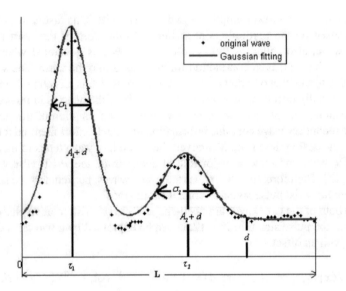

Fig. 12.6 Gaussian model fitting parameters for a typical single-period waveform

             algorithm is selected because it can solve difficult nonlinear problems
             more efficiently than the other algorithms.

Step 4.   Iterate the process by returning to step 2 until the fit reaches the specified
             convergence criteria.

    As an example, Fig. 12.6 shows an original wrist pulse signal in a single-period
and its Gaussian fitting result. It can be seen that the fitted curve using the two-term
Gaussian model is in good agreement with the original signal.

    Except for the above Gaussian parameters, the length of the single-period wave-
form L is also calculated. After we separate a wrist pulse signal into single periods,
the length of each single period can be determined (i.e., L is the number of points
between two consecutive start points V_i and V_{i+1}). To summarize, the obtained
parameters can be divided into the ones associated with magnitude, like A_1, A_2, and
d, and the ones associated with time, like r_1, r_2, a_1, a_2, and L. These parameters are
illustrated in Fig. 12.6 as well.

    By using the curve fitting technology, the models of the primary wave and sec-
ondary wave in the pulse signal can be obtained. Obtaining parameters by Gaussian
curve fitting has two advantages. First, the noise contained in the original pulse
signal can be reduced. Second, the information contained in the primary wave and
the secondary wave can be obtained in a straightforward way. Particularly, even
when the primary wave and secondary wave contained in a pulse signal cannot be
easily distinguished either because of noise or because of the intrinsic characteristic
of the pulse signal, this curve fitting using Gaussian model can still reliably extract
related parameters.

    After the Gaussian model has been identified, the parameters $\{A_i, r_i, a_i, L\}$ ($i = 1$,
2), which represent the amplitude, phase, and shape information of the two waves

Table 12.1 Feature candidates for wrist pulse signals

Relative parameter	Parameter value
Ratio of the amplitude of the primary wave to the amplitude of the secondary waves	A_2/A_1
Ratio of the phase of the primary wave to the phase of the secondary waves	τ_2/τ_1
Ratio of the shape of the primary wave to the shape of the secondary waves	σ_2/σ_1
Ratio of the phase of the primary wave to the length of a single-period waveform	τ_1/L
Ratio of the phase of the secondary wave to the length of a single-period waveform	τ_2/L
Ratio of the shape of the primary wave to the length of a single-period waveform	σ_1/L
Ratio of the phase of the secondary wave to the length of a single-period waveform	σ_2/L

as well as the length information, can be obtained. Generally, the relative values between these two waves can provide more reliable information and therefore are taken as feature candidates. The seven relative values used in this research are illustrated in Table 12.1. A feature vector, which represents the characteristics of a single-period waveform, is then constructed using these relative values.

12.3.2   Feature Selection

In the previous section, we have used a Gaussian model to extract a feature vector for a single-period of a wrist pulse signal. However, there may be some closely correlated parameters in the feature vector, and these parameters need to be eliminated. Since a typical wrist pulse signal contains many periods, a "pool" of feature vectors, each corresponds to one period of the pulse signal, is obtained. The feature vectors for a typical pulse signal are illustrated in Fig. 12.7. It can be seen that the feature will vary with the period. The correlation coefficient matrix of these features is shown in Table 12.2. It can be seen that there exist three tightly correlated feature pairs: $(\tau_2/\tau_1, \tau_1/L)$, $(\sigma_2/\sigma_1, \sigma_2/L)$, and $(\tau_2/L, \tau_1/L)$. Since these pairs of features provide similar information, using only one feature from each pair is enough for classification. The redundant features, such as τ_1/L, τ_2/L, and τ_2/L, can then be eliminated from the feature vector.

So far a feature vector has been obtained which contains no tightly correlated elements. However, the remaining elements in this feature vector are still subject to further selection. Since the purpose of the study is for disease diagnosis, only the disease-sensitive features are required. A statistical difference based approach is used here to select the disease-sensitive features. Assuming a training dataset is available which contains N_1 wrist pulse signals from the healthy persons and N_2 pulse signals from the patients. For a given feature ˌ as an example, a group of this

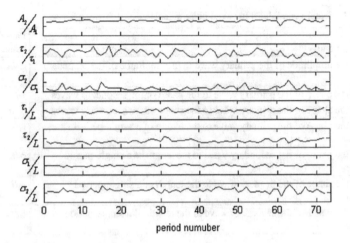

Fig. 12.7 Variability of the Gaussian fitting parameters of a wrist pulse waveform

Table 12.2 Cross-correlation coefficients for the features

	A_2/A_1	τ_2/τ_1	σ_2/σ_1	τ_1/L	τ_2/L	σ_1/L	σ_2/L
A_2/A_1	1.00	0.16	0.19	−0.28	−0.39	−0.17	0.35
τ_2/τ_1	0.16	1.00	−0.25	−0.90	−0.33	0.36	−0.04
σ_2/σ_1	0.19	−0.25	1.00	0.02	−0.35	−0.30	0.86
τ_1/L	−0.28	−0.90	0.02	1.00	0.79	−0.16	−0.13
τ_2/L	−0.39	−0.33	−0.35	0.79	1.00	0.31	−0.30
σ_1/L	−0.17	0.36	0.36	−0.16	0.31	1.00	0.15
σ_2/L	0.35	−0.04	0.86	−0.13	−0.30	0.15	1.00

feature for the healthy person, denoted as $\{\alpha\}_H = \{\{\alpha\}_{H,1}, \{\alpha\}_{H,2}, \ldots, \{\alpha\}_{H,N1}\}$, is established, where $\{\alpha\}_{H,i}$ ($i = 1, \ldots, N_1$) is the features extracted from the ith healthy person. Similarly, a group of this feature for patients with a certain decease is established and is denoted as $\{\alpha\}_P = \{\{\alpha\}_{P,1}, \{\alpha\}_{P,2}, \ldots, \{\alpha\}_{P,N2}\}$, where $\{\alpha\}_{P,i}$ ($i = 1, \ldots, N_2$) is the features extracted from the ith patients. The statistical difference between these two groups can be calculated as:

$$\text{statistical difference of } \alpha = \frac{\#\overline{\{\alpha\}}_H - \overline{\{\alpha\}}_P\#}{S_{\overline{\{\alpha\}}_H, \overline{\{\alpha\}}_P}}, \tag{12.3}$$

where $\overline{\{\alpha\}}_H$ and $\overline{\{\alpha\}}_P$ are the means of $\{\alpha\}_H$ and $\{\alpha\}_P$, respectively. $S_{\overline{\{\alpha\}}_H, \overline{\{\alpha\}}_P}$ is defined as:

$$S_{\overline{\{\alpha\}}_H, \overline{\{\alpha\}}_P} = \sqrt{\frac{S_1^2}{N_1} + \frac{S_2^2}{N_2}}, \tag{12.4}$$

where S_1^2 and S_2^2 are the variances of $\{\alpha\}_H$ and $\{\alpha\}_P$, respectively.

For each feature, its statistical difference between the healthy persons and patients with a certain disease reflects the sensitivity of this feature to the disease; therefore, the statistical difference determines whether this feature should be selected. If the statistical difference of a feature is relatively large, then this feature is a good indicator for this disease and should be selected for classification. Otherwise, the feature is not good enough and should not be used.

12.4 FCM Clustering

The selected features are then used as inputs to the classifier for further pattern classification, which is to determine from these features that whether the pulse signals are from healthy persons or from patients with certain disease. In this study, a FCM classifier is adopted.

Clustering is a common technique for statistical data analysis. It aims to cluster data points into clusters so that items in the same class are as similar as possible and items in different classes are as dissimilar as possible [27]. There are many algorithms for fuzzy clustering, and the FCM is one of the most widely used ones [28]. In this study, after selecting the disease-sensitive features, we use the FCM to make the pattern classification. The FCM is used in this study due to it ability to classify data belonging to two or more groups. Moreover, another aspect of the FCM is the use of membership function, which means an object can belong to several clusters at the same time but with different degrees. Such characteristic is important for the disease diagnosis.

12.5 Experimental Result

By collaborating with the Harbin 211 hospital (Harbin, Heilongjiang Province, China), we collected the wrist pulse signals using a Doppler ultrasonic blood analyzer from both healthy persons (100 samples) and patients with different diseases (88 samples). Half of these data, which are randomly selected, are used for the training purpose, and the remaining data are used for testing. The testing dataset includes 50 signals from healthy persons (Group H), 23 signals from patients with pancreatitis (Group P), and 21 signals from patients with duodenal bulb ulcer (Group DBU).

As was described previously, these signals are first partitioned into single-period waveforms. Then the modified Gaussian model is used to fit each single-period waveform. As an example, Fig. 12.8 illustrates three pulse signals (single-period), which are from Group H, Group P, and Group DBU, respectively, as well as the corresponding fitting results using Gaussian models. The values of the Gaussian fitting

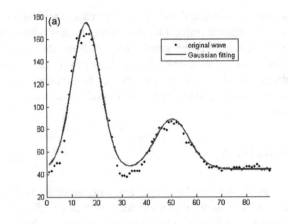

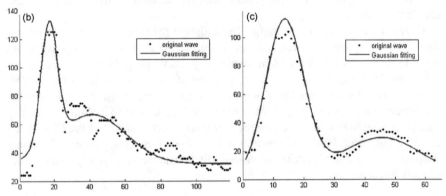

Fig. 12.8 Gaussian curve fitting results for (**a**) a healthy person, (**b**) a pancreatitis patient, and (**c**) a DBU patient, respectively, where the dots represent the single-period wrist pulse waveform and the solid line is its Gaussian fitting result

Table 12.3 Gaussian fitting parameters for a healthy person (Group H), a pancreatitis patient (Group P), and a DBU patient (Group DBU)

Gaussian fitting parameters	A_1	A_2	τ_1	τ_1	σ_1	σ_2	L
Group H	130.4	44.6	15.8	50.3	8.0	9.6	90
Group P	85.7	34.7	17.0	41.5	6.7	26.6	120
Group DBU	110.2	27.8	13.8	45.4	8.7	18.7	63

parameters A_1, A_2, r_1, r_2, a_1, a_2 and the length of each waveform L are calculated (see Table 12.3).

As was discussed in Sect. 12.3.2, the cross-correlation analysis is used to find out the tightly correlated features. Tables 12.4, 12.5, and 12.6 show the mean value of the cross-correlation coefficients for Group H (Table 12.4), Group P (Table 12.5), and Group DBU (Table 12.6). All these calculations are based on the training data-set. Two observations can be reached from these tables: first, the magnitude-related

Table 12.4 Mean cross-correlation coefficients for Group H

	A_2/A_1	τ_2/τ_1	σ_2/σ_1	τ_1/L	τ_2/L	σ_1/L	σ_2/L
A_2/A_1	1.00	0.24	0.08	−0.38	−0.27	−0.34	−0.03
τ_2/τ_1	0.24	1.00	−0.41	−0.88	0.13	0.42	−0.23
σ_2/σ_1	0.08	−0.41	1.00	0.24	−0.40	−0.43	0.91
τ_1/L	−0.38	−0.88	0.24	1.00	0.34	−0.19	0.15
τ_2/L	−0.27	0.13	−0.40	0.34	1.00	0.46	−0.24
σ_1/L	−0.34	0.42	−0.43	−0.19	0.46	1.00	−0.02
σ_2/L	0.03	−0.23	0.91	0.15	−0.24	−0.02	1.00

Table 12.5 Mean cross-correlation coefficients for Group P

	A_2/A_1	τ_2/τ_1	σ_2/σ_1	τ_1/L	τ_2/L	σ_1/L	σ_2/L
A_2/A_1	1.00	0.43	0.62	0.35	0.29	0.07	0.68
τ_2/τ_1	0.43	1.00	−0.29	0.89	0.22	0.37	0.85
σ_2/σ_1	0.62	−0.29	1.00	−0.43	−0.10	0.08	0.10
τ_1/L	0.35	0.89	−0.43	1.00	0.77	0.25	0.79
τ_2/L	0.29	0.22	−0.10	0.77	1.00	0.01	0.38
σ_1/L	0.07	0.37	0.08	0.25	0.01	1.00	0.33
σ_2/L	0.68	0.85	0.10	0.79	0.38	0.33	1.00

Table 12.6 Mean cross-correlation coefficients for Group DBU

	A_2/A_1	τ_2/τ_1	σ_2/σ_1	τ_1/L	τ_2/L	σ_1/L	σ_2/L
A_2/A_1	1.00	−0.09	−0.10	0.18	0.24	−0.12	−0.06
τ_2/τ_1	−0.09	1.00	−0.14	−0.84	−0.39	0.47	−0.02
σ_2/σ_1	−0.10	−0.14	1.00	−0.30	−0.70	−0.85	0.94
τ_1/L	0.18	−0.84	−0.30	1.00	0.82	−0.08	−0.43
τ_2/L	0.24	−0.39	−0.70	0.82	1.00	0.41	−0.79
σ_1/L	−0.12	0.47	−0.85	−0.08	0.41	1.00	−0.78
σ_2/L	−0.06	−0.02	0.94	−0.43	−0.79	−0.78	1.00

feature, for example, $A2/A1$, is not correlated with the time-relevant features, such as τ_2/τ_1 and σ_2/σ_1, and second, for all the three groups, two tightly correlated pairs can be detected: $(\tau_2/\tau_1, \tau_1/L)$ and $(\sigma_2/\sigma_1, \sigma_2/L)$.

As a result, two features can be eliminated because of the two tightly correlated pairs. The resulted feature vector contains five features: A_2/A_1 τ_2/τ_1, σ_2/σ_1, τ_2/L, and σ_1/L. The statistical differences of the selected features are calculated and the results are shown in Table 12.7. Again, the calculation is based on the training dataset. It can be seen that the feature σ_2/σ_1, which has the largest statistical difference, is the best parameter to be used in order to distinguish between Group H and Group P. Similarly, the other two features τ_2/L and A_2/A_1 can also be selected due to their relatively large statistical difference for all these three groups. In conclusion, three

Table 12.7 The statistical differences of the selected features for the three groups

	Group H vs. Group P	Group H vs. Group DBU	Group P vs. Group DBU
A_2/A_1	7.01	5.65	8.98
τ_2/τ_1	3.71	2.15	4.62
σ_2/σ_1	14.29	7.79	9.47
τ_2/L	8.64	8.61	10.36
σ_1/L	1.53	2.96	4.01

Table 12.8 Classification result using FCM

Sample class	Testing samples	Classification results	Accuracy (%) (Gaussian model)		Accuracy (%) (AR model [18])		Accuracy (%) (WT method [13])	
Group H	50	48(2)	96.0	94.5	88.9	86.3	86.7	84.8
Group P	23	21(2)	91.3		80.6		80.5	
Group H	50	42(8)	84.0	85.9	85.7	82.3	88.9	85.4
Group DBU	21	19(2)	90.4		74.3		77.1	
Group P	23	21(2)	91.3	90.9	85.7	87.3	80.6	82.2
Group DBU	21	19(2)	90.4		88.9		83.7	
Group H	50	48(2)	84.0	85.1	86.0	78.9	82.0	71.7
Group DBU	21	21(2)	76.2		77.1		72.7	
Group P	23	42(8)	95.7		73.5		60.0	

features (σ_2/σ_1, τ_2/L, and A_2/A_1) with relatively large statistical difference for all the three groups are selected as the features for classification.

The classification results on the testing dataset using the FCM classifier are shown in Table 12.8. It can be seen that an accuracy of 94.5% is obtained in distinguishing the Group H and Group P using feature a2/a1 alone, which means only 2 of the 50 healthy persons and 2 of the 23 pancreatitis patients are misclassified. The classification result for the healthy person and DBU patients is relatively low, which confirms the previous results of statistical difference in Table 12.7. By mixing all these three groups together, the accuracy of the classification can still reach 85%, which is quite encouraging because no previous work has been done in distinguishing more than two groups. In Table 12.8, the classification results of the proposed method are compared with the previous wavelet transform method [13] and the auto-regressive method [18]. It can be found that the proposed method can provide a better classification accuracy (i.e., about 8% higher than the AR model for distinguishing healthy person and patients with pancreatitis). This result indicates that the proposed method has a great potential in pulse diagnosis for the current situation.

12.6 Summary

A modified Gaussian model was proposed in this chapter to extract useful features from each single-period waveform of a wrist pulse signal. The features were then selected by using the cross-correlation analysis and the statistical difference calculation. The performance of the selected parameters was evaluated using the established testing dataset, including both healthy persons and patients. The experimental results demonstrate that the proposed method performs well for the current research: an accuracy of over 90% can be reached in distinguishing the healthy person from the patients with some specific types of diseases. Moreover, an accuracy of over 85% can be reached in distinguishing healthy persons from the mixed kinds of diseases.

References

1. Lukman S, He Y, Hui S. "Computational methods for traditional Chinese medicine: a survey," Computer Methods and Programs in Biomedicine 2007;88:283–94.
2. Hammer L. Chinese pulse diagnosis—contemporary approach. Eastland Press; 2001.
3. Zhu L, Yan J, Tang Q, Li Q. "Recent progress in computerization of TCM," Journal of Communication and Computer 2006;3(7).
4. Wang K, Xu L, Zhang D, Shi C. "TCPD based pulse monitoring and analyzing," In: Proceedings of the 1st ICMLC conference. 2002.
5. Wang H, Cheng Y. "A quantitative system for pulse diagnosis in Traditional Chinese Medicine," In: Proceedings of the 27th IEEE EMB conference. 2005.
6. Lau E, Chwang A. "Relationship between wrist-pulse characteristics and body conditions," In: Proceedings of the EM2000 conference. 2000.
7. Lu W, Wang Y, Wang W. "Pulse analysis of patients with severe liver problems," IEEE Engineering in Medicine and Biology Magazine 1999;18(January/February (1)):73–5.
8. Wang B, Luo J, Xiang J, Yang Y. "Power spectral analysis of human pulse and study of traditional Chinese medicine pulse-diagnosis mechanism," Journal of Northwestern University (Natural Science Edition) 2001;31(1):22–5.
9. Wang Y, Wu X, Liu B, Yi Y. "Definition and application of indices in Doppler ultrasound sonogram," Journal of Biomedical Engineering of Shanghai 1997;18:26–9.
10. Ruano M, Fish P. "Cost/benefit criterion for selection of pulsed Doppler ultrasound spectral mean frequency and bandwidth estimators," IEEE Transactions on BME 1993;40:1338–41.
11. Leonard P, Beattie TF, Addison PS, Watson JN. "Wavelet analysis of pulse oximeter waveform permits identification of unwell children," Journal of Emergency Medicine 2004;21:59–60.
12. Zhang Y, Wang Y, Wang W, Yu J. "Wavelet feature extraction and classification of Doppler ultrasound blood flow signals," Journal of Biomedical Engineering 2002;19(2):244–6.
13. Zhang D, Zhang L, Zhang D, Zheng Y. "Wavelet based analysis of Doppler ultrasonic wrist-pulse signals," In: Proceedings of the ICBBE 2008 conference, vol. 2. 2008. p. 539–43.
14. Chen B, Wang X, Yang S, McGreavy C. "Application of wavelets and neural networks to diagnostic system development, 1, feature extraction," Computers and Chemical Engineering 1999;23:899–906.
15. Heral A, Hou Z. "Application of wavelet approach for ASCE structural health monitoring benchmark studies," Journal of Engineering Mechanics 2004;1:96–104.

16. Burges C. "A tutorial on support vector machines for pattern recognition," Data Mining and Knowledge Discovery 1998;2:121–67.
17. Chiu C, Yeh S, Yu Y. "Classification of the pulse signals based on self-organizing neural network for the analysis of the autonomic nervous system," Chinese Journal of Medical and Biological Engineering 1996;16: 461–76.
18. Chen Y, Zhang L, Zhang D, Zhang D. "Pattern classification for Doppler ultrasonic wrist pulse signals," In: 5th ICBBE conference. 2009.
19. Yoon Y, Lee M, Soh K. "Pulse type classification by varying contact pressure," IEEE Engineering in Medicine and Biology Magazine 2000;19:106–10.
20. Xu L, Zhang D, Wang K. "Wavelet-based cascaded adaptive filter for removing baseline drift in pulse waveforms," IEEE Transactions on Biomedical Engineering 2005;52(11):1973–5.
21. Xia C, Li Y, Yan J, Wang Y, Yan H, Guo R, et al. "A practical approach to wrist pulse segmentation and single-period average waveform estimation," In: The ICBEI conference. 2008. p. 334–8.
22. Walsh S, King E. Pulse diagnosis: a clinical guide. Elsevier; 2007.
23. Shu J, Sun Y. "Developing classification indices for Chinese pulse diagnosis," Complementary Therapies in Medicine 2007;15:190–8.
24. More JJ. "Recent developments in algorithms and software for trust region methods," In: Mathematical programming. NY: Springer-Verlag; 1983. p. 258–87.
25. Mor JJ. The Levenberg–Marquardt algorithm: implementation and theory. Berlin/Heidelberg: Springer; 2006.
26. Jorge N, Stephen W. Numerical optimization. New York: Springer; 1999.
27. Bezdek JC. Pattern recognition with fuzzy objective function algorithms, New York: Plenum Press; 1981.
28. Wang X, Wang Y, Wang L. "Improving fuzzy c-means clustering based on feature weight learning," Pattern Recognition Letters 2004;25:1123–32.

Chapter 13
Modified Auto-regressive Models

Abstract This chapter aims to present a novel time series analysis approach to analyze wrist pulse signals. First, a data normalization procedure is proposed. This procedure selects a reference signal that is "closest" to a newly obtained signal from an ensemble of signals recorded from the healthy persons. Second, an auto-regressive (AR) model is constructed from the selected reference signal. Then, the residual error, which is the difference between the actual measurement for the new signal and the prediction obtained from the AR model established by reference signal, is defined as the disease-sensitive feature. This approach is based on the premise that if the signal is from a patient, the prediction model previously identified using the healthy persons would not be able to reproduce the time series measured from the patients. The applicability of this approach is demonstrated using a wrist pulse signal database collected using a Doppler ultrasound device. The classification accuracy is over 82% in distinguishing healthy persons from patients with acute appendicitis and over 90% for other diseases. These results indicate a great promise of the proposed method in telling healthy subjects from patients of specific diseases.

13.1 Introduction

Wrist pulse signals contain vital information of health activities and can reflect the pathologic changes of a person's body condition. Therefore, the practitioners can tell the health conditions of a patient by feeling his wrist pulses, and this method has been used in traditional Chinese medicine for thousands of years. Modern clinical studies demonstrate that there is premature loss of arterial elasticity and endothelial function for patients with certain diseases, such as hypertension, hypercholesterolemia, and diabetes [1]. Such loss will eventually decrease the flexibility of vasculature while increasing the stress to the circulatory system. As a result, the shape, amplitude, and rhythm of patient wrist pulses will also alter in correspondence with the hemodynamic characteristics of blood flow [1].

Although traditional Chinese pulse diagnosis has been attracting more attention in recent years, the wrist pulse assessment is a matter of technical skill and subjective

© Springer Nature Singapore Pte Ltd. 2018   247
D. Zhang et al., *Computational Pulse Signal Analysis*,
https://doi.org/10.1007/978-981-10-4044-3_13

experience [2]. The intuitional accuracy mainly depends upon the individual's persistent practice and quality of sensitive awareness. Different practitioners may not give identical diagnosis results for the same patient. Therefore, it is necessary to develop computational pulse signal analysis techniques to standardize and objectify the pulse diagnosis method. A couple of methods have been proposed to analyze the digitized pulse signals [3–7]. For example, Leonard et al. [3] revealed that it is possible to distinguish healthy and unwell children by using wavelet power features and wavelet entropy of the pulse signal. Zhang et al. [4] proposed a wavelet transform-based method to extract features from carotid blood flow signals and used a back-propagation (BP) neural network to make the classification among 30 samples. Some other researchers [5, 6] also proved that it is possible to identify human sub-health status based on pulse signals by using linear discriminant classifier. Moreover, Zhang et al. [7] used the wavelet method to extract different pulse features, including wavelet powers, wavelet packet powers, and Doppler ultrasonic diagnostic parameters. Although some of the above methods have achieved encouraging results, their effectiveness are still subject to further assessment due to the limited number of samples and types of diseases. For example, in Leonard's research [3], only 20 samples are used to distinguish well and unwell children, while in Zhang's research [7], two kinds of diseases are investigated.

In this chapter, an auto-regressive (AR)-based method is proposed to extract the pulse signal features. Since a wrist pulse signal is in essence a time series, using AR model can help to describe the characteristic of this signal and therefore to capture its important features. This AR model is first trained based on the healthy samples and then it is used to predict the input signal. The mean and variance of the prediction error are calculated and selected as features. Except for the AR features, some Doppler ultrasonic diagnosis parameters are also investigated in order to see if they can be helpful to improve the classification accuracy. The selected features are then taken as inputs to a support vector machine (SVM) for pattern classification because the SVM performs well on problems with low training set sizes. The applicability of the proposed method is tested on the established dataset including 100 healthy persons and 148 patients of diseases. There are four kinds of diseases investigated in this chapter, i.e., 46 patients with pancreatitis (P), 42 with duodenal bulb ulcer (DBU), 22 with appendicitis (A), and 38 with acute appendicitis (AA). It can be seen that both the sample numbers and disease types are much larger than those of previous researches mentioned above.

The rest of the chapter is organized as follows. "The Proposed Method" section presents the proposed method. The "Experimental Results" section performs experiments to validate the developed technique. The "Conclusions and Future Work" section concludes the chapter and makes some discussion.

13.2   The Proposed Method

13.2.1   Feature Extraction via AR Modelling

AR models [8] are widely used in time series analysis, control, and signal prediction. Considering the fact that wrist pulse signals are naturally a time series, the AR model can be used to analyze the time series and then extract the disease-sensitive features. Then, one branch of statistical hypothesis tests called support vector machine (SVM) is applied to the aforementioned features to classify the current subject to either a patient or a healthy person.

When one attempts to apply the time series analysis to the real-world data, it is important to normalize these data in an effort to account for operational and environmental variability. For the wrist pulse signals collected by using the Doppler ultrasound device, the ability to normalize the measured data with respect to varying operational and environmental conditions is essential if one is to avoid false-positive classification. Therefore, each wrist pulse signal $f(t)$ is normalized prior to fitting an AR model:

$$\hat{f}(t) = \frac{f(t) - m_f}{\delta_f}, \tag{13.1}$$

where m_f and δ_f are the mean and standard deviation of $f(t)$, respectively. The reference signal, denoted as $\bar{f}(t)$, is obtained by averaging the normalized pulse signals $\hat{f}(t)$ from all the available training samples from healthy persons. The reference AR model with n terms is then constructed as:

$$\bar{f}(t) = \sum_{i=1}^{n} a_i \bar{f}(t-i) + \varepsilon_f(t), \tag{13.2}$$

where a_i $(i = 1,2,\ldots,n)$ is the ith AR coefficient and $\varepsilon_f(t)$ is a term representing the modelling error. The order of this AR model can be determined by the Akaike information criteria (AIC) [9] and the AR coefficients are calculated using the least square method [10].

After the reference AR model is identified, it is used to fit the input normalized pulse signals. For a given wrist pulse signal $g(t)$, which is obtained from a person with unknown healthy status, it is fitted by the reference AR model as follows:

$$\varepsilon_g(t) = g(t) \partial \sum_{i=t}^{n} a_i g(t-i), \tag{13.3}$$

where $\varepsilon_g(t)$ is the prediction error, representing the discrepancy between the input pulse signal and the reference AR model. The mean and standard deviation of $\varepsilon_g(t)$, denoted by mean_ε_g and std_ε_g, can then be calculated.

Factors like age, gender, and the environment of collecting the data may also affect the sampled wrist pulse waveforms. However, it has been validated in traditional Chinese medicine that these factors mainly affect the amplitude and rhythm, while the waveform shapes, which are used in this chapter, are less affected [11]. Moreover, the shape of a wrist pulse waveform is mainly dependent on the type of the disease. It can be expected that when a pulse signal is from a healthy person, the reference model which is trained from healthy persons will accurately predict the signal. As a result, the mean and the standard deviation of the prediction error are relatively small. Otherwise, when a pulse signal is from a patient, the reference AR model will not be able to well predict the signal, and the mean and the standard deviation of the prediction error are expected to increase. Therefore, for a given wrist pulse signal $g(t)$, the associate mean_ε_g and std_ε_g values are significant features for the classification of $g(t)$.

13.2.2   SVM Classification

After the pulse signal features have been extracted, an SVM [12] is employed to classify this signal as being from either healthy persons or patients. Particularly, a soft-margin SVM is adopted in this study. SVM is a supervised learning method for classification. Given a set of points of the form:

$$D = \left\{ \left(\mathbf{x}_i, y_i \right) \middle| \mathbf{x}_i \in R^P, y_i \in \left\{ -1, 1 \right\} \right\}_{i=1}^n ,$$

(13.4)

where y_i is either 1 or -1, indicating the class to which the point x_i belongs. Each x_i is a p-dimensional real vector. The aim of the SVM is to find a separating hyperplane which maximizes the margin between the points having $y_i = 1$ and those having $y_i = -1$. This hyperplane can be expressed as:

$$\mathbf{w} \cdot \mathbf{x} - b = 0,$$

(13.5)

where w is a vector and perpendicular to the hyperplane and b is the offset. It can be found that the width of the margin is $2/\|w\|$, where $\|\cdot\|$ represents the Euclidean norm. In case there is no hyperplane that can split the two data sets, the soft-margin SVM will choose a hyperplane that splits the two data sets as cleanly as possible while maximizing the distance to the nearest cleanly split examples [12]. The soft-margin SVM introduces slack variables ξ_i which measure the degree of misclassification of the datum x_i:

$$y_i \left(\mathbf{w} \cdot \mathbf{x} - b \right) \geq 1 - \xi_i, 1 \leq i \leq n.$$

(13.6)

The objective function then becomes:

$$\min_{w,b,\xi} \frac{1}{2}\mathbf{w}^2 + C\sum_{i-1}^{n}\xi_i$$

$$s.t. \ y_i\left(\mathbf{w}^T \cdot x_i - b\right) \geq 1 - \xi_i, \text{and } \xi \geq 0,$$

(13.7)

where C is the trade-off parameter. Standard quadratic programming technique is used to solve this constrained optimization problem [12].

13.2.3   The Selection of Doppler Ultrasonic Diagnostic Parameters

In this research, the wrist pulse signals are collected by using a Doppler ultrasonic device. Compared with detecting pulse signal by using the pressure sensor, which is heavily interfered by the artery blood flowing in the wrist [13], capturing pulse signal through ultrasound scanning is more accurate by locating the probe directly on the styloid processes. In addition, ultrasound scanning can provide new information, which is not available by using the pressure sensor, because it can reflect the deep radial artery changes beneath the skin. Therefore, it would be interesting to see if the Doppler ultrasonic diagnosis parameters can be helpful to improve the classification accuracy. Some previous researchers have found that there are relationships between the Doppler ultrasonic parameters (which can be calculated from the Doppler spectrogram) and the status of blood flow, after applying the Doppler ultrasound technique to clinical diagnosis [14]. These ultrasonic parameters have been taken as the evidence of medical diagnosis [7, 15].

Some widely used Doppler ultrasonic diagnostic parameters are defined as follows as illustrated in Fig. 13.1 [15]:

- Time interval between onset and peak of primary wave: RT.
- Time interval between half-peak points of the ascent and decent parts of primary wave: SW.
- Spectrum broadening index (SBI): SBI = $(F_{avpk} - F_{mean})/F_{avpk}$, where F_{avpk} means frequency excursion of peak systolic velocity and F_{mean} means frequency excursion of mean velocity.
- Stenosis index (STI): STI = $0.9^*(1 - V_m/S)$, where V_m is the mean velocity.
- Resistance index(RI):RI = $(S - D)/S$.
- Ratio of systolic by diastolic velocity (S/D), where S and D are the systolic peak (maximum velocity) and the end of diastolic velocity.

It should be noted that the sensitivities of the Doppler parameters to different diseases are different. Therefore, in order to increase the accuracy of diagnosis, only the Doppler parameters which are sensitive to the diseases are selected as additional features [16]. The procedures of selecting Doppler parameters are described as follows.

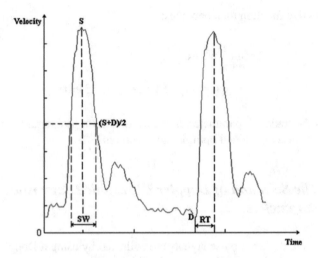

Fig. 13.1 A typical Doppler signal and some Doppler parameters

Assume that the training database contains a total of m sets of pulse signals from healthy persons and n sets of pulse signals from patients. For each pulse signal, a certain Doppler parameter can be extracted. The Doppler parameters estimated from healthy persons are denoted as $\left\{ DP_1^H ,, DP_2^H ,, \ldots DP_m^H \right\}$, and those estimated from patients, where $DP_i^H \left(i = 1, \ldots m \right)$ and $DP_i^P \left(j = 1, \ldots n \right)$, refer to the Doppler parameters estimated from a healthy person and a patient, respectively. The upper level limit (ULL) and lower level limit (LLL) of $\left\{ DP_1^H ,, DP_2^H ,, \ldots DP_m^H \right\}$ are estimated as:

$$ULL = mean\_DP^H + std\_DP^H , \tag{13.8}$$

$$LLL = mean\_DP^H - std\_DP^H , \tag{13.9}$$

where mean_DP^H and std_DP^H are the mean and standard deviation of $\left\{ DP_1^H ,, DP_2^H ,, \ldots DP_m^H \right\}$.

The obtained ULL and LLL are taken as the thresholds which discriminate patients from healthy persons. If, for example, the DP of an unknown pulse signal is within the range defined by the ULL and LLL, the signal is then classified as from a healthy person. Otherwise, we have some confidence to conclude that the signal is from a patient. Based on the above criteria, the percentage of false-positive classification (indication of a disease for a healthy person) can be estimated by counting the number of DP^H which falls outside the range defined by ULL and LLL. Similarly, the percentage of false-negative classification (no indication of disease for a patient) can be calculated by the number of DP^p which falls inside the range. If the percentages of these two false classifications are kept low, the Doppler parameter has a potential to be an effective feature to distinguish healthy persons from patients. After the Doppler parameters have been selected, these parameters are adopted as the features to the pulse signals. These features, combined with those estimated by the AR method, constitute the inputs to the SVM.

13.3 Experimental Results

13.3.1 Data Description

The wrist pulse signals used in this chapter were collected by a Doppler ultrasonic blood analyzer module (Edan Instruments, Inc.) from both healthy persons and patients who had been previously diagnosed with certain diseases. There are three steps in each measurement. First, find the rough position where the fluctuation of pulse is bigger than other positions using the probe, second move the probe slowly and carefully around the rough location, and third change the angle of the probe against the skin in order to get the most significant signals; finally, these Doppler spectrograms of wrist pulses were recorded and saved. These steps were repeated several times for each measurement to reduce the measurement errors.

By collaborating with the Harbin 211 Hospital (Harbin, Heilongjiang Province, China), an experimental database was established, including 248 wrist pulse Doppler ultrasonic blood images for testing. These pulses were collected from people at different ages and with different kinds of diseases, i.e., 100 healthy persons, 46 patients with pancreatitis (P), 42 with duodenal bulb ulcer (DBU), 22 with appendicitis (A), and 38 with acute appendicitis (AA). In this study, the experimental database is split into a training dataset and a testing dataset. For each group (healthy persons and patients), half of the data are randomly selected for the training use and the remaining are for the testing use. Table 13.1 summarizes the composition of the testing database.

The collected wrist pulse samples are preprocessed before extracting features. First, the maximum velocity envelope of each pulse waves is extracted and normalized. Then the noise and baseline drift are removed from the normalized signal. In this chapter, the wavelet transform is used to remove the noise and baseline drift [17]. Figure 13.2 shows the Doppler spectrogram of a wrist pulse signal and the extracted velocity envelope.

Table 13.1 Sample distribution of the testing database

Diseases	Age				Total
	0–20	20–40	40–60	60 and older	
Healthy	4	23	15	8	50
DBU	2	13	3	3	21
Pancreatitis	8	13	2	0	23
Appendicitis	0	11	0	0	11
Acute appendicitis	10	4	5	0	19

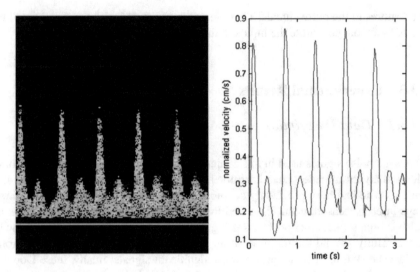

Fig. 13.2 The Doppler spectrogram of a wrist pulse signal (left) and its maximum velocity envelope after denoising (right)

13.3.2 Experimental Results by Using the AR Features

The method described in the "The proposed method" section is applied to the experimental data. As was discussed, the mean and standard deviation of the AR model prediction error $\varepsilon_g(t)$ can be used to distinguish healthy persons from patients. Therefore, these two features are taken as the inputs to the SVM for classification. Figure 13.3a–d illustrates the classification results for healthy persons versus patients with four kinds of diseases, respectively. In this figure, the estimated support vectors are marked with "o." The classification accuracies using these AR features are listed in Table 13.2. The classification accuracy corresponding to the healthy people is defined as the percentage of healthy people who are identified as not having the condition (i.e., specificity). The classification accuracy for the patients is defined as the proportion of actual patients which are correctly identified as such (i.e., sensitivity). Moreover, the average of specificity and sensitivity is also calculated as the total classification rate. It can be seen from Table 13.2 that the features extracted by the AR model work well for wrist pulse signal classification.

To demonstrate the effectiveness of normalization procedure when estimating AR features, the classification results using AR features obtained without normalization are shown in Fig. 13.4 a–d. Furthermore, the receiver operating characteristic (ROC) curve of the classifiers using normalized AR features (in Fig. 13.3) and un-normalized ones (in Fig. 13.4) is illustrated in Fig. 13.5. It can be seen from Fig. 13.5 the classifiers using normalized AR features yield 4 points in the upper left corner of the ROC space, representing high sensitivity (low false negatives) and high specificity (low false positives). On the contrary, classifiers using unnormalized AR features cannot provide comparable classification results.

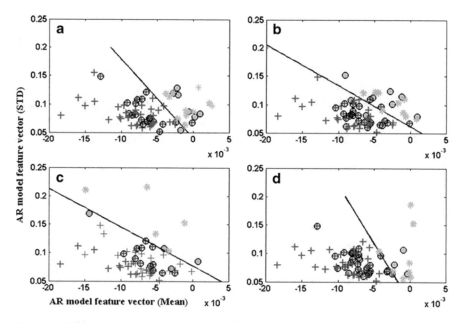

Fig. 13.3 SVM classification results using the normalized AR model: (**a**) for pancreatitis patients and the healthy persons; (**b**) for the DBU patients and the healthy persons; (**c**) for the appendicitis patients and the healthy persons; (**d**) for the acute appendicitis patients and the healthy persons

Table 13.2 Experimental results to distinguish patients from healthy people

Sample	Sample number	Accuracy (%) (AR features only)		Accuracy (%) (AR and SW features)		Accuracy (%) (WPT method [7])	
Healthy	50	73	88.9	86.3	94.4	90.9	86.7	84.8
Pancreatitis	23		80.6		83.3		80.5	
Healthy	50	71	85.7	82.3	91.4	88.0	88.9	85.4
DBU	21		74.3		80		77.1	
Healthy	50	61	90.0	88.2	93.3	91.2	76.7	76.1
Appendicitis	11		80.0		81.8		73.3	
Healthy	50	69	79.4	77.8	82.4	80.8	77.1	72.4
Acute appendicitis	19		73.5		76.5		60.6	
Healthy	50	124	86.0	83.7	89.7	87.3	82.4	80
All kinds of diseases	74		77.1		80.4		72.7	

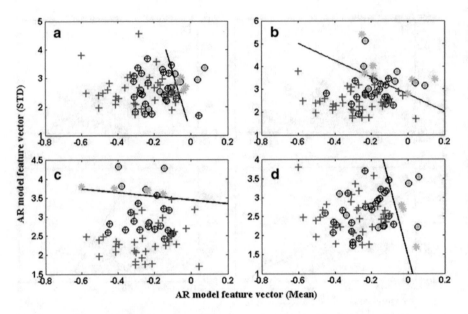

Fig. 13.4 SVM classification results using the unmoralized AR model: (**a**) for pancreatitis patients and the healthy persons; (**b**) for the DBU patients and the healthy persons; (**c**) for the appendicitis patients and the healthy persons; (**d**) for the acute appendicitis patients and the healthy persons

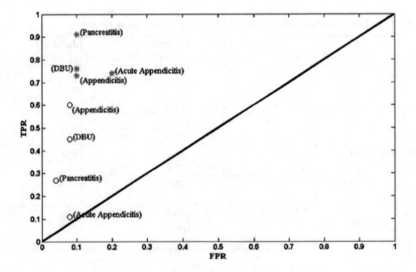

Fig. 13.5 ROC curve of the four classifiers (asterisks classifiers using normalized AR features, open circles classifiers using un-normalized AR features)

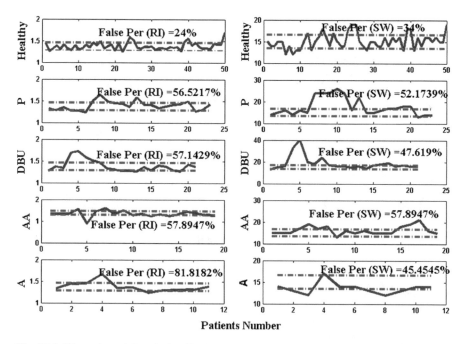

Fig. 13.6 Illustration of the misclassification percentage of the Doppler parameter RI (left) and SW (right) for healthy persons and patients with pancreatitis (P), duodenal bulb ulcer (DBU), appendicitis (A), and acute appendicitis (AA)

Table 13.3 False classification rates (%) of four Doppler parameters for different diseases

	RI	SW	RT	SD
Healthy	24.00	34.00	32.00	32.00
Pancreatitis	56.52	52.17	65.22	52.17
DBU	57.14	47.62	47.62	42.86
Appendicitis	57.89	57.89	52.63	47.37
Acute appendicitis	81.82	45.45	45.45	63.64
Average	55.48	47.43	48.58	47.61

13.3.3   Experimental Results by Using the Doppler Parameters as Additional Features

As described in the "The selection of Doppler ultrasonic diagnostic parameters" section, the sensitivities of different Doppler parameters may vary for different kinds of diseases. Choosing Doppler parameters which can distinguish healthy persons from patients would help us for further classification. As an example, Fig. 13.6 illustrates the results of the false classification test for Doppler parameters RI and SW. The ULL and LLL (dashed lines) were determined using the pulse signals from the healthy persons. Table 13.3 lists the false classification rates of four Doppler

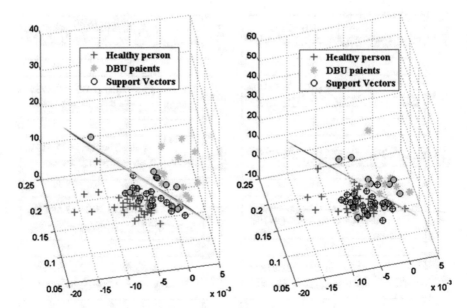

Fig. 13.7 SVM classification result to distinguish the healthy people from patients with pancreatitis (left) and healthy persons from DBU patients (right), using the AR model feature vectors (mean and standard deviation) as well as the Doppler parameter (SW)

parameters for different diseases. It can be seen that the Doppler parameter SW has lower false classification rates on average compared with other parameters and therefore is selected as a feature.

It should be noted that the false classification percentages of SW are still high, which implies that it cannot be used alone for classification. Therefore, the Doppler parameter SW should be combined with other features in order to obtain a satisfactory result.

The Doppler parameter SW was selected as the additional feature to the AR features for SVM classification. As an example, Fig. 13.7 illustrates the classification results for healthy persons versus patients with pancreatitis and DBU, respectively, and the experimental results are listed in Table 13.2. Compared with the results by using only the AR features, it is clear that the selected Doppler features further improve the classification results. In Table 13.2, we also listed the classification results in distinguishing between healthy persons and unhealthy persons (i.e., all the patients with four kinds of disease). Moreover, the results by using the wavelet packet transform (WPT) method introduced in [7] are also shown in Table 13.2 for comparison. It can be seen the proposed method outperforms much the WPT method in most of the cases.

13.4   Conclusions and Future Work

An auto-regressive (AR) modeling method was proposed to extract features from the wrist pulse signals. The extracted distinctive features were adopted as inputs to a soft margin support vector machine (SVM) for classification. The applicability and performance of this method were evaluated using wrist pulse signals, including both healthy persons and patients. Moreover, some Doppler ultrasonic diagnostic parameters were selected and used as the additional inputs to the SVM. The experimental results showed that, by using the AR method, an accuracy of over 82% in telling the healthy persons from the patients can be reached. A higher accuracy (about 90%) can be achieved by using the combination of the AR method with the Doppler parameters. These results demonstrate the proposed methods have great potentials for computation pulse diagnosis.

References

1. Shu, J., and Sun, Y., "Developing classification indices for Chinese pulse diagnosis," Complement. Ther. Med. 15 (3)190–198, 2007.
2. Hammer, L., Chinese pulse diagnosis—Contemporary approach. Eastland, Vista, 2001.
3. Leonard, P., Beattie, T., Addison, P., and Watson, J., "Wavelet analysis of pulse oximeter waveform permits identification of unwell children," Emerg. Med. J. 21:59–60, 2004.
4. Zhang, Y., Wang, Y., Wang, W., and Yu, J., "Wavelet feature extraction and classification of Doppler ultrasound blood flow signals," J. Biomed. Eng. 19 (2)244–246, 2002.
5. Lu, W., Wang, Y., and Wang, W., "Pulse analysis of patients with severe liver problems," IEEE Eng. Med. Biol. Mag. 18 (1)73–75, 1999.
6. Zhang, A., and Yang, F., "Study on recognition of sub-health from pulse signal," Proceedings of the ICNNB Conference. 3:1516–1518, 2005.
7. Zhang, D., Zhang, L., Zhang, D., and Zheng, Y., "Wavelet-based analysis of Doppler ultrasonic wrist-pulse signals," Proceedings of the ICBBE Conference, Shanghai. 2:589–543, 2008.
8. Sohn, H., and Farrar, C., "Damage diagnosis using time series analysis of vibration signals," Smart Mater. Struct. 10:446–451, 2001.
9. Akaike, H., "A new look at the statistical model identification," IEEE Trans. Automat. Contr. 19 (6)716–723, 1974.
10. Ljung, L., "System identification: Theory for the user. Prentice-Hall PTR, Upper Saddle River, 1999.
11. Lukman, S., He, Y., and Hui, S., "Computational methods for traditional Chinese medicine: A survey," Comput. Methods Programs Biomed. 88:283–294, 2007.
12. Burges, C., A tutorial on support vector machines for pattern recognition," Data Min. Knowl. Discov. 2:121–167, 1998.
13. Yoon, Y., Lee, M., and Soh, K., "Pulse type classification by varying contact pressure," IEEE Eng. Med. Biol. Mag. 19:106–110, 2000.
14. Powis, R., and Schwartz, R., "Practical Doppler ultrasound for the clinician," Williams and Wilkins, Baltimore, 1991.
15. Wang, Y., Wu, X., Liu, B., and Yi, Y., "Definition and application of indices in Doppler ultrasound sonogram," J. Biom. Eng. (Shanghai). 18:26–29, 1997.
16. Leeuwen, G., Hoeks, A., and Reneman, R., "Simulation of real- time frequency estimators for pulsed Doppler systems," Ultrason. Imag. 8 (4)252, 1986.
17. Xu, L., Zhang, D., and Wang, K., "Wavelet-based cascaded adaptive filter for removing baseline drift in pulse waveforms," IEEE Trans. Biomed. Eng. 52 (11)1973–1975, 2005.

Chapter 14
Combination of Heterogeneous Features for Wrist Pulse Blood Flow Signal Diagnosis via Multiple Kernel Learning

Abstract A number of feature extraction methods have been proposed to extract linear and nonlinear and time and frequency features of wrist pulse signal. These features are heterogeneous in nature and are likely to contain complementary information, which highlights the need for the integration of heterogeneous features for pulse classification and diagnosis. In this chapter, we propose a novel effective method to classify the wrist pulse blood flow signals by using the multiple kernel learning (MKL) algorithm to combine multiple types of features. In the proposed method, seven types of features are first extracted from the wrist pulse blood flow signals using the state-of-the-art pulse feature extraction methods and are then fed to an efficient MKL method, SimpleMKL, to combine heterogeneous features for more effective classification. Experimental results show that the proposed method is promising in integrating multiple types of pulse features to further enhance the classification performance.

14.1 Introduction

Wrist pulse signal contains rich physiological and pathologic information and is of great importance in the analysis of the health status and pathologic changes of a person. In traditional Chinese medicine (TCM), for thousands of years, the practitioners use the fingers to feel the pulse fluctuations as a measure of the pulse signal and then analyze the health condition of the person. Studies on modern medicine also show that pulse signal can also be used as signs of several cardiac diseases, such as ventricular tachycardia or atrial fibrillation.

Traditional pulse diagnosis method, however, suffers from several intrinsic limitations. First, pulse diagnosis is a skill that requires considerable training and experience. Second, the results sincerely depend on the subjective analysis of the practitioner and sometimes may be unreliable and inconsistent. To overcome these limitations, computational pulse signal diagnosis techniques have been recently studied to acquire quantitative pulse signal using various types of sensors and to obtain objective and consistent analysis results using signal processing and pattern recognition approaches [1–4].

© Springer Nature Singapore Pte Ltd. 2018
D. Zhang et al., *Computational Pulse Signal Analysis*,
https://doi.org/10.1007/978-981-10-4044-3_14

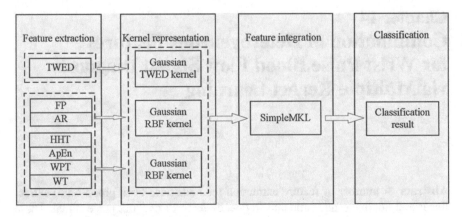

Fig. 14.1 Schematic diagram of the proposed integration method of heterogeneous features for pulse signal classification

Generally speaking, computational pulse signal diagnosis involves the following three modules: data acquisition, feature extraction, and pattern classification. In the first module, pulse signals are first acquired using a pressure, a photoelectric, or a Doppler ultrasound sensor and then preprocessed for denoising, baseline drift removal [5, 6], and segmentation [7].

In the feature extraction module, a number of feature extraction methods have been proposed to extract the features from the pulse signals, which can be roughly grouped into two categories according to the usage of the frequency transform or not. In the first category, fiducial points usually are first required to be detected [8]. Spatial features, elastic similarity measures, autoregressive [9], and Gaussian mixture models [10] are then adopted to derive appropriate feature description of pulse signal. In the second category, pulse signal is first transformed to the transform domain using Fourier wavelet [11] or Hilbert-Huang transform (HHT) [8]. Energy or other statistical features are then extracted for pulse feature representation.

In the classification module, various classifiers have been developed for different classification tasks, e.g., diagnosis of diseases, pulse waveform classification, and analysis of health conditions. Several classifiers, e.g., Bayesian networks classifier [12], support vector machine (SVM) [13, 34, 38], and artificial neural network [14], have been adopted for pulse signal classification.

Although the feature extraction and classification methods are heterogeneous in nature, different feature representations may reflect different aspects of pulse signal and are likely to contain complementary information for pulse diagnosis. Thus, appropriate combination of these heterogeneous features would benefit the classification performance. Moreover, it is also interesting to investigate the redundancy of the features and what types of features would contribute more to pulse diagnosis.

In this chapter, using multiple kernel learning (MKL), we proposed a framework for integrating heterogeneous pulse features to enhance the classification accuracy of pulse diagnosis. As shown in Fig. 14.1, the proposed framework consists of three major stages. First, we extract seven types of pulse features using the following feature extraction methods developed by our research group: fiducial point-based spatial features (FP), auto-regressive model (AR), time warp edit distance (TWED), Hilbert-Huang transform (HHT), approximate entropy (ApEn), wavelet packet transform (WPT), and wavelet transform (WT). Second, we design suitable kernel function (basis kernel) for each type of features, i.e., we adopt Gaussian time warp edit distance kernel [15] for a single-period pulse signal and adopt a Gaussian RBF kernel for the other types of features. Finally, an MKL algorithm, SimpleMKL [16], is used to integrate the heterogeneous features by simultaneously learning an optimal linear combination of the basis kernels and a kernel classifier. SimpleMKL [16] is an efficient algorithm recently developed for solving the MKL problem. Compared with other MKL algorithms [17, 18], SimpleMKL [16] is more efficient, especially for large-scale problems with many data points and multiple kernels. By combining the heterogeneous features of pulse signal using SimpleMKL, we expect that such a framework would further enhance the pulse signal classification accuracy.

Recent studies have verified the effectiveness of Doppler ultrasonic blood flow signal for computational pulse diagnosis [9, 10, 19]. In this chapter, we first evaluate the proposed method using our Doppler wrist blood flow signal dataset. Naturally, the proposed method can be directly extended to the classification of pressure or photoelectric pulse signals and other pulse classification tasks. To verify this, using the pressure pulse signals, we further test the proposed method for pulse waveform classification.

The remainder of this chapter is organized as follows. Section 14.2 describes the seven feature extraction and matching methods for pulse signals. Section 14.3 introduces the SimpleMKL algorithm for learning the linear combination of basis kernels and the kernel classifier. Section 14.4 provides the experimental results. Finally, Sect. 14.5 ends this chapter with a few concluding remarks.

14.2 Pulse Signal Feature Extraction

Before pulse signal feature extraction, a preprocessing step usually is required for denoising, baseline drift removal, and segmentation. As shown in Fig. 14.2a, the raw data acquired by the Doppler ultrasonic device are in the form of Doppler spectrogram, where the up envelope corresponds to the blood flow velocity signal. In the preprocessing step, we first detect the maximum velocity envelope of the Doppler spectrogram to extract wrist pulse blood flow signal. Using the seven-level "db6" wavelet transform, we remove the baseline drift by suppressing the seventh-level "db6" wavelet approximation coefficients and reduce the first-level wavelet detail coefficients for denoising. Figure 14.2b shows an example of the wrist pulse blood flow signal after drift and noise removal. Considering that pulse signals are quasiperiodic signals, we finally adopt an automatic method to locate the onset of each period, as shown in Fig. 14.2b.

Pulse signal feature extraction approaches can be roughly grouped into two categories: nontransform-based and transform-based methods. In this section, we

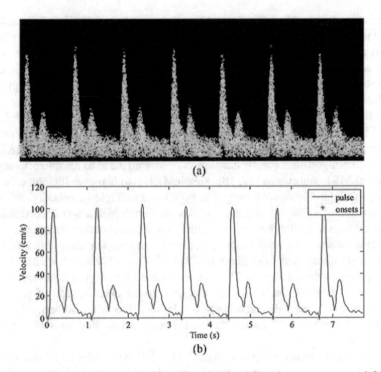

Fig. 14.2 Preprocessing of wrist pulse blood flow signal: (**a**) Doppler spectrogram and (**b**) location of the onsets and wrist pulse blood flow signal after denoising and drift removal

describe seven feature extraction methods, which involve three nontransform-based methods, i.e., fiducial point-based features, AR model, and time series matching, and four transform-based methods, i.e., HHT, ApEn, WPT, and WT.

14.2.1   Nontransform-Based Feature Extraction

The fiducial point-based feature [7, 8, 20, 21] that we have discussed in Chaps. 1 and 9 is one of the nontransform-based pulse signal feature extraction methods; in this section, we introduce another two nontransform-based pulse signal feature extraction methods, i.e., AR model and time series matching.

14.2.1.1   AR Model

In [9], Chen et al. proposed an AR model-based feature extraction method. In the training stage, an AR model is constructed from the reference signal obtained by pulse signals from healthy persons. During feature extraction, given a test wrist pulse signal, one can compute the residual error to the AR model and then calculate the mean and the standard deviation of the residual error as features of the test signal. According to [1], the residual error feature is disease sensitive and is promising in distinguishing healthy persons from patients with specific diseases.

In the following, we describe the procedure of the AR model-based method in more detail. First, each pulse signal $f(t)$ in the training set is normalized by:

$$\hat{f}(t) = \frac{f(t) - m_f}{\delta_f}, \tag{14.1}$$

where m_f and δ_f are the mean and the standard deviation of the original signal $f(t)$, respectively. The reference signal $\overline{f}(t)$ is defined as the average of all the normalized pulse signals of healthy persons in the training set.

In an AR model, the current observation $f(t)$ can be predicted as a linear function of the previous observations, $f(t-1), f(t-2), ..., f(t-p)$. Given the reference signal $\overline{f}(t)$, the AR model with p terms is then given by:

$$\overline{f}(t) = \sum_{i=1}^{p} a_i \overline{f}(f-i) + \varepsilon_f(t), \tag{14.2}$$

where a_i is the ith AR coefficient and $\varepsilon_f(t)$ denotes the modeling error. Using the reference signal $\overline{f}(t)$, all the model parameters can be estimated, where the coefficients a_i are obtained using the least-squares method and the order p is determined by the Akaike information criteria.

For a given wrist pulse signal of a person with unknown healthy status $g(t)$, its residual error can be calculated as:

$$\varepsilon_g(t) = g(t) - \sum_{i=1}^{p} a_i g(t-i). \tag{14.3}$$

We further calculate two features, the mean and the standard deviation of $\varepsilon_g(t)$, to characterize the diagnostic parameters of the pulse signal.

14.2.1.2   Time Series Matching

Wrist pulse signals actually are time series data, and thus, time series matching algorithms can be used for pulse signal classification. To date, various time series matching methods have been developed, e.g., edit distance, dynamic time warping [22], edit distance with real penalty [23], and TWED [24]. In [25], Liu et al. applied TWED for the diagnosis of wrist blood flow signals.

TWED satisfies the triangular inequality property and is an elastic metric for time series matching. Let A and B be the two time series $A = \{a'_1, ..., a'_n\}$ and $B = \{b'_1, ..., b'_m\}$ with $a'_i = (a_i, t_{a_i})$, where a_i is the ith sample value and t_{ai} is the corresponding time label. TWED introduces a stiffness parameter ν to control the elasticity of the distance of the two elements a_i' and b_j', $d\left(a_i',b_j'\right)=d\left(a_i,b_j\right)+v*d\left(t_{a_i},t_{b_j}\right)$, and introduces a parameter λ to penalize the delete operation. Then the TWED $\delta_{\lambda,v}$ of A and B is recursively defined as:

$$\delta_{\lambda,v}\left(A_1^P,B_1^q\right)=\min\begin{cases}\delta_{\lambda,v}\left(A_1^{p-1},B_1^q\right)+\Gamma\left(a_p'\to\Lambda\right) & \text{delete}_A\\ \delta_{\lambda,v}\left(A_1^{p-1},B_1^{q-1}\right)+\Gamma\left(a_p'\to b_q'\right) & \text{match}\\ \delta_{\lambda,v}\left(A_1^p,B_1^{q-1}\right)+\Gamma\left(\Lambda\to b_q'\right) & \text{delete}_B\end{cases} \quad (14.4)$$

with:

$$\Gamma\left(a_p'\to\Lambda\right)=d\left(a_p,a_{p-1}\right)+v\cdot\left(t_{a_p}-t_{a_{p-1}}\right)+\lambda$$

$$\Gamma\left(a_p'\to b_q'\right)=d\left(a_p,b_q\right)+d\left(a_{p-1},b_{q-1}\right)+v\cdot\left(\left|t_{a_p}-t_{b_q}\right|+\left|t_{a_{p-1}}-t_{b_{q-1}}\right|\right) \quad (14.5)$$

$$\Gamma\left(\Lambda\to b_q'\right)=d\left(b_q,b_{q-1}\right)+v\cdot\left(t_{b_q}-t_{b_{q-1}}\right)+\lambda,$$

where A_1^P denotes a time subseries with discrete time index varying between 1 and p. The TWED $\delta_{\lambda,v}$ can be calculated efficiently using dynamical programming. To further improve the efficiency, one can incorporate the Sakoe-Chiba band to prune the paths required to be considered [25].

14.2.2   Transform-Based Feature Extraction

In this section, we introduce four transform-based pulse signal feature extraction methods, i.e., HHT, ApEn, WPT, and WT.

HHT In [11], Zhang et al. proposed an HHT-based method for wrist blood flow signal feature extraction. Let $g(t)$ be a pulse signal. First, empirical mode decomposition EMD [26] is used to decompose $g(t)$ into a series of intrinsic mode functions (IMFs), $\text{IMF}_n(t)$, and a residue, $r(t)$. For simplicity, the residue $r(t)$ is treated as the last IMF, resulting in:

$$g(t)=\sum_{n=1}^{N}\text{IMF}_N(t), \quad (14.6)$$

where N is the number of IMFs. Then, Hilbert transform [26] of $\text{IMF}_n(t)$ is defined as:

$$Y_n(t) = \frac{1}{\pi} P \int_{-\infty}^{\infty} \frac{\mathrm{IMF}_n(\tau)}{t-\tau} d\tau, \tag{14.7}$$

where P denotes the Cauchy principal value [26]. Using $\mathrm{IMF}_n(t)$ and $Y_n(t)$, one can define a complex analytic signal $Z_n(t)$ as:

$$Z_n(t) = \mathrm{IMF}_n(t) + iY_n(t) = a_n(t)e^{j\phi_n(t)}, \tag{14.8}$$

where $a_n(t)$ and $\phi_n(t)$ defined as follows:

$$a_n(t) = \sqrt{\left(\mathrm{IMF}_n(t)\right)^2 + \left(Y_n(t)\right)^2}, \tag{14.9}$$

$$\phi_n(t) = \arctan\left(\frac{Y_n(t)}{\mathrm{IMF}_n(t)}\right), \tag{14.10}$$

where $a_n(t)$ and $\phi_n(t)$ are the instantaneous amplitude and phase of $Z_n(t)$, respectively. Furthermore, the frequency $f_n(t)$ of $Z_n(t)$ is defined as:

$$f_n(t) = \frac{1}{2\pi} \frac{d\phi_n(t)}{dt}. \tag{14.11}$$

Finally, given $a_n(t)$, $f_n(t)$, and $\mathrm{IMF}_n(t)$, we calculate three kinds of features, i.e., the average amplitude $\bar{h}_n$, the average frequency $\bar{\omega}_n$, and the energy p_n:

$$\bar{h}_n = \frac{\sum_{t=1}^{m} a_n(t)}{m}, \tag{14.12}$$

$$\bar{\omega}_n = \frac{\sum_{t=1}^{m} a_n(t) f_n(t)}{\sum_{t=1}^{m} a_n}(t), \tag{14.13}$$

$$P_n = \frac{\sum_{t=1}^{m} \left|\mathrm{IMF}_n(t)\right|^2}{\sqrt{\sum_{n=1}^{N} \sum_{t=1}^{m} \left|\mathrm{IMF}_n(t)\right|^2}}, \tag{14.14}$$

where m is the length of $g(t)$. However, the number of IMFs N differs for different signals. To obtain features with fixed dimension, we empirically observe $N \geq 5$ and thus only use the first five lower-order IMFs to derive a 15-D feature vector.

ApEn It is a measure of the complexity and predictability of a time series [27] and thus can be used to describe the nonlinear characteristics of pulse signal [28]. We choose the pattern length m = 2 and the measure of similarity r = 25%. By treating a pulse signal as a time series $A = [a_1, a_2, …, a_n]$, a pattern $P_m(i)$ is defined as a subsequence $[a_i, …, a_{i+m-1}]$ of length m beginning at location i. Two patterns $P_m(i)$ and $P_m(j)$ are similar if the following equation holds:

$$\left| a_{i+k} - a_{j+k} \right| \le r, \; k = 0, …, m-1. \tag{14.15}$$

Let $n_{im}(r)$ denote the number of patterns of length m which are similar to $P_m(i)$. We then define ApEn as:

$$\mathrm{ApEn}\left(m,,r,,A\right) = \phi^{m+1}\left(r\right) - \phi^m\left(r\right), \tag{14.16}$$

$$\phi^m\left(r\right) = \frac{1}{n-m+1} \sum_{i=1}^{n-m+1} \ln C_i^m\left(r\right), \tag{14.17}$$

$$C_i^m\left(r\right) = \frac{n_{im}\left(r\right)}{n-m+1}. \tag{14.18}$$

Different from [28], we calculate ApEn in the transform domain, where EMD is first used to decompose a pulse signal into seven IMFs; ApEn is then calculated for each IMF to derive a 5-D feature vector of the pulse signal.

WPT In [11], pulse signal $f(t)$ is decomposed as follows:

$$\begin{cases} p_0^1\left(t\right) = f\left(t\right) \\ … \\ p_j^{2i-1}\left(t\right) = \sum_k H\left(k-2t\right) p_{j-1}^i\left(t\right), \\ p_j^{2i}\left(t\right) = \sum_k G\left(k-2t\right) p_{j-1}^i\left(t\right) \end{cases} \tag{14.19}$$

where $i = 1,2,…,2^j$; $H(k)$ and $G(k)$ are the low-pass and high-pass filters, respectively; and $p_j^i\left(t\right)$ is the coefficient of the decomposed subband. Here, we choose the "db3" wavelet and the decomposition level of 5. Using the Shannon entropy criterion, we obtain the optimal WT decomposition tree together with the corresponding coefficients of the pulse signal. For each subband of the optimal decomposition tree, the energy of coefficients is computed as follows:

$$E_j^i = \sum_n \left| p_j^i\left(t\right) \right|^2. \tag{14.20}$$

Then we use energies as the features of the pulse signal.

WT According to [11], we use WT to decompose pulse signal and extract the energy feature of each subband. Using the 7-level "db6" WT, we decompose the pulse signal into seven subbands, one coarse subband, and seven detailed subbands. Finally, we define the energies of coefficients as follows:

$$E_{cA_7} = \sum_{k=1}^{L\_cA_7} cA_7^2(k),$$ (14.21)

$$E_{cDi} = \sum_{k=1}^{L\_cD_i} cD_i^2(k), \; i=1,\dots,7,$$ (14.22)

where cA_7 and cD_i are the coarse and the ith detailed wavelet subbands, respectively, and L_cA_7 and L_cD_i denote the length of cA_7 and cD_i, respectively.

14.3   Pulse Signal Classification Based on MKL

In this section, we proposed an MKL framework to integrate heterogeneous features extracted from the pulse signal. First, we choose suitable kernel function for each feature extraction or matching method, resulting in kernel-based representation of features or matching methods. Second, we use a recently proposed MKL algorithm, SimpleMKL [16], to learn a linear combination of kernels together with an SVM classifier to integrate heterogeneous features for enhanced classification accuracy.

14.3.1   Kernel Functions

Normalization usually is required to address the difference in distribution of heterogeneous features extracted by different methods. For the TWED method, we normalize each time series to have zero mean with standard deviation of 1. For the features extracted by other methods, each feature is normalized to have zero mean with standard deviation of 1.

Kernel functions are used to implicitly embedding features or matching methods into a higher indefinite-dimensional feature space [29]. By far, kernel classifiers, e.g., SVM, have been widely adopted in many classification applications [30–32]. For different feature extraction methods, the feature vectors vary in feature dimension. Moreover, TWED should be regarded as a matcher rather than a feature extraction method. Thus, the design of appropriate kernel function [33] for each feature extraction or matching method is essential for building kernel classifier.

For different features extracted from pulse signal, we adopt two kinds of kernel functions. By referring to [15], we can represent TWED by means of a Gaussian TWED kernel function:

Table 14.1 Feature dimensions of different methods

Method	Feature dimension
Fiducial point-based (FP)	10
Auto-regressive model (AR)	2
Hilbert-Huang transform (HHT)	15
ApEn	6
Wavelet packet transform (WPT)	14
Wavelet transform (WT)	8
TWED	Unfixed

$$K_{\text{GTWED}}(A,B) = \exp\left(-\frac{\delta_{\lambda,\nu}^2(A,B)}{2\sigma^2}\right), \tag{14.23}$$

where A and B are two time series and σ is the kernel parameter. Besides, the Gaussian RBF kernel is adopted for the features extracted by other feature extraction methods:

$$K_{\text{GRBF}}(\mathbf{x},\mathbf{y}) = \exp\left(-\frac{\mathbf{x}-\mathbf{y}_2^2}{2\sigma^2}\right), \tag{14.24}$$

where $\mathbf{x}$ and $\mathbf{y}$ are two feature vectors and σ is the kernel parameter.

As a summary, Table 14.1 lists the dimension of features extracted by each method. If we use one kernel function to represent the features extracted by each method, we have seven kernel functions. Except TWED, the number of features extracted by the other methods is 55 in total. More aggressively, we can construct four kernels for each of these 55 features with four different values of σ. To automatically select the kernel parameter, for each feature, we construct four Gaussian RBF kernel functions with $\sigma = 10, 15, 20,$ and 25. For TWED, we construct seven Gaussian TWED kernel functions with $\sigma = 5, 10, 15, 20, 25, 30,$ and 35. Finally, we use MKL to adaptively learn the optimal kernel parameter or linear combination. Taking both Gaussian RBF kernels and Gaussian TWED kernels into account, we construct 227 basis kernels in total.

14.3.2   SimpleMKL

Compared with other MKL algorithms, e.g., the quadratically constrained quadratical programming method by Lanckriet et al. [29] and the semi-infinite linear programming method by Sonnenburg et al. [18], SimpleMKL [16] is much more efficient for large-scale classification problems with many data points and multiple kernels. Thus, we adopt SimpleMKL to integrate the heterogeneous features extracted from pulse signal.

Given M basis kernels $K_m(\mathbf{x}, \mathbf{y})$ ($m = 1, \ldots, M$), MKL intends to learn an optimal combination of basis kernels:

$$K(\mathbf{x}, \mathbf{y}) = \sum_{m=1}^{M} d_m K_m(\mathbf{x}, \mathbf{y}), \text{subject to } d_m \geq 0, \sum_{m=1}^{M} d_m = 1, \qquad (14.25)$$

together with an SVM classifier:

$$f(\mathbf{x}) = \sum_{i=1}^{l} \alpha_i^* K(\mathbf{x}, \mathbf{x}_i) + b^*, \qquad (14.26)$$

where d_m denotes the weight of kernel $K_m(\mathbf{x}, \mathbf{y})$, $\mathbf{x}_i$ denotes the ith support vector, l is the number of support vectors, and α_i^* and b^* are coefficients of SVM. If the basis kernels $K_m(\mathbf{x}, \mathbf{y})$ satisfy the Mercer criterion, one can easily verify that $K(\mathbf{x}, \mathbf{y})$ also satisfies the Mercer criterion.

In MKL, the coefficients and weights can be simultaneously learned by solving the following convex optimization problem:

$$\min_{a,b,\xi,d} \frac{1}{2} \sum_i \alpha_i K(\cdot, \mathbf{x}_i)^2 + C \sum_i \xi_i$$
$$s.t. \ y_i \sum_i \alpha_i K(\mathbf{x}, \mathbf{x}_i) + y_i b \geq 1 - \xi_i$$
$$\xi_i \geq 0 \qquad (14.27)$$
$$\sum_m d_m = 1, d_m \geq 0.$$

To enforce fast MKL learning, simple MKL adopts an equivalent constrained optimization of (14.27):

$$\min_d J(\mathbf{d}), \ s.t. \sum_m d_m = 1, d_m \geq 0 \forall m, \qquad (14.28)$$

where:

$$J(\mathbf{d}) = \begin{cases} \min_{a,b,\xi} \dfrac{1}{2} \sum_i \alpha_i K(\cdot, \mathbf{x}_i)^2 + C \sum_i \xi_i \\ s.t. \ y_i \sum_i \alpha_i K(\mathbf{x}, \mathbf{x}_i) + y_i b \geq 1 - \xi_i . \\ \xi_i \geq 0 \end{cases} \qquad (14.29)$$

One can use a state-of-the-art SVM solver to solve the problem to obtain the optimal solutions of α_i^* and b^*. Actually, this problem can be solved more efficiently by using the "warm-start" strategy [16]. The function $J(\mathbf{d})$ can be rewritten as:

$$J(\mathbf{d}) = -\frac{1}{2}\sum_{i,j}\alpha_i^*\alpha_j^*y_iy_j\sum_{m=1}^{M}d_mK_m\left(\mathbf{x}_i,\mathbf{x}_j\right)+\sum_i\alpha_i^*. \tag{14.30}$$

Using (14.30), one can obtain the partial derivative of $J(\mathbf{d})$ with respect to d_m:

$$\frac{\partial J}{\partial d_m} = -\frac{1}{2}\sum_{i,j}\alpha_i^*\alpha_j^*y_iy_j\sum_{m=1}^{M}K_m\left(x_i,x_j\right). \tag{14.31}$$

By taking into account the equality constraint $\sum_m d_m = 1$, the reduced gradient of $J(\mathbf{d})$ is represented as:

$$\begin{cases} \left[\nabla_{red}J\right]_m = \dfrac{\partial J}{\partial d_m} - \dfrac{\partial J}{\partial d_\mu}, \forall m \neq \mu \\[3mm] \left[\nabla_{red}J\right]_m = \displaystyle\sum_{m\neq\mu}\dfrac{\partial J}{\partial d_\mu} - \dfrac{\partial J}{\partial d_m}, \text{else} \end{cases}, \tag{14.32}$$

where μ is chosen to be the index of the largest component of vector $\mathbf{d}$ for the sake of the numerical stability. Furthermore, to satisfy the non-negativity constraint $d_m \geq 0$, rather than directly use $-\nabla_{red}J$, the descent direction should be modified for updating d:

$$D_m = \begin{cases} 0, & \text{if } d_m = 0 \text{ and } \dfrac{\partial J}{\partial d_m} - \dfrac{\partial J}{\partial d_s} > 0 \\[3mm] -\dfrac{\partial J}{\partial d_m} - \dfrac{\partial J}{\partial d_\mu}, & \text{if } d_m > 0 \text{ and } m \neq \mu \\[3mm] \displaystyle\sum_{v\neq\mu, d_v>0}\left(\dfrac{\partial J}{\partial d_v} - \dfrac{\partial J}{\partial d_\mu}\right), & \text{for } m = \mu \end{cases}. \tag{14.33}$$

Given the descent direction D_m, SimpleMKL uses the greedy and line search methods to further enhance the efficiency. For more details on the implementation of SimpleMKL, refer to [16, Algorithm 1].

14.4   Experimental Results and Discussion

The proposed method is implemented in MATLAB. All the experiments are carried out on a computer with a Core 2 Quad Q6600 processor running at 2.40 GHz.

Table 14.2 Sample distribution of our dataset

Diseases	Age				
	0~20	21~40	41~60	>61	Total
Healthy	2	89	4	0	95
SD	0	3	20	13	36
Nephropathy	10	20	9	11	50
GD	15	53	46	7	121

14.4.1 Classification Experimental of Wrist Blood Flow Signal

In this subsection, we evaluate the classification performance of the proposed MKL framework using our wrist blood flow signal dataset and compare MKL with the individual classifiers and other classifier fusion approaches.

Using EDAN's CBS 2000 Transcranial Doppler Flow Analyzer, we construct a wrist blood flow signal dataset of 302 samples. Specifically, the samples in dataset are grouped into 4 categories, which include 95 samples of healthy persons, 36 samples of patients with sugar diabetes (SD), 50 with nephropathy (N), and 121 with gastrointestinal diseases (GD). The healthy persons are chosen from the staff and students from the Harbin Institute of Technology who have been diagnosed as healthy persons in their yearly physical examination. The patients are collected from Harbin Binghua Hospital where the diseases are diagnosed by the doctors according to the clinical data. The sampling frequency of CBS 2000 is 110 Hz. For each subject, only the pulse signal of the left hand is acquired, and we select a stable segment of 1200 points for subsequent feature extraction and classification. In addition, in our dataset, 205 persons are male. The age distribution and the number of subjects of each category are summarized in Table 14.2.

In order to verify the effectiveness of the proposed MKL method, using the wrist blood flow signal dataset, we test the classification methods for classifying healthy persons and patients with three kinds of diseases. Specifically, we adopt the tenfold cross-validation method to evaluate the diagnostic accuracy of the proposed MKL method, where the proposed method achieves the classification accuracy of 66.89%.

We further compare the proposed method with SVM with individual feature extractor. For each of the seven feature extraction methods, we constructed an individual SVM classifier [13], resulting in seven SVM classifiers, SVM-FP, SVM-AR, SVM-HHT, SVM-ApEn, SVM-WPT, and SVM-WT, and then adopted the tenfold cross-validation method to assess the classification accuracy. Tables 14.3 and 14.4 list the classification accuracy and false-positive rate of different methods, respectively. From Tables 14.3 and 14.4, one can see that the proposed method could obtain much higher classification accuracy and lower false-positive rate than any individual classifier, which verifies that the integration of the heterogeneous features would enhance the classification accuracy and reduce false-positive rate. Besides, we adopt the McNemar test [36] to evaluate the statistical significance of the difference between the proposed method and SVM-TWED. The result shows

Table 14.3 Classification accuracy of different classification methods

Methods	Accuracy (%)
SVM-FP	49.34
SVM-AR	40.07
SVM-HHT	50.66
SVM-ApEn	47.68
SVM-WPT	52.32
SVM-WT	50.66
SVM-TWED	55.63
SimpleMKL with all kernels	66.89
SVM-MVR [35]	52.32
SVM-BSR [35]	53.31
INN-TWED [24]	51.66

Table 14.4 False-positive rate (%) of different classification methods

Methods	H	N	SD	GD
SVM-FP	25.12	8.33	3.82	36.46
SVM-AR	28.99	10.71	6.02	43.09
SVM-HHT	24.15	7.93	5.26	35.91
SVM-ApEn	25.6	9.12	5.64	37.02
SVM-WPT	30.43	5.56	1.50	34.81
SVM-WT	28.99	5.56	2.26	32.60
SVM-TWED	24.15	9.01	2.26	32.04
SimpleMKL with all kernels	16.43	4.37	1.88	27.62
SVM-MVR	31.88	4.37	0.75	35.91
SVM-BSR	24.15	8.33	2.26	35.36
INN-TWED	26.09	6.35	2.26	38.67

Table 14.5 Classification time of different classifier combination methods

Methods	MKL	MVR	BSR
CPU time(s)	67.56	89.65	97.78

that the statistic value of the McNemar test is 20.04, which indicates that the performance difference is statistically significant at $\alpha = 0.05$.

We compare the classification accuracy obtained using the proposed method and other conventional classification combination methods, e.g., major vote rule (MVR) and Bayes sum rule (BSR). From Tables 14.3 and 14.4, one can see that the proposed method is superior to these classification combination methods. Table 14.5 lists the classification time of these methods. Again, the proposed method can achieve a proper balance between the classification accuracy and the computational cost and is more computationally efficient than the conventional combination

Table 14.6 The confusion matrix of the proposed method

		Predicted			
		H	N	SD	GD
Actual	H	**72**	2	0	21
	N	7	**25**	2	16
	SD	4	3	**16**	13
	GD	23	6	3	**89**

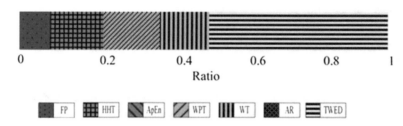

Fig. 14.3 Contributions of the feature extraction methods for pulse signal classification

methods. Moreover, we also compare the proposed method with another pulse signal classification method, nearest neighbor classifier using TWED (1NN-TWED) [24], and the proposed method can also achieve higher classification accuracy than 1NN-TWED.

The wrist blood flow signal dataset is class imbalanced, where the number of samples for different classes is different. Thus, we list the confusion matrices of the proposed method in Table 14.6. From Table 14.6, the proposed method can achieve comparable classification accuracy for each class.

Finally, we show the weight of each feature extraction method in Fig. 14.3. From Fig. 14.3, the weights of the ApEn and AR methods are zero in the final combined kernel. Specifically, most features have nonzero weights which only include a small number 33 of kernels in the combined kernel. Since only part of the basis kernels and feature extraction methods are needed in the classification stage, it is reasonable that the proposed method would be more computationally efficient than conventional combination methods.

14.4.2 Other Pulse Classification Application

In this section, in order to verify this method, we could extend to other pulse classification tasks using the pressure or photoelectric pulse signals; we test the proposed method for pulse waveform classification using the pressure pulse signal dataset [37]. Specifically, we selected 800 samples of five typical pulse patterns, moderate, smooth, taut, unsmooth, and hollow, where the number of samples of each pulse pattern is 160. The confusion matrix and the classification results are

Table 14.7 Confusion matrix of the proposed method for pulse waveform classification

		Predicted			
		M	S	T	H
Actual	M	**150**	6	4	0
	S	15	**142**	0	3
	T	0	3	**155**	1
	H	2	1	1	**156**

Table 14.8 The classification rate of the proposed method

Methods	Dataset		
	Size	Classes	Accuracy (%)
Simple MKL with all kernels	800	5	94.13

shown in Tables 14.7 and 14.8, respectively. One can see that the proposed method can achieve high accuracy for this pulse classification task.

14.5   Summary

In this chapter, we propose an MKL framework for integrating heterogeneous features extracted from pulse signals. By designing appropriate kernel function for the features extracted by each feature extraction method, MKL provides a flexible way to combining information from different feature extraction and matching methods. We adopt six pulse feature extraction methods, i.e., HHT, ApEn, WPT, WT, AR, and fiducial point-based method, and one pulse matching method, i.e., TWED. In our MKL framework, we use 7 Gaussian TWED kernels for the representation of the TWED method and 220 Gaussian RBF kernels for the representation of features extracted by the other methods. Finally, we adopt the SimpleMKL algorithm to integrate the heterogeneous features of pulse signals.

We first evaluate the classification performance of the proposed MKL framework on our wrist blood flow signal dataset. Experimental results show that compared with other classification fusion approaches and individual SVM classifiers, the proposed MKL framework is very effective in enhancing the classification accuracy of pulse signal. To further verify the proposed method, we test the proposed method for pulse waveform classification.

References

1. K. Wang, L. Xu, D. Zhang, and C. Shi, "TCPD based pulse monitoring and analyzing," in Proc. IEEE Mach. Learning Cybern. Conf., vol. 3, Beijing, China, 2002, pp. 1366–1370.
2. H. Wang and Y. Cheng, "A quantitative system for pulse diagnosis in traditional Chinese medicine," in Proc. IEEE Eng. Med. Biol. Soc. Conf., Shanghai, China, 2005, pp. 5676–5679.
3. S. Lukman, Y. He, and S.-C. Hui, "Computational methods for traditional Chinese medicine: A survey," Comput. Methods Programs Biomed., vol. 88, no. 3, pp. 283–294, 2007.
4. L. Zhu, J. Yan, Q. Tang, and Q. Li, "Recent progress in computerization of TCM, " J. Commun. Comput., vol. 3, no. 7, pp. 78–81, 2006.
5. L. Xu, D. Zhang, and K. Wang, "Wavelet-based cascaded adaptive filter for removing baseline drift in pulse waveforms," IEEE Trans. Biomed. Eng., vol. 52, no. 11, pp. 1973–1975, Nov. 2005.
6. L. Xu, D. Zhang, K. Wang, N. Li, and X. Wang, "Baseline wander correction in pulse waveforms using wavelet-based cascaded adaptive filter," Comput. Biol. Med., vol. 37, no. 5, pp. 716–731, May 2007.
7. L. Xu, M. Q.-H. Meng, R. Liu, and K. Wang, "Robust peak detection of pulse waveform using height ratio," in Proc. IEEE Eng. Med. Biol. Soc. Conf., 2008, pp. 3856–3859.
8. D. Zhang, W. Zuo, D. Zhang, H. Zhang, and N. Li, "Wrist blood flow signal-based computerized pulse diagnosis using spatial and spectrum features," J. Biomed. Sci. Eng., vol. 3, no. 4, pp. 361–366, 2010.
9. Y. Chen, L. Zhang, D. Zhang, and D. Zhang, "Computerized wrist pulse signal diagnosis using modified auto-regressive models," J. Med. Syst., vol. 35, no. 3, pp. 321–328, 2011.
10. Y. Chen, L. Zhang, D. Zhang, and D. Zhang, "Wrist pulse signal diagnosis using modified Gaussian models and fuzzy C-means classification," J. Med. Eng. Phys., vol. 31, no. 10, pp. 1283–1289, 2009.
11. D. Zhang, L. Zhang, D. Zhang, and Y. Zheng, "Wavelet-based analysis of Doppler ultrasonic wrist-pulse signals," in Proc. BioMed. Eng. Informatics Conf., 2008, vol. 2, pp. 539–543.
12. H. Wang and Y. Cheng, "A quantitative system for pulse diagnosis in Traditional Chinese Medicine," in Proc. IEEE Eng. Med. Biol. Conf., 2005, pp. 5676–5679.
13. C. J. C. Burges, "A tutorial on support vector machines for pattern recognition," J. Data Mining Knowl. Discovery, vol. 2, pp. 121–167, 1998.
14. C. Chiu, S. Yeh, and Y. Yu, "Classification of the pulse signals based on self-organizing neural network for the analysis of the autonomic nervous system," Chin. J. Med. Biol. Eng., vol. 16, pp. 461–476, 1996.
15. D. Zhang, W. Zuo, D. Zhang, and H. Zhang, "Time series classification using support vector machine with Gaussian elastic metric kernel," in Proc. Int. Conf. Pattern Recog, 2010, pp. 29–32.
16. A. Rakotomamonjy, F. R. Bach, S. Canu, and Y. Grandvalet, "SimpleMKL, " J. Mach. Learning Res., vol. 9, pp. 2491–2521, 2008.
17. F. R. Bach, G. R. G. Lanckriet, and M. I. Jordan, "Multiple kernel learning, conic duality, and the SMO algorithm," in Proc. 21st Int. Conf. Mach. Learning, 2004, pp. 41–48.
18. S. Sonnenburg, G. Rätsch, C. Schäfer, and B. Schölkopf, "Large scale multiple kernel learning," J. Mach. Learning Res., vol. 7, pp. 1531–1565, 2006.
19. Y.-J. Lee, J. Lee, and J.-Y. Kim, "A study on characteristics of radial arteries through ultrasonic waves," in Proc. IEEE Eng. Med. Biol. Soc. Conf., 2008, pp. 2453–2456.
20. L. Xu, M. Q.-H. Meng, K. Wang, L. Wang, and N. Li, "Pulse image recognition using fuzzy neural network," Expert Syst. Appl., vol. 36, pp. 3805–3811, 2009.

21. Y. Wang, X. Wu, B. Liu, and Y. Yi, "Definition and application of indices in Doppler ultrasound sonogram, " Shanghai J. Biomed. Eng., vol. 18, pp. 26–29, 1997.
22. H. Sakoe and S. Chiba, "A dynamic programming approach to continuous speech recognition," in Proc. Acoust. Conf. 1971, pp. 65–68.
23. L. Chen and R. Ng, "On the marriage of LP-norm and edit distance," Proc. Very Large Data Bases Conf., pp. 792–801, 2004.
24. P.-F. Marteau, "Time warp edit distance with stiffness adjustment for time series matching," IEEE Trans. Pattern Anal. Mach. Intell., vol. 31, no. 2, pp. 306–318, Feb. 2009.
25. L. Liu, W. Zuo, D. Zhang, H. Zhang, and N. Li, "Classification of wrist pulse blood flow signal using time warp edit distance," in Proc. Int. Conf. Med. Biometrics, 2010, vol. 6165, pp. 137–144.
26. N. E. Huang, Z. Shen, S. R. Long, M. C. Wu, H. H. Shih, Q. Zheng, N. C. Yen, C. C. Tung, and H. H. Liu, "The empirical mode decomposition and the Hilbert spectrum for nonlinear and non-stationary time series analysis," in Proc. R. Soc. Lond. A, Math. Phys. Eng. Sci., 1998, vol. 454, pp. 903–995.
27. S. M. Pincus, "Approximate entropy as a measure of system complexity," Proc. Nat. Acad. Sci., vol. 88, no. 6, pp. 2297–2301, 1991.
28. L. Xu, M. Q.-H. Meng, X. Qi, and K. Wang, "Morphology variability analysis of wrist pulse waveform for assessment of arteriosclerosis status, " J. Med. Syst., vol. 34, no. 3, pp. 331–339, 2010.
29. G. R. G. Lanckriet, T. D. Bie, N. Cristianini, M. I. Jordan, and W. S. Noble, "A statistical framework for genomic data fusion, " J. Bioinformatics, vol. 20, pp. 2626–2635, 2004.
30. A. Kampouraki, G. Manis, and C. Nikou, "Heartbeat time series classification with support vector machines, " IEEE Trans. Inf. Technol. Biomed., vol. 13, no. 4, pp. 512–518, Jul. 2009.
31. A.-M. Zou, J. Shi, J. Ding, and F.-X. Wu, "Charge state determination of peptide tandem mass spectra using support vector machine (SVM), " IEEE Trans. Inf. Technol. Biomed., vol. 14, no. 3, pp. 552–558, May 2010.
32. J. Shawe-Taylor and N Cristianini, Kernel Methods for Pattern Analysis. Cambridge, U.K.: Cambridge Univ. Press, 2004.
33. J. T. L. Wang and X. Wu, "Kernel design for RNA classification using Support Vector Machines," J. Data Mining Bioinformatics, vol. 1, no. 1, pp. 57–76, 2006.
34. D. Tao, X. Tang, X. Li, and X. Wu, "Asymmetric bagging and random subspace for support vector machines-based relevance feedback in image retrieval, " IEEE Trans. Pattern Anal. Mach. Intell., vol. 28, no. 7, pp. 1088–1099, Jul. 2006.
35. D. Jia, N. Li, S. Liu, and S. Li, "Decision level fusion for pulse signal classification using multiple features, " in Proc. BioMed. Eng. Informatics Conf., 2010, pp. 843–847.
36. Q. McNemar, "Note on the sampling error of the difference between correlated proportions or percentages," Psychometrika, vol. 12, pp. 153–157, 1947.
37. D. Zhang, W. Zuo, D. Zhang, Y. Li, and N. Li, "Gaussian ERP kernel classifier for pulse waveforms classification, " in Proc. Int. Conf. Pattern Recog., 2010, pp. 2736–2739.
38. M. A. Davenport, R. G. Baraniuk, and C. D. Scott, "Tuning support vector machines for minimax and Neyman–Pearson classification, " IEEE Trans. Pattern Anal. Mach. Intell., vol. 32, no. 10, pp. 1888–1898, Oct. 2010.

Part VI
Comparison and Discussion

Chapter 15
Comparison of Three Different Types of Wrist Pulse Signals

Abstract By far, a number of sensors have been employed for pulse signal acquisition, which can be grouped into three major categories, i.e., pressure, photoelectric, and ultrasonic sensors. To guide the sensor selection for computational pulse diagnosis, in this chapter, we analyze the physical meanings and sensitivities of signals acquired by these three types of sensors. The dependency and complementarity of the different sensors are discussed from both the perspective of cardiovascular fluid dynamics and comparative experiments by evaluating disease classification performance. Experimental results indicate that each sensor is more appropriate for the diagnosis of some specific disease that the changes of physiological factors can be effectively reflected by the sensor, e.g., ultrasonic sensor for diabetes and pressure sensor for arteriosclerosis, and improved diagnosis performance can be obtained by combining three types of signals.

15.1 Introduction

Pulse diagnosis has played an important role in traditional Chinese medicine (TCM) and traditional Ayurvedic medicine (TAM) for thousands of years [1–3]. Generally, the wrist pulse signals are mainly produced by cardiac contraction and relaxation and are also affected by the movement of blood and changes in the vessel diameter, making them effective for analyzing both cardiac and non-cardiac diseases.

However, pulse diagnosis is a subjective skill which needs years of training and practice to master [4]. Moreover, the diagnosis result relies on the personal experience of the practitioner. With different practitioners, the diagnosis results may then be inconsistent. To overcome these limitations, computational pulse diagnosis has been recently studied to objectify and quantify pulse diagnosis, and researchers have verified the connection of pulse signals with several certain diseases [5–12].

During the development of computational pulse diagnosis, a number of sensors and systems have been developed for acquiring pulse signals. Sorvoja et al. [13] reported a pressure pulse sensor based on electromechanical film. Kaniusas et al. [14] used a magnetoelastic skin curvature sensor to design a mechanical electrocardiography system for non-disturbing measurement of blood pressure signals. Chen

© Springer Nature Singapore Pte Ltd. 2018
D. Zhang et al., *Computational Pulse Signal Analysis*,
https://doi.org/10.1007/978-981-10-4044-3_15

et al. [15] presented a liquid sensor system that measures pulse signals. Wu et al. [16] proposed an air pressure system that measures pulse signals. Renevey et al. [17] proposed an infrared (IR) pulse detection system. Wang et al. [18] proposed a multichannel pressure pulse signal acquisition system with a linear sub-sensor array. Hu et al. [19] proposed a pulse measurement system based on a polyvinylidene fluoride (PVDF) pressure sensor array. Zhang and Wang [20] proposed a photoelectric system that measures pulse signals on fingers.

Among these systems, the three major types of sensors for pulse signal acquisition are pressure, photoelectric, and ultrasonic sensors. The pressure sensor is adopted in pulse diagnosis to imitate the TCM procedure of pulse taking [18], the photoelectric sensor is mainly adopted because it is inexpensive and easy to make [21], and the ultrasonic sensor is usually adopted for its robustness to interference [6]. As for pulse diagnosis, pressure signals have been investigated for pulse waveform classification and the diagnosis of cholecystitis, nephrotic syndrome, and diabetes [18, 22–24]. Lee et al. found that the photoplethysmogram (PPG) variability is related to sympathetic vasomotor activity, and photoelectric signal (i.e., PPG) had been combined with routine cardiovascular measurements (i.e., heart rate and mean arterial pressure) for the diagnosis of low systemic vascular resistance (SVR) [25]. Finally, ultrasonic signals have been investigated for the diagnosis of arteriosclerosis, pancreatitis, duodenal bulb ulcers, cholecystitis, and nephritis [5, 9, 26].

In this chapter, by conducting a comparative study, we analyze the physical meanings, correlations, sensitivities to physiological and pathological factors, and diagnosis performance of pulse signals acquired by these three types of sensors. With these studies, we intend to reveal the relative advantages of each type of pulse signal, which can guide us to choose a proper sensor for the diagnosis of specific diseases and to combine different types of pulse signals for improved diagnosis accuracy.

The remainder of the chapter is organized as follows. Section 15.2 is a discussion on the acquisition method and physical meaning of the signals sampled by the three types of sensors. Section 15.3 provides an analysis on the relationship between different pulse signals and sensitivities of these pulse signals with respect to different physiological and pathological factors. Section 15.4 provides the experimental results that demonstrate the relative advantages of different types of pulse signals and improved performance by combining different sensors. Finally, Sect. 15.5 gives several concluding remarks.

15.2   Measurement Mechanism

In this section, we introduce the measurement mechanism of the three major types of sensors to reveal the physical meaning of the acquired pulse signals. As shown in Fig. 15.1, one typical pulse acquisition hardware system usually involves three parts, the sensor, amplifier, and digitizer units, and the major difference between

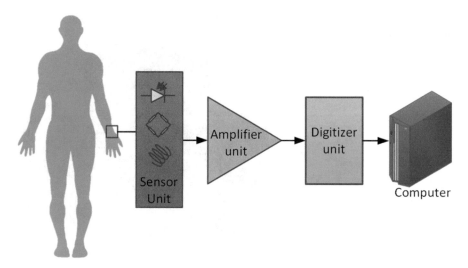

Fig. 15.1 Pulse signal acquisition framework

Fig. 15.2 Measurement
mechanism of a pressure
sensor

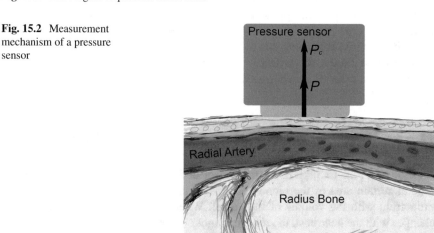

these pulse systems is the sensor unit. Thus, by analyzing the sensor units, we discuss the measurement mechanism of different pulse signal acquisition systems.

15.2.1 Measurement Mechanism of Pressure Sensors

As shown in Fig. 15.2, pressure sensor is designed to measure the transmural pressure at certain positions of the blood vessel. Pulse waves are generated by the expulsion of blood with heart contraction into the aorta, resulting in the dilatation of the vessel [27]. Blood flow takes place in a closed system of vessels, and any generated

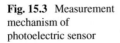

Fig. 15.3 Measurement
mechanism of
photoelectric sensor

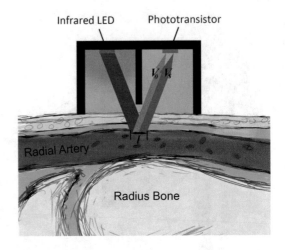

pressure affects the entire system. The wrist radial artery is close to the skin surface and thus changes in pressure can be noninvasively measured.

The measured pressure p_m is composed of the counterforce of the hold-down pressure p_c and transmural pressure from blood vessel p, i.e., $p_m = p_c + p$. Usually p is smaller than its true value due to the damping of the skin and tissue. Since the radial artery is close to the surface of the skin, the damping usually is slight, and that is why a TCM practitioner chooses the wrist as the position for pulse diagnosis.

15.2.2 Measurement Mechanism of Photoelectric Sensors

As shown in Fig. 15.3, photoelectric sensor is designed to measure the blood volume at certain area of the blood vessel. The intensity of the reflected light is in proportion with the volume of the vessel. When the blood volume in the vessel changes with the heartbeat, the reflected light will change accordingly, and thus the volume variation can be recorded by measuring the intensity of the reflected light from the vessel. Infrared light is usually employed in photoelectric sensor because it can penetrate deeper into the vessel than visible light while being absorbed/reflected less by epidermal melanin [28].

The measured volume signal V_m is composed of the light reflected from tissue V_0 and the reflected light from vessel V_s, i.e., $V_m = V_s + V_0$, where V_0 is almost constant for the same person and V_s is time-dependent and changes with the vessel volume. As shown in Fig. 15.3, for photoelectric sensor the phototransistor can only receive the reflected infrared light from a certain area. The measured volume is the integral of the cross-sectional area over the length l determined by the sensor size. Since l is constant, the measured volume by photoelectric sensor would depend on the change of cross-sectional area within the measure area.

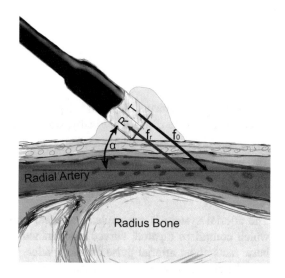

Fig. 15.4 Measurement mechanism of ultrasonic sensor

15.2.3 Measurement Mechanism of Ultrasonic Sensors

Ultrasonic sensor is employed to measure the blood velocity at certain positions along the blood vessel. As shown in Fig. 15.4, velocity information can be obtained by measuring the frequency shifting between the ultrasonic wave emitted by the transmitter (T) and that returned to the receiver (R). The ultrasonic signals reflect the velocities of red blood cells in the vessel, where the relationship of the frequency shift and velocity can be formulated as:

$$u = \frac{c\left(f_r - f_0\right)}{2f_0 \cos \alpha},$$
(15.1)

where f_0 is the emitted frequency, f_r is the reflected frequency, u is the flow velocity, and c is the speed of sound in soft tissue (about 1540 m/s) [29]. Usually, the angle α should be between 30° and 60° [27]. In this work, we assume that the speed u is the speed of blood at the center of the vessel because this scenario can be applicable by locating the position with maximum blood speed u_{max}, and this strategy is commonly used in practice [29].

15.3 Dependency and Complementarity

In this section, we first analyze the dependence between the different types of pulse signals. The analysis and discussion begun with some ideal simplifying assumptions to deduce the basic facts of the relationship between signals acquired by

Table 15.1 Physical
meaning of the measured
signals

Sensor	Physical meaning
Pressure	p
Photoelectric	A (or R^2)
Ultrasonic	u_{max}

different types of sensors. Then, the diagnostic factors that affect each type of measured signal will be discussed. Finally, we will consider their complementarities.

15.3.1   Assumptions

The arterial system is a complex nonlinear anisotropic and viscoelastic system, which comprises tapered, curved, and branching tubes. In order to obtain some basic facts about arterial pulse characteristics, we put forth some assumptions on both the arterial system and the sensors to simplify the analysis.

First, we assume that the blood composition, blood density, and the elasticity of the vessel wall are uniform and that the flow in the sampling window is laminar as indicated by most physiological fluid dynamic theories. We also assume that the vessel is a straight cylindrical tube and has a circular cross section and the distortion of the vessel is minimal. Therefore, for photoelectric signals we have:

$$V_m = V_s + V_0 = Al + V_0 = l\pi R^2 + V_0, \tag{15.2}$$

where R is the radius of the vessel. The length is fixed, and thus photoelectric signals are in proportion with the square of the radius under this assumption. Table 15.1 summarizes the physical meaning of measured signals. For simplicity purposes, the p_c in the measured pressure signals and V_0 in the measured photoelectric signals are not taken into consideration. Since these signals were continuously recorded, both the values and time derivatives of these signals can be easily obtained.

15.3.2   Relationship Among Blood Velocity, Radius, and Pressure in Steady Laminar Flow

In this section, we analyze the relationship of the blood velocity, area (radius), and pressure in steady laminar and pulsatile flows to reveal their relationship.

We first provide a cylindrical coordinate system (r, θ, z) which will be used in this section. As shown in Fig. 15.5, the coordinate is set along the vessel, the Z-axis is in the center of the vessel and toward the direction of the blood flow, and the r-axis is perpendicular to the skin.

In order to determine the basic arterial pulse characteristics, we first consider the simplest model: steady laminar flow in which the radius R, density ρ, viscosity η,

Fig. 15.5 Cylindrical coordinates and flow in the vessel

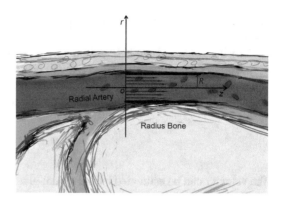

velocity u, volume V, and pressure p are all constant. The pressure gradient is also uniform. The general time-dependent governing equations can be given by the continuity and the Navier-Stokes equations. For steady laminar flow, the solution is [30, 31]:

$$u = \frac{R^2 - r^2}{4\eta} \frac{\partial p}{\partial z}. \tag{15.3}$$

The pressure gradient along the Z-axis is hard to measure with only one sensor, considering that the pulse wave is a wave that is traveling without distortion with velocity c. Then the pressure will have the form of [32]:

$$p = p_0 + f\left(t - \frac{z}{c}\right). \tag{15.4}$$

By differentiating Eq. (15.4) with respect to t and z, we get:

$$\frac{\partial p}{\partial z} = -\frac{1}{c} \frac{\partial p}{\partial t}. \tag{15.5}$$

Therefore, a good approximation to the pressure gradient along the Z-axis is the time derivative of the measured pressure signal.

The measured ultrasonic signals are the velocity at the center of the vessel and thus $r = 0$. By inserting $r = 0$ and Eq. (15.5) into Eq. (15.3), we obtain:

$$u_{max} = -\frac{1}{4\eta c} \frac{\partial p}{\partial t} R^2. \tag{15.6}$$

One can see that the measured velocity u_{max}, radius R, and time derivative of the measured pressure p are highly correlated with each other. Under the simplifying assumptions described in Sect. 15.3.1, if we have parameters η and c, the continuous pressure and photoelectric signals, respectively, we can get the velocity by using Eq. (15.6). If we have three types of measured signals, we can estimate the parameter ηc.

The discussion above is based on several strong assumptions in order to determine the basic relationship between the three types of measured signals. If we consider more realistic conditions, the relationship will become more complicated. For example, if we let the pressure gradient be in a pulsatile form:

$$\frac{\partial p}{\partial z} = ae^{i\omega t},$$

(15.7)

the velocity can be estimated by the model given by Womersley [32],

$$u = \frac{ae^{i\omega t}}{\rho i\omega}\left(1 - \frac{J_0\left(r\sqrt{\frac{\rho\omega}{\eta}i^{\frac{3}{2}}}\right)}{J_0\left(R\sqrt{\frac{\rho\omega}{\eta}i^{\frac{3}{2}}}\right)}\right),$$

(15.8)

where $J_0(xi^{3/2})$ is a Bessel function of the order zero with a complex argument. If we insert $r = 0$ and Eq. (15.5) into Eqs. (15.7) and (15.8), we can obtain a more complicated model on the measured blood velocity, volume, and pressure. If we let the radius R be a time-dependent variable, the model would be more difficult to obtain. Moreover, for real pulse signals, the parameters ρ and η are also time-dependent, and all of these parameters would vary with individual, health conditions, and many other factors. Thus, although the three types of signals are closely related, it is difficult to obtain an explicit model that uses two signals to estimate the other while using multiple types of signals to estimate some of the circulatory parameters that are still available which we will discuss in the next section.

15.3.3   Influence of Physiological and Pathological Factors

Different types of sensors have different physical meanings and thus would be influenced by different circulatory parameters. In this section, we analyze the influence of physiological and pathological factors on the different types of pulse signals.

Pressure signals are associated with the elasticity of the vessel wall and the radius. From the definition of incremental elastic modulus:

$$E_{inc} = \frac{\sigma_{inc}}{\varepsilon_{inc}} = \frac{\bar{R}\partial p}{h\partial t} / \frac{\partial R}{\bar{R}\partial t},$$

(15.9)

Table 15.2 Influence from circulatory parameters

	Pressure	Photoelectric	Ultrasonic
Radius of vessel	●	●	●
Wall elastic property	●		
Wall thickness	●		
Blood composition		●	
Blood flow status			●
Blood viscosity			●

we can get

$$\frac{\partial p}{\partial t} = \frac{Eh}{\overline{R}^2}\frac{\partial R}{\partial t}, \tag{15.10}$$

where E_{inc} is the incremental elastic modulus, σ_{inc} is the incremental stress, ε_{inc} is the incremental strain, $\overline{R}$ is the mean radius of the blood vessel, and h is the thickness of the blood wall.

From these equations, one can see that pressure signals are sensitive to changes in the radius, the elastic property, and the thickness of the blood vessel.

Photoelectric signals can be used to measure the volume changes of the blood in the vessel and are primarily sensitive to radius changes. Moreover, physically the photoelectric signals are measurements of the intensity of reflected infrared light and influenced by blood composition. The infrared absorption spectra of blood elements are also different, i.e., water, oxyhemoglobin, and deoxyhemoglobin exhibit different absorption spectra, and thus the composition ratio may influence the infrared absorption rate [33]. Actually, the blood oxygen monitor is designed by using this principle to measure blood oxygen saturation.

Ultrasonic signals represent the velocity of the blood flow. From Eqs. (15.6) and (15.8), one can see that the ultrasonic signals are associated with the pressure gradient, blood density, and viscosity. The velocity also reflects the flow statement. For example, the Reynolds number [30]:

$$\text{Re} = \frac{2u\rho R}{\eta}, \tag{15.11}$$

where ρ is a measure of the tendency for turbulence to occur. The viscosity of blood is normally about 1/30 poise, and the density is only slightly greater than 1. When the Reynolds number rises above 200–400, turbulent flow will occur in some branches of vessels; when the Reynolds number rises above approximately 2000, turbulence will usually occur even in straight and smooth vessels [27].

Table 15.2 summarizes the sensitiveness of different types of signals to changes in physiological parameters. Pressure signals mainly represent the transmural pressure and are sensitive to the parameter changes of the vessel wall, such as the wall elastic modulus and its thickness. Photoelectric signals represent the volume information of the vessel and are sensitive to the area of the cross section. Moreover, volume information is measured by the intensity of the reflected infrared light, and thus photoelectric signals are also sensitive to blood composition. Ultrasonic signals represent the blood velocity and are sensitive to the parameters associated with blood flow, such as viscosity and blood flow state. All three signals are sensitive to the changes of the vessel radius. As discussed above, the complex nonlinear aniso-tropic and viscoelastic properties of the arterial system and the relationship between different parameters are mostly nonlinear. Thus, the analysis results in Table 15.2 are obtained based on some common assumptions used in most physiological fluid dynamic theories. Except for these basic circulatory parameters, some other impor-tant diagnosis parameters are also associated with pressure, volume and velocity, such as the blood flow, and vascular compliance and resistance. The diagnostic validity of these parameters reveals the complementarity of the different measured signals.

Blood flow is the quantity of blood that passes through a given point in circula-tion in a given period. Blood flow Q can be calculated by $Q = uA$. Since photoelec-tric signals are in proportion to area A, blood flow is related to both ultrasonic and photoelectric signals.

Vascular compliance is of particular significance in cardiovascular physiology and has been reported to be sensitive to hypertension, congestive heart failure, and aging [34, 35]. Vascular compliance is defined as:

$$C = \frac{\Delta V}{\Delta p}, \tag{15.12}$$

which is a measure of the tendency of the arteries to stretch in response to pressure. Blood vessels with a higher compliance deform easier than those of lower compli-ance under the same pressure and volume conditions. From its definition, ΔV has a fixed length, and we can replace ΔV with ΔA, and Eq. (15.18) becomes:

$$C = \frac{\Delta A}{\Delta p} = \frac{\partial A}{\partial t} / \frac{\partial p}{\partial z} = -c \frac{\partial A}{\partial t} / \frac{\partial p}{\partial t}. \tag{15.13}$$

From Eqs. (15.12) and (15.13), one can see that vascular compliance is related to photoelectric and pressure signals and can be calculated by using their time derivatives.

Vascular resistance is defined as:

$$Res = \frac{\Delta p}{Q} = \frac{1}{uA} \frac{\partial p}{\partial t}. \tag{15.14}$$

Several documented conditions are associated with low vascular resistance, such as sepsis, pancreatitis, cirrhosis, and so on [36]. From the definitions, we can see that the resistance parameter is related to all three types of signals.

15.3.4 Summary

Signals measured by three popular sensors are closely related but have different physical meanings and are sensitive to different circulatory parameters. By combining different types of signals, some useful diagnostic parameters, such as blood flow, and vascular compliance and resistance can be inferred, which demonstrate the complementarity of different signals. Since they have different sensitivity parameters to diseases that may be associated with a certain parameter, the use of a sensor which is sensitive to that certain parameter may achieve better diagnosis performance.

From Table 15.2, one can see that all types of signals are sensitive to the radius of the vessel, and thus a disease that is associated with radius change may be detected by these sensors. As pressure signals are more sensitive to changes in the elastic property and the thickness of the vessel wall, they should be more effective than signals from the other types of sensors in the diagnosis of the related disease (e.g., arteriosclerosis). With a similar rationale, photoelectric sensors should be more effective than the other sensors in the diagnosis of diseases related to the area of the vessel cross section and blood composition, and ultrasonic sensors should be more effective than the other sensors in the diagnosis of the blood flow-related disease, e.g., diabetes which has been reported to be related to viscosity. Moreover, since the different signals are complementary, the combination of these signals may further reveal other diagnostic parameters, like vascular compliance and resistance which are related to many kinds of diseases. Thus, the combination of all of these signals may further increase diagnosis performance.

15.4 Case Studies

In the case studies, the pulse signals are acquired by using the pressure and photo-electric systems designed by our lab [18] and the CBS 2000 ultrasonic system provided by EDAN Instruments, Inc. Figure 15.6 shows the pulse signals sampled from a healthy volunteer using different systems, where Fig. 15.6a shows the pressure signals, Fig. 15.6b the photoelectric signals, and Fig. 15.6c the ultrasonic signals. From these figures one can see that different types of pulse signals are similar in terms of waveform, which demonstrated that these signals are dependent. However their difference is also obvious which may be because of their different physical attributes and influential factors. Thus, it is natural to suppose that the diagnosis of

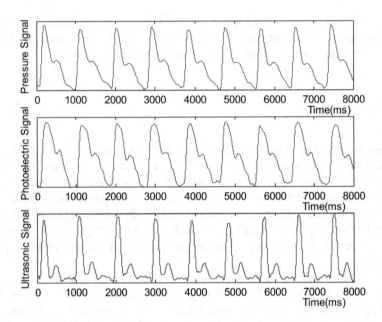

Fig. 15.6 Three types of pulse signals from a healthy volunteer: (**a**) pressure signals, (**b**) photo-electric signals, and (**c**) ultrasonic signals

different disease using the three types of pulse signals may also have different performance.

Diabetes and arteriosclerosis diagnoses are used as two examples in the experiments because diabetes is reported to be associated with blood viscosity [37] and arteriosclerosis refers to the thickening and hardening of the arteries [38]. Using these two diseases, experiments were conducted to compare the diagnosis performance of the three types of pulse sensors and to validate the effectiveness of combining three types of measured signals.

15.4.1 Method

In this subsection we introduced the preprocessing, feature extraction, and classification methods. In preprocessing, the high-frequency noise and baseline drift coupled with pulse signal were removed. These two interferences are mainly introduced by the power line interference and breathing, respectively. The wavelet denoising method was adopted to remove the noise, and the wavelet-based cascaded adaptive filter [39] was adopted to correct the baseline drift.

In feature extraction, three kinds of features were extracted to characterize the pulse signal. First, the time domain fiducial point-based feature was extracted. Fiducial point-based feature describes the shape of an average pulse cycle; it includes the position of the primary peak, dicrotic notch, and secondary peak which is the most common feature used in pulse signal classification [7, 40–44]. Second, the multi-scale sample entropy of the pulse signal was calculated. Sample entropy can be used to measure the unpredictability of pulse signal, and multi-scale sample entropy can reveal unpredictability with long-range correlations on multiple spatial and temporal scales which had been successfully applied for pulse signal classification [45–47]. The last feature was the TWED feature. TWED is an elastic metric to measure the distance between time series, which is reported effective and efficient in pulse signal classification [7, 48].

In the classification we adopted the composite kernel learning (CKL) method to combine these features since it is more flexible than SVM in combining features from different sources [49]. For each type of pulse signal, we extract three kinds of features, i.e., time domain fiducial point-based feature, multi-scale sample entropy (SampEn), and TWED feature. Thus, nine basis kernels $K_{1,1}\sim K_{3,3}$ are built that correspond to three types of signals and three kinds of features, where $K_{1,m}$, $K_{2,m}$, and $K_{3,m}$ are the basis kernels for pressure, photoelectric, and ultrasonic signals, respectively, and $K_{1,1}$, $K_{1,2}$, and $K_{1,3}$ are the basis kernels for time domain fiducial point-based feature, SampEn, and TWED feature, respectively.

To combine the basis kernels, we adopt the composite kernel learning (CKL) model [7] which defines a tree structure to guide the selection and removal of kernels. In pulse classification, as shown in Fig. 15.7, the basis kernels are structured into three groups based on the types of sensors, i.e., $G_1 = \{K_{1,1}, K_{1,2}, K_{1,3}\}$, $G_2 = \{K_{2,1}, K_{2,2}, K_{2,3}\}$, and $G_3 = \{K_{3,1}, K_{3,2}, K_{3,3}\}$. In CKL [7], the combination of the kernels is defined by:

$$K(\mathbf{x},\mathbf{y}) = \sum_l \sigma_l \sum_m \sigma_{lm} K_{lm}(\mathbf{x},\mathbf{y}), \tag{15.15}$$

where σ_{lm} and σ_l are the nonnegative coefficients for kernel K_{lm} and group G_l, respectively. For kernel selection/removal, the following constraints are imposed on σ_{lm} and σ_l,

$$\sum_l d_l \sigma_l^{2/p} \leq 1, \sigma_l \geq 0, \tag{15.16}$$

$$\sum_{lm} \sigma_{lm}^{2/q} \leq 1, \sigma_{lm} \geq 0, \tag{15.17}$$

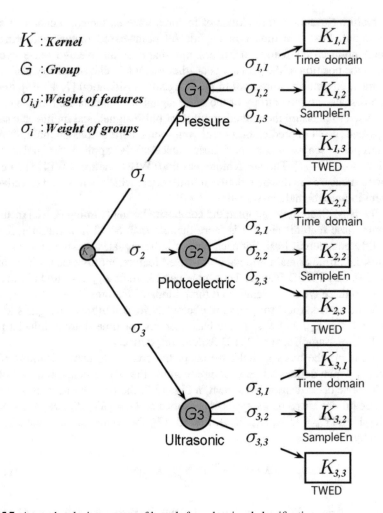

Fig. 15.7 A tree that depicts groups of kernels for pulse signal classification.

where p and q are two hyper-parameters for tuning sparsity within or between groups, and d_l is the number of basis kernels in group G_l. Let $\gamma_{lm} = \sigma_l^p \sigma_{lm}^q$ and $f_{lm}(\mathbf{x}) = \sum_i \alpha_i K_{lm}(\mathbf{x}_i, \mathbf{x})$, the CKL model [7] is formulated as,

$$\min_{\gamma} J(\gamma) \ \text{s.t.} \sum_l \left(d_l^p \left(\sum_m \gamma_{lm}^{1/q} \right)^q \right)^{1/(p+q)} \leq 1, \gamma_{lm} \geq 0 \qquad (15.18)$$

with

$$J(\gamma) = \min_{f_{lm},b,\xi} \frac{1}{2} \sum_{lm} \frac{1}{\gamma_{lm}} f_{lm\mathcal{H}_{lm}}^2 + C\sum_i \xi_i$$

$$\text{s.t.} y_i \left(\sum_{lm} f_{lm}(\mathbf{x}_i) + b \right) \geq 1 - \xi_i, \xi_i \geq 0.$$

(15.19)

As introduced in [7], the model above can be efficiently solved by iterating between (1) updating flm with the standard SVM solver and (2) updating γ with the fixed point algorithm. In this work we set $p = q = 0.5$ and set $C = 100$.

The tenfold cross-validation method is used to evaluate the classification performance. Three performance indicators, i.e., classification accuracy, sensitivity, and specificity, are adopted for quantitative evaluation. The accuracy is defined as the percentage of all the correctly identified samples, the sensitivity is defined as the percentage of patients who are correctly identified as sick, and specificity was defined as the percentage of healthy people who are correctly identified as healthy [50].

15.4.2   Diabetes Experiment

In the diabetes experiment, we constructed a dataset of 392 volunteers, including 191 healthy and 201 diabetic volunteers by collaborating with the Yao Chung Kit Diabetes Assessment Centre in Hong Kong. Each volunteer provided three different types of sample data for the dataset. To avoid the potential influence of biological factors, we also ensured that the distributions of gender and age of volunteers with diabetes are similar to those of the healthy volunteers. Table 15.3 lists the basic information of the dataset.

In the experiment, we used the preprocessing, feature extraction, and classification methods described in Sect. 15.4.1. In the classification of signals from single source, we have only one group in CKL model, and in the classification of pulse signals from multiple sources, we have three groups in CKL model as shown in Fig. 15.7. The classification results of the signals from the different types of sensors are listed in Table 15.4. One can see that the ultrasonic pulse signal is more effective in the diagnosis of diabetes than the other types of pulse signals. The

Table 15.3 Summary of diabetes datasets

	Age distribution				Gender distribution	
	1 ~ 40	40 ~ 50	50 ~ 60	>60	Male	Female
Healthy	9	41	69	72	119	72
Diabetes	3	35	67	96	131	70

result is consistent with a previous study in which diabetes is reported to be associated with viscosity [37]. Note that the ultrasonic sensor is more sensitive to the changes in the viscosity. The results also show that the combination of the three types of signals can obtain improved classification accuracy, which indicates that the three types of signals contain some complementary information for the diagnosis of diabetes. The result of the McNemar's test [51] shows that in the diabetes classification, the performance difference between ultrasonic and other types of signals are statistically significant at $\alpha = 0.05$. The performance difference between the group of combined signals and any single signal group are also statistically significant at $\alpha = 0.05$.

15.4.3   Arteriosclerosis Experiment

In the arteriosclerosis experiment, we constructed a dataset of 184 volunteers, including 95 healthy and 89 arteriosclerosis volunteers by collaborating with the Guangzhou Hospital of TCM. The principle of the constructing the dataset and the format of the samples are the same as those of the diabetes dataset. Table 15.5 lists the basic information of the arteriosclerosis dataset.

The results are listed in Table 15.6. From Table 15.6, it can be observed that the pressure pulse signal outperforms the other types of pulse signal in the arterioscle-

Table 15.4 Diabetics diagnosis performance

	Accuracy (%)	Sensitivity (%)	Specificity (%)
Pressure	84.2	86.1	82.2
Photoelectric	79.8	82.6	77.0
Ultrasonic	87.0	88.6	85.3
Combination of three types of signals	91.6	92.5	90.6

Table 15.5 Summary of arteriosclerosis datasets

	Age distribution				Gender distribution	
	1 ~ 40	40 ~ 50	50 ~ 60	>60	Male	Female
Healthy	19	22	23	31	60	35
Diabetes	15	18	24	32	59	30

Table 15.6 Arteriosclerosis diagnosis performance

	Accuracy (%)	Sensitivity (%)	Specificity (%)
Pressure	86.4	87.6	85.2
Photoelectric	79.3	83.1	75.8
Ultrasonic	83.7	85.4	82.1
Combination of three types of signals	89.7	91.0	88.4

rosis experiment. This may because it is more sensitive to the changes in vessel hardness and thickness which are related to arteriosclerosis [38]. The ultrasonic group also obtained good performance because the hardness of the vessel will also influence the blood speed. Moreover, in the arteriosclerosis experiment, the classification performance can also be improved by combining all three types of signals. The result of the McNemar's test [51] shows that in the arteriosclerosis classification, the performance difference between the pressure and photoelectric signals is statistically significant at $\alpha = 0.1$. The performance difference between the group of combined signals and any single signal group is also statistically significant at $\alpha = 0.1$. The higher α-value can be partially explained by that the dataset size in the arteriosclerosis experiment is lower than that in the diabetes experiments.

15.5 Summary

In this chapter, we study the dependency and complementarity among three major types of sensors, i.e., pressure, photoelectric, and ultrasonic sensors, for pulse signal diagnosis. Our analysis on their physical meanings, relationships, and sensitivity factors shows that (1) the changes in the elastic property and thickness of the vessel wall can be more readily detected using pressure signals; (2) the changes in the area of the cross section and blood composition can be more readily captured using photoelectric signals; and (3) the changes in the blood viscosity and the blood flow state can be more effectively characterized using ultrasonic signals. Thus, we state that each sensor is more appropriate for the diagnosis of some specific disease that the changes of physiological factors can be effectively reflected by the sensor, and different types of signals are complementary.

Case studies have been conducted to validate these statements. The experimental results show that, in terms of accuracy, sensitivity, and specificity, the ultrasonic sensor is superior to the others for the diagnosis of diabetes, while the pressure sensor outperforms the others for the diagnosis of arteriosclerosis. These results can be explained by that the onset of diabetes is usually accompanied by the changes in blood flow viscosity [37] which can be well depicted by ultrasonic signals and arteriosclerosis usually results in the changes in the hardness and thickness of wrist radial artery [38] which can be well characterized by pressure signals. Moreover, the combination of the three types of signals further improves the diagnosis performance, which can be explained by the complementarity among sensors.

References

1. S. Walsh and E. King, Pulse Diagnosis: A Clinical Guide. Sydney Australia: Elsevier, 2008.
2. V. D. Lad, Secrets of the Pulse. Albuquerque, New Mexico: The Ayurvedic Press, 1996.
3. E. Hsu, Pulse Diagnosis in Early Chinese Medicine. New York, American: Cambridge University Press, 2010.

4. R. Amber and B. Brooke, Pulse Diagnosis: Detailed Interpretations For Eastern & Western Holistic Treatments. Santa Fe, New Mexico: Aurora Press, 1993.
5. Y. Chen, L. Zhang, D. Zhang, and D. Zhang, "Wrist pulse signal diagnosis using modified Gaussian Models and Fuzzy C-Means classification," Medical Engineering & Physics, vol. 31, pp. 1283–1289, Dec 2009.
6. Y. Chen, L. Zhang, D. Zhang, and D. Zhang, "Computerized wrist pulse signal diagnosis using modified auto-regressive models," Journal of Medical Systems, vol. 35, pp. 321–328, Jun 2011.
7. L. Liu, W. Zuo, D. Zhang, N. Li, and H. Zhang, "Combination of heterogeneous features for wrist pulse blood flow signal diagnosis via multiple kernel learning," IEEE Transactions on Information Technology in Biomedicine, vol. 16, pp. 599–607, Jul 2012.
8. L. Liu, W. Zuo, D. Zhang, N. Li, and H. Zhang, "Classification of wrist pulse blood flow signal using time warp edit distance," Medical Biometrics, vol. 6165, pp. 137–144, 2010.
9. D. Y. Zhang, W. M. Zuo, D. Zhang, H. Z. Zhang, and N. M. Li, "Wrist blood flow signal-based computerized pulse diagnosis using spatial and spectrum features," Journal of Biomedical Science and Engineering, vol. 3, pp. 361–366, 2010.
10. Q. L. Guo, K. Q. Wang, D. Y. Zhang, and N. M. Li, "A wavelet packet based pulse waveform analysis for cholecystitis and nephrotic syndrome diagnosis," in IEEE International Conference on Wavelet Analysis and Pattern Recognition, Hong Kong, China, 2008, pp. 513–517.
11. S. Charbonnier, S. Galichet, G. Mauris, and J. P. Siche, "Statistical and fuzzy models of ambulatory systolic blood pressure for hypertension diagnosis," IEEE Transactions on Instrumentation and Measurement, vol. 49, pp. 998–1003, 2000.
12. H.-T. Wu, C.-H. Lee, C.-K. Sun, J.-T. Hsu, R.-M. Huang, and C.-J. Tang, "Arterial Waveforms Measured at the Wrist as Indicators of Diabetic Endothelial Dysfunction in the Elderly," IEEE Transactions on Instrumentation and Measurement, vol. 61, pp. 162–169, 2012.
13. H. Sorvoja, V. M. Kokko, R. Myllyla, and J. Miettinen, "Use of EMFi as a blood pressure pulse transducer," IEEE Transactions on Instrumentation and Measurement, vol. 54, pp. 2505–2512, 2005.
14. E. Kaniusas, H. Pfutzner, L. Mehnen, J. Kosel, C. Tellez-Blanco, G. Varoneckas, et al., "Method for continuous nondisturbing monitoring of blood pressure by magnetoelastic skin curvature sensor and ECG," IEEE Sensors Journal, vol. 6, pp. 819–828, Jun 2006.
15. C. Lianyi, H. Atsumi, M. Yagihashi, F. Mizuno, H. Narita, and H. Fujimoto, "A preliminary research on analysis of pulse diagnosis," in IEEE International Conference on Complex Medical Engineering, Beijing,China, 2007, pp. 1807–1812.
16. H.-T. Wu, C.-H. Lee, and A.-B. Liu, "Assessment of endothelial function using arterial pressure signals," Journal of Signal Processing Systems, vol. 64, pp. 223–232, 2011.
17. P. Renevey, R. Vetter, J. Krauss, P. Celka, and Y. Depeursinge, "Wrist-located pulse detection using IR signals, activity and nonlinear artifact cancellation," in Annual International Conference of the IEEE Engineering in Medicine and Biology Society, 2001, pp. 3030–3033 vol.3.
18. P. Wang, W. Zuo, H. Zhang, and D. Zhang, "Design and implementation of a multi-channel pulse signal acquisition system," in IEEE International Conference on Biomedical Engineering and Informatics, ChongQing, China, 2012, pp. 1063–1067.
19. C.-S. Hu, Y.-F. Chung, C.-C. Yeh, and C.-H. Luo, "Temporal and Spatial Properties of Arterial Pulsation Measurement Using Pressure Sensor Array," Evidence-Based Complementary and Alternative Medicine, vol. 2012, pp. 1–9, 2012.
20. A. Zhang and H. Wang, "Real-time detection system For photoelectric pulse signals," in IEEE International Conference on Business Management and Electronic Information Guangzhou,China, 2011, pp. 498–501.
21. N. Selvaraj, K. H. Shelley, D. G. Silverman, N. Stachenfeld, N. Galante, J. P. Florian, et al., "A Novel Approach Using Time Frequency Analysis of Pulse-Oximeter Data to Detect Progressive Hypovolemia in Spontaneously Breathing Healthy Subjects," IEEE Transactions on Biomedical Engineering, vol. 58, pp. 2272–2279, 2011.

22. Q. Guo, K. Wang, D. Zhang, and N. Li, "A wavelet packet based pulse waveform analysis for cholecystitis and nephrotic syndrome diagnosis," in IEEE International Conference on Wavelet Analysis and Pattern Recognition, Hong Kong, China, 2008, pp. 513–517.

23. I. Wakabayashi and H. Masuda, "Association of pulse pressure with fibrinolysis in patients with type 2 diabetes," Thrombosis Research, vol. 121, pp. 95–102, 2007.

24. N. Arunkumar and K. M. M. Sirajudeen, "Approximate entropy based ayurvedic pulse diagnosis for diabetics – a case study," in IEEE International Conference on Trendz in Information Sciences and Computing, Chennai,India, 2011, pp. 133–135.

25. Q. Y. Lee, G. S. H. Chan, S. J. Redmond, P. M. Middleton, E. Steel, P. Malouf, et al., "Classification of low systemic vascular resistance using photoplethysmogram and routine cardiovascular measurements," in Annual International Conference of IEEE Engineering in Medicine and Biology Society, Buenos Aires, Argentina, 2010, pp. 1930–1933.

26. R. Murata, H. Kanai, N. Chubachi, and Y. Koiwa, "Measurement of local pulse wave velocity on aorta for noninvasive diagnosis of arteriosclerosis," in IEEE Annual International Conference of the Engineering in Medicine and Biology Society, Baltimore, MD, 1994, pp. 83–84 vol.1.

27. A. C. Guyton and J. E. Hall, Textbook of medical physiology. Philadelphia, Pennsylvania: Elsevier, 2006.

28. ICNIRP, "ICNIRP Statement on Far Infrared Radiation Exposure," Health Physics, vol. 91, pp. 630–645, 2006.

29. W. Schèaberle, Ultrasonography in Vascular Diagnosis: A Therapy-oriented Textbook and Atlas. Germany: Springer, 2005.

30. G. E. Mase, Schaum's outline of theory and problems of continuum mechanics: McGraw-Hill New York, 1970.

31. M. Kutz, Biomedical Engineering and Design Handbook: Biomedical Engineering Fundamentals. United States: McGraw-Hill Professional, 2009.

32. J. R. Womersley, "Method for the calculation of velocity, rate of flow and viscous drag in arteries when the pressure gradient is known," The Journal of physiology, vol. 127, pp. 553–563, 1955.

33. L. V. Wang and H.-i. Wu, Biomedical optics: principles and imaging. New Jersey: Wiley & Sons, 2012.

34. S. M. Finkelstein, W. Feske, J. Mock, P. Carlyle, T. Rector, S. Kubo, et al., "Vascular compliance in hypertension," in Annual International Conference of the IEEE Engineering in Medicine and Biology Society, New Orleans, LA, USA, 1988, pp. 241–242 vol.1.

35. S. M. Finkelstein, G. E. McVeigh, D. E. Burns, P. F. Carlyle, and J. N. Cohn, "Arterial Vascular Compliance In Heart Failure," in 12th Annual International Conference of the IEEE Engineering in Medicine and Biology Society, Michigan,American, 1990, pp. 548–549.

36. J. Melo and J. I. Peters, "Low systemic vascular resistance: differential diagnosis and outcome," Critical Care, vol. 3, pp. pp.71–77, 1999.

37. D. A. Fedosov, W. Pan, B. Caswell, G. Gompper, and G. E. Karniadakis, "Predicting human blood viscosity in silico," Proceedings of the National Academy of Sciences, vol. 108, pp. 11772–11777, 2011.

38. W. A. N. Dorland, Illustrated medical dictionary. WB Saunders Company, 2011.

39. L. Xu, D. Zhang, and K. Wang, "Wavelet-based cascaded adaptive filter for removing baseline drift in pulse waveforms," IEEE Transactions on Biomedical Engineering, vol. 52, pp. 1973–1975, Nov 2005.

40. L. Xu, M. Q. H. Meng, R. Liu, and K. Wang, "Robust peak detection of pulse waveform using height ratio," in International Conference of the IEEE Engineering in Medicine and Biology Society, Vancouver, BC, Canada, 2008, pp. 3856–3859.

41. D. Zhang, W. Zuo, D. Zhang, H. Zhang, and N. Li, "Wrist blood flow signal-based computerized pulse diagnosis using spatial and spectrum features," Journal of Biomedical Science and Engineering, vol. 3, pp. 361–366, 2010.

42. C. Xia, Y. Li, J. Yan, Y. Wang, H. Yan, R. Guo, et al., "Wrist Pulse Waveform Feature Extraction and Dimension Reduction with Feature Variability Analysis," in International Conference on Bioinformatics and Biomedical Engineering, Shanghai, China, 2008, pp. 2048–2051.
43. L. Xu, M. Q. H. Meng, K. Wang, W. Lu, and N. Li, "Pulse images recognition using fuzzy neural network," Expert systems with applications, vol. 36, pp. 3805–3811, 2009.
44. Y. Wang, X. Wu, B. Liu, Y. Yi, and W. Wang, "Definition and application of indices in Doppler ultrasound sonogram," Shanghai Journal of Biomedical Engineering, vol. 18, pp. 26–29, Aug 1997.
45. M. Costa, A. L. Goldberger, and C. K. Peng, "Multiscale entropy analysis of biological signals," Physical Review E, vol. 71, pp. 1–18, Feb 2005.
46. M. Costa, A. L. Goldberger, and C. K. Peng, "Multiscale entropy analysis of complex physiologic time series," Physical Review Letters, vol. 89, pp. 1–4, Aug 5 2002.
47. L. Liu, N. Li, W. Zuo, D. Zhang, and H. Zhang, "Multiscale sample entropy analysis of wrist pulse blood flow signal for disease diagnosis," in Sino-foreign-interchange Workshop on Intelligence Science and Intelligent Data Engineering, NanJing China, 2012, pp. pp.475–482.
48. L. Liu, W. Zuo, D. Zhang, N. Li, and H. Zhang, "Classification of Wrist Pulse Blood Flow Signal Using Time Warp Edit Distance," Medical Biometrics. Springer Berlin Heidelberg, pp. pp. 137–144, 2010.
49. M. Szafranski, Y. Grandvalet, and A. Rakotomamonjy, "Composite kernel learning," Machine learning, vol. 79, pp. 73–103, 2010.
50. A. G. Lalkhen and A. McCluskey, "Clinical tests: sensitivity and specificity," Continuing Education in Anaesthesia, Critical Care & Pain, vol. 8, pp. 221–223, 2008.
51. Q. McNemar, "Note on the sampling error of the difference between correlated proportions or percentages," Psychometrika, vol. 12, pp. 153–157, June 1947.

Chapter 16
Comparison Between Pulse and ECG

Abstract Both wrist pulse and electrocardiogram (ECG) signals are mainly caused by cardiac activities and are valuable in analyzing heart rhythms and cardiac diseases. For noninvasive monitoring, recent studies indicate that ECG and wrist pulse signal can be adopted for the diagnosis of several non-cardiac diseases and reflect the movement of blood and the change of vessel diameter. To reveal the complementarities between pulse signal and ECG, a comparative study of these two signals is conducted for the diagnosis of non-cardiac diseases. The two types of signals are compared based on two classes of indicators: information complexity and classification performance. The results show that wrist pulse blood flow signal is more informative by complexity measure and can achieve higher classification accuracy. Some examples of non-cardiac diseases, e.g., diabetes, liver, and gallbladder diseases, are given to illustrate the strengths of wrist pulse signal.

16.1 Introduction

Both electrocardiogram (ECG) [1–4] and wrist pulse signals [5, 6] are mainly driven by cardiac contraction and relaxation and are valuable in the clinical analysis of heart rhythms and cardiac diseases [7]. Considering that wrist pulse and ECG signals can be noninvasively acquired and continuously measured, they are suitable to be adopted for the diagnosis and monitoring of both cardiac [1–3, 7] and non-cardiac [8–13] diseases. As to ECG, Ling et al. [8, 9, 14] used ECG signal for noninvasive monitoring of hypoglycemic episodes in type 1 diabetes mellitus patients (T1DM). Based on nocturnal ECG signals, Khandoker et al. [10] applied support vector machine (SVM) for the recognition of obstructive sleep apnea syndrome (OSAS).

Compared with ECG, wrist pulse signal is some kind of bloodstream signal influenced by many other physiological or pathological factors, such as arterial walls, blood parameters, nerves, muscles, skin, etc. [5, 6, 15–17], making wrist pulse signal suitable for the analysis of non-cardiac diseases. Fedosov et al. revealed the relationship between and blood viscosity anomalies and the condition of several diseases, e.g., malaria, AIDS, and diabetes [18]. Lu et al. [11] showed that pulse analysis can be used to assess the liver problems, Zhang et al. [12] investigated the

© Springer Nature Singapore Pte Ltd. 2018
D. Zhang et al., *Computational Pulse Signal Analysis*,
https://doi.org/10.1007/978-981-10-4044-3_16

recognition of nephritis and cholecystitis, and Chen et al. [13] proposed an SVM-based method for the diagnosis of duodenal bulb ulcer and appendicitis. Using multiple kernel learning (MKL) to combine heterogeneous features, Liu et al. [19] adopted the pulse signal for classification of diabetes, nephropathy, and gastrointestinal diseases.

With the increasing interests on applying ECG and wrist pulse signals for non-cardiac diseases, to the best of our knowledge, so far no comparative studies were conducted for these two types of signals. By comparing ECG and wrist pulse signals, we can find which one is more suitable for noninvasive monitoring of the specific non-cardiac diseases and reveal the complementarities of pulse signal with respect to ECG.

In this chapter, we conduct a comparative study of ECG and pulse signals for the diagnosis of some specific non-cardiac diseases. We use Doppler ultrasound device to acquire wrist pulse blood flow signal. For the sake of fairness, the bipolar Lead I ECG signals, i.e., the voltage between the left arm (LA) and right arm (RA) electrodes, are adopted for comparison. We construct a dataset of ECG and wrist pulse blood flow signals captured from healthy persons and patients with three non-cardiac diseases, i.e., liver, gallbladder, and diabetes diseases. The reason for choosing these three diseases is that the conditions of these diseases are believed to be reflected more by pulse signals [5, 15] than by ECG. Our results show that wrist pulse blood flow signal is more informative by complexity measure and can achieve higher classification accuracy.

16.2 Methods

ECG is the signal of electrical activity of the heart, while wrist pulse signal is a bloodstream signal mainly driven by heart but affected by many other factors. In this section, we first discuss the characteristics of wrist pulse signal and ECG signal, introduce the signal acquisition and preprocessing of ECG and wrist pulse blood flow signal, and construct a dataset. Then, we introduce the complexity measures, provide the feature extraction and classification methods, and describe the McNemar test for the evaluation of the accuracy difference of two classifiers.

16.2.1 Analysis of ECG and Wrist Pulse Signals

ECG is a record of the electrical activity which is generated by cardiac depolarization and repolarization and spreads throughout the body. ECG is useful in analyzing the rate and regularity of heartbeats and has been widely investigated for the diagnosis of cardiac and cardiovascular diseases. Moreover, heart rate variability can also be used to analyze the activities of the autonomic nervous system (ANS) [20]. Considering the intensive applications of ECG in noninvasive monitoring, it is

Table 16.1   The different characteristics of ECG and wrist pulse signals

Signal	Signal type	Major cause	Other factors	Acquisition
ECG	Electrical activity	Heart	ANS	Invasive
Wrist pulse	Bloodstream	Heart	Blood parameters, ANS, muscle, etc.	Invasive

convenient to use ECG for the diagnosis of non-cardiac diseases, e.g., obstructive sleep apnea syndrome (OSAS) [8, 21].

Wrist pulse signal is some kind of bloodstream signal which is mainly caused by cardiac contraction and relaxation. Other physiological or pathological factors, such as blood parameters (blood pressure, velocity, and viscosity) and nerves, would also have influence on pulse signal [5, 15], making pulse signal suitable for the diagnosis of several non-cardiac diseases. Recent progress in biomedical engineering has shown that anomalies in blood pressure, velocity, and viscosity are useful in the analysis of many diseases, e.g., malaria, AIDS, diabetes, moyamoya, and pediatric sickle cell disease [18, 22, 23]. In TCM, pulse signal is viewed as the music of the body's symphony and is valuable in the analysis of health condition [5, 15, 24].

The characteristics of ECG and pulse signals are summarized in Table 16.1. Both ECG and wrist pulse signal can be invasively acquired and are mainly caused by cardiac activities. But ECG is a signal of electrical activity, while wrist pulse is a signal of bloodstream. Compared with ECG, wrist pulse signal can be affected by more other physiological or pathological factors. Thus, it is very likely that pulse signal would be more informative and be superior to ECG for the diagnosis of some specific non-cardiac diseases.

16.2.2   Acquisition of ECG and Wrist Pulse Signal

In this subsection, we introduce the device and procedure to acquire ECG and wrist pulse blood flow signals.

Wrist Pulse Blood Flow Signal Acquisition   As shown in Fig. 16.1 a, the blood would flow from the heart to the arteries along the body, and the abnormalities in blood pressure, velocity, and viscosity are useful in the analysis of human health conditions. Compared with the other arteries, wrist radial artery is relatively easy to be sensed and captured. Thus, in TCM, a doctor puts three fingers on the three positions (i.e., Cun, Guan, and Chi) of the patient's wrist to adaptively feel the fluctuations in the radial artery at the styloid processes.

By far, several devices have been developed to acquire wrist pulse signals by strain gauge, photoelectric, and Doppler ultrasonic sensors [12, 19, 25, 28]. Physiological modeling and experimental studies had shown that blood pressure, volume, and velocity have a close relationship [26, 27], and reliable estimation of blood pressure and volume information can be obtained based on the blood flow velocity. In this work, we use the Edan's CBS 2000 Doppler ultrasound

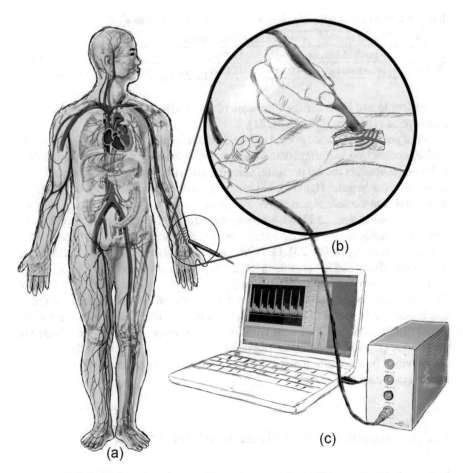

Fig. 16.1 Wrist pulse blood flow signal acquisition. (**a**) The blood would flow from the heart to the arteries along the body. For wrist pulse acquisition, (**b**) we put the probe at the Guan position of the wrist and tune the angle of the probe with respect to the wrist radial artery until the acquired signal is stable and satisfactory. (**c**) Finally, wrist pulse blood flow signal is recorded by the Doppler ultrasonic device and stored in the computer

device to acquire Doppler spectrogram, where the up-envelope is adopted as the blood flow signal.

To acquire pulse signal, as shown in Fig. 16.1 b, we first put the probe at the Guan position of the wrist and then tune the angle of the probe with respect to the wrist radial artery until the acquired signal is stable and satisfactory. As shown in Fig. 16.1 c, wrist pulse Doppler spectrogram signal is recorded by the Doppler ultrasonic device and stored in the computer.

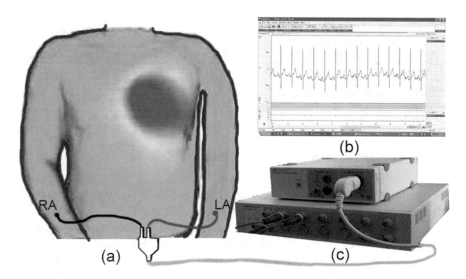

Fig. 16.2 ECG signal acquisition. (**a**) The electrical activity generated by cardiac depolarization and repolarization would spread throughout the body, and we place the electrodes to the left arm (LA) and right arm (RA) to obtain the bipolar Lead I ECG signals. (**b**) An example of the acquired ECG signal. (**c**) The acquired signal would be recorded and stored by the device

The acquired wrist pulse blood flow signals are preprocessed for denoising, baseline drift removal, and segmentation. We first detect the maximum velocity envelope of Doppler spectrogram to extract wrist pulse blood flow signal, use the seven-level "db6" wavelet transform to remove the baseline drift by suppressing the seventh level "db6" wavelet approximation coefficients, and then reduce the first level wavelet detail coefficients for denoising. Finally, we adopt the method in [29] to locate the onset of each period.

ECG Signal Acquisition As shown in Fig. 16.2a, the electrical activity generated by cardiac depolarization and repolarization would spread throughout the body [30]. To acquire ECG signal, we first place the electrodes to the proper positions on the patient's body (Please refer to [31] for more details on electrode placement). Then each lead of ECG can be recorded as the voltage between a pair of electrodes.

We use ADInstruments ML870 PowerLab 8/30 and ML408 Dual Bio Amp/ Stimulator for ECG signal acquisition. Based on grounded ECG acquisition method, the left arm (LA) and right arm (RA) electrodes are adopted to obtain the bipolar Lead I ECG signals with the right leg grounded. Figure 16.2b shows an example of the acquired ECG signal. For the preprocessing of ECG signal, we use the linear and nonlinear filtering scheme in [32] to detect the QRS complexes and T peak and remove the baseline drift and noise.

Table 16.2 Summary of the dataset

	Age (years)				Gender		
	20~40	40~50	50~60	>60	Male	Female	Number of volunteers
Healthy (H)	48	46	45	43	98	84	182
Diabetes (D)	45	50	56	54	97	108	205
Liver (L)	12	15	15	16	33	25	58
Gallbladder (G)	9	10	8	9	17	19	36

16.2.3 Construction of the Dataset

We construct a dataset of wrist pulse blood flow and ECG signals which contains 481 volunteers, including 182 healthy persons, 205 patients with diabetes, 58 patients with liver diseases, and 36 patients with gallbladder diseases. For each subject, we acquire both the ECG and wrist pulse blood flow signals. The distributions of gender and age of volunteers with different classes are similar. Table 16.2 lists a summary of the dataset. The reason to choose these three diseases is that both physiological modeling and experimental evidences had indicated the relationships between wrist bloodstream signal and the condition of these diseases [5, 15, 18, 19].

All the samples are collected from the volunteers from the Harbin Binghua Hospital, the Hong Kong Yao Chung Kit Diabetes Assessment Centre, and the Guangdong Provincial TCM Hospital. We categorized a volunteer to the class "healthy" if he/she was diagnosed as healthy person based on physical examination and categorized a volunteer to the class of one of the three diseases based on the diagnosis of the doctors.

For each volunteer, we collect both the ECG and the wrist pulse blood flow signals. After preprocessing, we select a 12-second stable segment of ECG signal and a 12-second stable segment of wrist pulse blood flow signal for subsequent comparative study.

16.2.4 Entropy-Based Complexity Analysis

Entropy-based complexity measure of physiologic signals is valuable in quantifying the regularity of physiologic signals. The increase in the dynamical complexity usually indicates the increase of information content of the physiologic signal. In this work, we adopt the multiscale entropy framework [33] and consider two complexity measures: approximation entropy (ApEn) [34] and sample entropy (SampEn) [35].

ApEn Given a time series of length N, for each pattern x_i of length m, ApEn [34, 36] first determines the occurrence of repetitive runs $n_{i,m}$ by calculating the number of patterns similar with x_i. Similarly, the occurrence of repetitive runs $n_{i+1,m}$ can be computed. Then, a measure of prevalence is calculated as the negative average natural logarithm of the frequency of the occurrence of repetitive runs. Finally, ApEn is defined the difference between the prevalence of length $m + 1$ and that of length m. ApEn can be used as a measure of the rate of generation of new information and is valuable in quantifying the complexity of dynamical models and physiologic signals.

SampEn   In the calculation of the occurrence of repetitive runs, ApEn always counts the pattern itself (self-matching) to avoid the logarithm of 0 and lead to the introduction of bias. To reduce bias, Richman and Moorman [35, 37] developed a modified ApEn method, i.e., SampEn, which excludes self-matching and precisely computes the negative logarithm of the conditional probability. Let A and B be the accumulated numbers of the occurrence of repetitive runs for length $m + 1$ and length m, respectively. SampEn can be expressed as $-\ln(A/B)$. SampEn is computationally efficient, relatively consistent, and more independent of time series length.

Multiscale Entropy   The original ApEn and SampEn performed only on the smallest scale. Since the influence of random noise and highly erratic fluctuations, for some diseases like atrial fibrillation, the pathologic signal would even have the higher entropy value. To address this, Costa et al. [33] proposed a multiscale entropy method to measure complexity on physiologic signals on multiple scales, which is robust in quantifying the complexity of physiologic signals and can separate long-range correlated noise from uncorrelated noise.

16.2.5   Classification Accuracy and Statistical Test

To compare the diagnosis accuracy, we follow the methods described in [19, 38] to extract ECG and pulse features, use MKL [19, 43] for classification, and finally adopt the McNemar test [39] to assess the accuracy difference.

16.2.5.1   Feature Extraction of Wrist Pulse Blood Flow Signal

In [19], Liu et al. grouped the pulse signal feature extraction methods in two classes: nontransform-based and transform-based approaches. Based on [19], we extract three nontransform-based features, i.e., fiducial point-based (FP) features [12, 40], auto-regressive (AR) model [13], and time warp edit distance (TWED) [41], and three transform-based features, i.e., Hilbert-Huang transform (HHT) [12], wavelet transform [42], and wavelet packet transform [42]. Table 16.3 lists the pulse features used in our study. In the HHT domain, we extract the amplitude, frequency, energy, and ApEn features. For TWED, we normalize each time series to have the mean of zero and the standard deviation (*std.*) of 1. For the other methods, each feature is normalized to have zero mean with *std.* of 1.

Table 16.3 Summary of feature extraction methods for wrist pulse blood flow signal

	Method	Feature dimension
Nontransform-based	Fiducial point-based	10
	Auto-regressive model	2
	TWED	Unfixed
Transform-based	HHT	21
	Wavelet packet transform	14
	Wavelet transform	8

16.2.5.2   Feature Extraction of ECG Signal

We locate the heartbeat fiducial points, detect the locations of the QRS onset and offset and T-wave offset, and extract three types of ECG features [31]:

RR-interval features: We extract four heartbeat fiducial point interval (i.e., RR-interval) features: (a) pre-RR-interval, the RR-interval between a given heartbeat and the previous heartbeat; (b) post-RR-interval, the RR-interval between a given heartbeat and the following heartbeat; (c) local average RR-interval of the ten neighbored RR-intervals; and (d) average RR-interval of the ECG signal.

Heartbeat interval features: Based on the QRS onset and offset and T-wave offset, we extract two heartbeat interval features: (a) QRS duration, the time interval between the QRS onset and the QRS offset, and (b) T-wave duration, the time interval between the QRS offset and the T-wave offset. Moreover, the third heartbeat interval feature is introduced as a Boolean variable to indicate whether a P-wave is presented.

Morphology features: We extract four types of morphology features. As described in [20], we extract nineteen-dimensional morphology features from the segmented ECG signal. Then, by scaling the signal to have the std. of 1, we perform the same process to extract another nineteen-dimensional morphology features. Similarly, we extract eighteen-dimensional fixed-interval morphology features by locating the sampling windows of the heartbeat fiducial point and fixing the sampling rate. Finally, by scaling the signal to have the std. of 1, we extract another eighteen-dimensional fixed-interval features.

To be consistent with pulse signal, we also extract all the other pulse features from ECG signals except the pulse fiducial point-based features.

16.2.5.3   Classifiers

Since the features extracted from ECG or pulse signals are heterogeneous, we use MKL for disease diagnosis. Given M basis kernels $K_m(x, y)$ ($m = 1, \ldots, M$), the linear combination of basis kernel would also be a kernel function:

$$K(\mathbf{x},\mathbf{y}) = \sum_{m=1}^{M} d_m K_m (\mathbf{x},\mathbf{y}), \text{ subject to } d_m \geq 0, \sum_{m=1}^{M} d_m = 1, \tag{16.1}$$

where d_m stands for the weight of $K_m(\mathbf{x}, \mathbf{y})$. We adopt the SimpleMKL algorithm [19, 43] to solve the following optimization problem:

$$\min_{\alpha,b,\mathbf{d},\xi} \frac{1}{2} \sum_m \frac{1}{d_m} \sum_i \alpha_i y_i d_m K_m (\mathbf{x}_i,\cdot)^2 + C\sum_i \xi_i$$

$$\text{s.t. } y_i \left(\left(\sum_i \alpha_i y_i \sum_m d_m K_m (\mathbf{x}_i,\cdot) \right) + b \right) \geq 1 - \xi_i \tag{16.2}$$

$$\xi_i \geq 0$$

$$d_m \geq 0, \sum_{m=1}^{M} d_m = 1, \ \forall i, \forall m.$$

Based on the learned $\mathbf{d}, \boldsymbol{\alpha}$, an b, we use the following kernel classifier to classify the test sample $\mathbf{x}$:

$$f(\mathbf{x}) = \sum_i \sum_{m=1}^{M} \alpha_i y_i d_m K_m (\mathbf{x},\mathbf{x}_i) + b. \tag{16.3}$$

16.2.5.4 McNemar Test

McNemar test [39] is used to answer the question: Is the difference in classification accuracy statistically significant? Our hypothesis H1 and the associated null hypothesis are formulated as:

H1: Classifier A is significantly better than classifier B.
H0: There is no difference in the classification accuracy between the two classifiers.

For each test sample, the classification results of the two classifiers should be an instance of one of the following four outcomes:

SS: Both classifier A and classifier B correctly classify the test sample.
SF: Classifier A correctly classifies the test sample while classifier B fails.
FS: Classifier B correctly classifies the test sample while classifier A fails.
FF: Both classifier A and classifier B fail to classify the test sample.

Given N test samples, we record the number of the times of the four outcomes as n_{SS}, n_{SF}, n_{FS}, and n_{FF}. In McNemar test, n_{SS} and n_{FF} are ignored, and a sign test is use to test the null hypothesis that the probability of SF is equal to that of FS. We are only interested in whether classifier A is better than classifier B and thus use the one-side McNemar test, where the probability of $H0$ is bounded by:

$$P_{H0} \leq \sum_{i=0}^{n_{FS}} \frac{(n_{SF} + n_{FS})!}{i!(n_{SF} + n_{FS} - i)!} 0.5^{(n_{SF} + n_{FS})}. \qquad (16.4)$$

If $P_{H0} \leq 0.05$, $H0$ will be rejected in favor of $H1$, and classifier A is significantly better than classifier B.

16.3 Results

We conducted two series of comparative experiments: complexity measure and classification performance. First, multiscale ApEn and multiscale SampEn are adopted to compare the complexity of ECG and wrist pulse blood flow signals. Second, we report the classification performance by using ECG and by using wrist pulse blood flow signals and employ McNemar test to evaluate the statistical significance of accuracy difference.

16.3.1 Comparison of Complexity Measures

In our experiments, we calculate the ApEn and SampEn values over eight scale factors, i.e., $\tau = 1, 5, 10, 15, 20, 25, 30,$ and 40 for each signal. Given a signal $\mathbf{x}$, the coarse signal $\mathbf{x}^{(\tau)}$ with the scale factor τ can be constructed by $\mathbf{x}^{(\tau)} = \{x_1^{(\tau)}, \cdots, x_j^{(\tau)}, \cdots x_{N/\tau}^{(\tau)} \mid x_j^{(\tau)} = 1/\tau \sum_{i=(j-1)\tau+1}^{j\tau} x_i\}$. For both ApEn and SampEn, we choose $r = 0.6$ and $m = 2$. For given complexity measure, the average and *std*. of the entropy values are computed among all the healthy ECG and all the healthy wrist pulse blood flow signals, respectively.

Figures 16.3 and 16.4 show the multiscale entropy results of ApEn and SampEn for healthy ECG and wrist pulse blood flow signals. When the scale factor $\tau \geq 5$, the average ApEn and SampEn values of wrist pulse blood flow signals are higher than those of ECG signals. For SampEn, the difference of entropy values is more distinct, which indicate that wrist pulse blood flow signal is more informative than ECG by complexity measures. Taking the error bars in account, ECG and wrist pulse blood flow signals have an overlap in terms of the distribution of entropy values, which might be explained by that both ECG and pulse signals are mainly caused by cardiac activities.

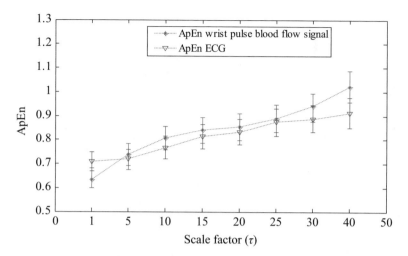

Fig. 16.3 Multiscale ApEn results for healthy ECG and wrist pulse blood flow signals. The symbols and the error bars stand for the values of mean SampEn and the standard deviation, respectively

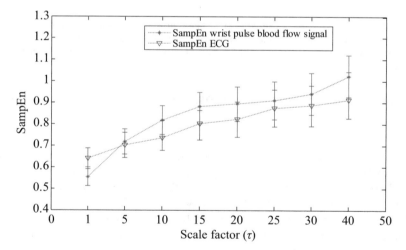

Fig. 16.4 Multiscale SampEn results for healthy ECG and wrist pulse blood flow signals. The symbols and the error bars stand for the values of mean SampEn and the standard deviation, respectively

16.3.2   Comparison of Classification Performance

Using the dataset described in Sect. 16.2, experiments are conducted to compare the classification accuracy, and McNemar test is adopted to evaluate the statistical significance of the performance difference.

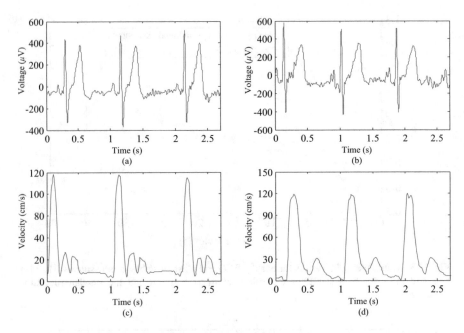

Fig. 16.5 Waveforms of ECG and wrist pulse blood flow signals of healthy person and patient with liver disease. (**a**) ECG signal of healthy person, (**b**) ECG signal of patient with liver disease, (**c**) wrist pulse blood flow signal of healthy person, (**d**) wrist pulse blood flow signal of patient with liver disease

16.3.3   *Typical Examples of Wrist Pulse Blood Flow and ECG Signals*

Using liver and gallbladder diseases, we analyze the typical waveforms of wrist pulse blood flow and ECG signals. Figure 16.5a, b shows the waveforms of ECG signals of a healthy person and a patient with liver disease, while Fig. 16.5c, d shows the waveforms of wrist pulse blood flow signals. The waveform of ECG signal of healthy person is similar with that of the patient with liver disease. The waveform of pulse signal of healthy person usually has three peaks in each period, while that of patient with liver disease only has two peaks.

Figure 16.6a, b shows the waveforms of ECG signals of a healthy person and a patient with gallbladder disease, while Fig. 16.6c, d shows the waveforms of wrist pulse blood flow signals. Again the waveform of ECG signal of healthy person is similar with that of the patient with gallbladder disease. The tidal wave of pulse signal of healthy person is distinctly different from that of patient with gallbladder disease. The possible explanation might be that the liver and gallbladder diseases would cause the anomalies of blood viscosity and velocity [18] and then could be reflected as the change of the waveforms of wrist pulse blood flow signal.

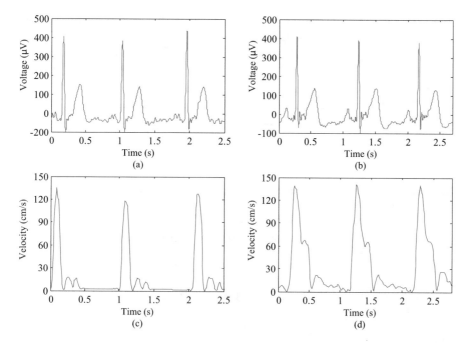

Fig. 16.6 Waveforms of wrist pulse blood flow and ECG signals of healthy person and patient with gallbladder disease. ECG signal of (**a**) healthy person and (**b**) of patient with gallbladder disease and wrist pulse blood flow signal of (**c**) healthy person and (**d**) of patient with gallbladder disease

Table 16.4 Classification performance of wrist pulse blood flow signal and ECG signal for the two-class problem: the healthy vs. disease problem

Performance indicators	Wrist pulse blood flow signal	ECG signal
Accuracy (%)	83.78	72.97
Sensitivity (%)	80.22	69.78
Specificity (%)	85.95	74.92

16.3.4   Classification Accuracy and McNemar Test

Experiments are conducted to compare the classification accuracy obtained using wrist pulse blood flow and ECG signals. The strategy in [44] is adopted to address the class imbalance problem. We use the tenfold cross-validation method to evaluate the classification accuracy.

We compare the classification accuracy for three classification tasks: healthy vs. disease, healthy vs. each disease, and multiclass classification (healthy, liver, gallbladder, and diabetes). To study the healthy vs. disease problem, we use the samples from the 182 healthy and 299 diseased persons. Table 16.4 lists the classification accuracy, sensitivity, and specificity based on wrist pulse blood flow signal and ECG signal. The classification accuracy of wrist pulse blood flow signal is 83.78%, which is 10% higher than that of ECG signal (72.97%). Table 16.5 lists the numbers

Table 16.5 The numbers of misclassified samples and classification accuracy of the four classes

		Wrist pulse blood flow signal		ECG signal	
Category	Size	Misclassified samples	Accuracy (%)	Misclassified samples	Accuracy (%)
Liver (L)	58	8	86.21	15	74.14
Gallbladder (G)	36	3	91.67	9	75.00
Diabetes (D)	205	31	84.88	51	75.12
Healthy (H)	182	36	80.22	55	69.78

Table 16.6 Classification performance of wrist pulse blood flow signal and ECG signal: the healthy vs. each disease

	Wrist pulse blood flow signal			ECG signal		
Task	Accuracy (%)	Sensitivity (%)	Specificity (%)	Accuracy (%)	Sensitivity (%)	Specificity (%)
Healthy (H) vs. liver (L)	85.65	86.81	84.48	75.81	77.47	74.14
Healthy (H) vs. gallbladder (G)	85.35	87.36	83.33	75.96	76.92	75.00
Healthy (H) vs. diabetes (D)	86.73	85.16	88.29	78.22	76.92	79.51

Table 16.7 Classification performance of wrist pulse blood flow signal and ECG signal: the multiclass classification problem

Performance indicators	Wrist pulse blood flow signal	ECG signal
Accuracy (%)	70.48	57.80

of misclassified samples and classification accuracy for each of the four categories (healthy, diabetes, liver disease, and gallbladder disease). Wrist pulse blood flow signal is much better for the classification of healthy persons from patients with diabetes, liver, and gallbladder diseases.

For healthy vs. each disease, we study three two-class tasks: healthy vs. diabetes, healthy vs. liver, and healthy vs. gallbladder. Table 16.6 lists the classification accuracy, sensitivity, and specificity based on wrist pulse blood flow signal and ECG signal. Again, wrist pulse blood flow signal can significantly outperform ECG signal.

For multiclass classification, we list the classification accuracy and the confusion matrices in Tables 16.7 and 16.8, respectively. Wrist pulse blood flow signal can achieve more than 12% higher classification accuracy than ECG, which demonstrates the superiority of wrist pulse blood flow signal.

Finally, we use McNemar test to verify whether wrist pulse blood flow signal is statistically better than ECG for multiclass classification. Table 16.9 lists the values of n_{SS}, n_{SF}, n_{FS}, and n_{FF}, where n_{SF} denotes the number of samples that are correctly

Table 16.8 The confusion matrices obtained based on (a) wrist pulse blood flow signal and (b) ECG signal, where L, G, D, and H denote liver, gallbladder, diabetes, and healthy, respectively

(a)

		Predicted			
		L	G	D	H
Actual	L	39	1	10	8
	G	0	23	8	5
	D	12	4	149	40
	H	11	4	39	128

(b)

		Predicted			
		L	G	D	H
Actual	L	29	2	16	11
	G	1	18	11	6
	D	16	6	124	59
	H	14	7	54	107

Table 16.9 The results of McNemar test on the multiclass classification problem

Outcome	n_{SS}	n_{SF}	N_{FS}	n_{FF}
Value	175	164	103	39

classified by wrist pulse signal but wrongly classified by ECG, and n_{FS} denotes the number of samples that are wrongly classified by wrist pulse signal but correctly classified by ECG. Based on the one-side McNemar test, the upper bound of the probability of $H0$ is $P_{H0} = 1.14 \times 10^{-4}$, which is much lower than 0.05. Therefore, wrist pulse blood flow signal is statistically better than ECG for the diagnosis of diabetes, liver, and gallbladder diseases.

16.4 Summary

This chapter conducts a comparative study of ECG and pulse signals for the diagnosis of non-cardiac diseases from two aspects: complexity measures and classification performance evaluation. Based on the multiscale entropy framework, the results clearly show that wrist pulse blood flow signal is more informative in terms of complexity measures. The experimental results on classification indicate that, for the diagnosis of diabetes, liver, and gallbladder diseases, wrist pulse blood flow signal is statistically better than ECG. In summary, at least for the diagnosis of some specific diseases, pulse signal is valuable and can outperform ECG signal. Considering its noninvasive property, pulse signal would be a suitable complementarity of ECG for some noninvasive monitoring applications.

References

1. Braunwald E, "Heart Disease: A Textbook of Cardiovascular Medicine," 5th ed. Philadelphia, PA: Saunders, 1997.
2. Meo M, Zarzoso V, Meste O, Latcu DG and Saoudi N. "Spatial variability of the 12-lead surface ECG as a tool for noninvasive prediction of Catheter ablation outcome in persistent atrial fibrillation," IEEE Trans Biomed Eng, 60: 20–27, 2013.
3. Liu X, Zheng Y, Phyu MW, Zhao B, Je M and Yuan X. "Multiple functional ECG signal is processing for wearable applications of long-term cardiac monitoring," IEEE Trans Biomed Eng, 58: 380–389, 2011.
4. Liu X, Zheng Y, Phyu MW, Zhao B, Je M and Yuan X. "A miniature on-chip multi-functional ECG signal processor with 30 µW ultra-low power consumption," IEEE Engineering in Medicine and Biology Society (EMBC), 2577–2580, 2010.
5. Lee CT and Wei LY. "Spectrum analysis of human pulse," IEEE Trans. Biomed Eng, BME-30: 348–352, 1983.
6. Wei LY and Chow P. "Frequency distribution of human pulse spectra," IEEE Trans. Biomedical Engineering, BME-32: 245–246, 1985.
7. Xu L, Zhang D, Wang K and Wang L. "Arrhythmic pulses detection using Lempel-Ziv complexity analysis," EURASIP Journal on Advances in Signal Processing, 1-12, 2006.
8. Nuryani N, Ling SSH and Nguyen HT. "Electrocardiographic signals and swarm-based support vector machine for hypoglycemia detection," Annals of Biomedical Engineering, 40: 934–945, 2012.
9. Ling SSH and Nguyen HT. "Genetic-algorithm-based multiple regression with fuzzy inference system for detection of nocturnal hypoglycemic episodes," IEEE Trans. Information Technology in Biomedicine, 15: 308–315, 2011.
10. Khandoker AH, Palaniswami M and Karmakar CK. "Support vector machines for automated recognition of obstructive sleep apnea syndrome from ECG recordings," IEEE Transactions on Information Technology in Biomedicine, 13(1): 37–48, 2009.
11. Lu WA, Lin Wang YY and Wang WK. "Pulse analysis of patients with severe liver problems: studying pulse spectrums to determine the effects on other organs," IEEE Engineering in Medicine and Biology Magazine, 18: 73–75, 1999.
12. Zhang DY, Zuo WM, Zhang D, Zhang HZ and Li NM. "Wrist blood flow signal-based computerized pulse diagnosis using spatial and spectrum features," Journal of Biomedical Science and Engineering, 3: 361–366, 2010.
13. Chen YH, Zhang L, Zhang D and Zhang DY. "Computerized wrist pulse signal diagnosis using modified auto-regressive models," Journal of Medical Systems, 35: 321–328, 2011.
14. Lai JCY, Leung FHF and Ling SSH. "Hypoglycaemia detection using fuzzy inference system with intelligent optimiser," Applied Soft Computing, 20: 54–65, 2014.
15. Walsh S, King E, Pulse Diagnosis: A Clinical Guide. Sydney Australia: Elsevier, 2008.
16. Wang YYL, Hsu TL, Jan MY and Wang WK. "Review: theory and applications of the harmonic analysis of arterial pressure pulse waves," Journal of Medical and Biological Engineering, 30.3: 125–131, 2010.
17. Baruch MC, Kalantari K, Gerdt DW and Adkins CM. "Validation of the pulse decomposition analysis algorithm using central arterial blood pressure," BioMedical Engineering OnLine, 13:96, 2014.
18. Fedosov DA, Pan W, Caswell B, Gompper G and Karniadakis GE. "Predicting human blood viscosity in silico," Proc National Academy of Sciences, 108: 11772–11777, 2011.
19. Liu L, Zuo W, Zhang D, Li N and Zhang H. "Combination of heterogeneous features for wrist pulse blood flow signal diagnosis via multiple kernel learning," IEEE Trans. Information Technology in Biomedicine, 16: 599–607, 2012.
20. Acharya UR, Joseph KP, Kannathal N, Lim CM and Suri JS. "Heart rate variability: a review," Med Bio Eng Comput, 44: 1031–1051, 2006.

21. Nuryani N, Ling S, and Nguyen H. "Hybrid particle swarm - based fuzzy support vector machine for hypoglycemia detection." *IEEE International Conference on Fuzzy Systems* IEEE, 2012

22. Lee M, Guzman R, Bell-Stephens T and Steinberg GK. "Intraoperative blood flow analysis of direct revascularization procedures in patients with moyamoya disease," J Cereb Blood Flow Metab, 31: 262–274, 2011.

23. Sanchez CE, Schatz J and Roberts CW. "Cerebral blood flow velocity and language functioning in pediatric sickle cell disease," Journal of the International Neuropsychological Society, 16: 326–334, 2010.

24. Hsu E, Pulse Diagnosis in Early Chinese Medicine. New York, American: Cambridge University Press, 2010.

25. Tyan CC, Liu SH, Chen JY, Chen JJ and Liang WM. "A novel noninvasive measurement technique for analyzing the pressure pulse waveform of the radial artery," IEEE Trans. Biomedical Engineering, 55: 288–297, 2008.

26. Chen Y, Wen C, Tao G, Bi M and Li G. "Continuous and noninvasive blood pressure measurement: a novel modeling methodology of the relationship between blood pressure and pulse wave velocity," Annals of Biomedical Engineering, 37: 2222–2233, 2009.

27. Butlin M, "Structural and functional effects on large artery stiffness: an in-vivo experimental investigation," PhD Thesis of the University of New South Wales, 2007.

28. Wang P, Zuo W and Zhang D. "A compound pressure signal acquisition system for multi-channel wrist pulse signal analysis," IEEE Trans Instrumentation and Measuremen, 63: 1556–1565, 2014.

29. Xu L, Zhang D, Wang K, Li N and Wang X. "Baseline wander correction in pulse waveforms using wavelet-based cascaded adaptive filter," Comput Biol Med, 37: 716–731, 2007.

30. Kilpatrick D and Johnston P. "Origin of the electrocardiogram," IEEE Engineering in Medicine and Biology Magazine, 13: 479–486, 1994.

31. Macfarlane PW and Coleman EN. "Resting 12-lead ECG electrode placement and associated problems," SCST Update 1995, online available at: http://www.scst.org.uk/ resources/ RESTING_12.pdf.

32. Hamilton PS and Tompkins WJ. "Quantitative Investigation of QRS Detection Rules Using the MIT/BIH Arrhythmia Database," IEEE Trans Biomedical Engineering, BME-33: 1157–1165, 1986.

33. Costa M, Goldberger AL and Peng CK. "Multiscale entropy analysis of complex physiologic time series," Physical Review Letters, 89: 1–4, 2002.

34. Pincus S, "Approximate entropy (ApEn) as a complexity measure," Chaos: An Interdisciplinary Journal of Nonlinear Science, 5: 110, 1995.

35. Richman JS and Moorman JR. "Physiological time-series analysis using approximate entropy and sample entropy," American Journal of Physiology-Heart and Circulatory Physiology, 278: H2039-H2049, 2000.

36. Pincus SM, "Approximate entropy as a measure of system complexity," Proc National Academy of Science, 88: 2297–2301, 1991.

37. Lake DE, Richman JS, Griffin MP and Moorman JR. "Sample entropy analysis of neonatal heart rate variability,"Am J Physiology-Regulatory, Integrative and Comparative Physiology, 283: R789-R797, 2002.

38. P. De Chazal, M. O'Dwyer and R. B. Reilly. "Automatic classification of heartbeats using ECG morphology and heartbeat interval features," IEEE Trans. Biomedical Engineering, vol. 51, pp. 1196–1206, Jul. 2004.

39. McNemar Q. "Note on the sampling error of the difference between correlated proportions or percentages," Psychometrika, 12: 153–157, 1947.

40. Xu L, Meng MQH, Wang K, Wang L and Li N. "Pulse image recognition using fuzzy neural network," Expert Syst Appl, 36: 3805–3811, 2009.

41. Zhang D, Zuo W, Zhang D and Zhang H. "Time series classification using support vector machine with Gaussian elastic metric kernel," Proc Int Conf Pattern Recognition, 29-32, 2010.

42. Zhang D, Zhang L, Zhang D and Zheng Y. "Wavelet-based analysis of Doppler ultrasonic wrist-pulse signals," Proc BioMed Eng Informatics Conf, 2: 539–543, 2008.
43. Rakotomamonjy A, Bach FR, Canu S and Grandvalet Y. "SimpleMKL," Journal of Machine Learning Research, 9: 2491–2521, 2008.
44. Ferrario M, Signorini MG, Magenes G and Cerutti S. "Comparison of entropy-based regularity estimators: application to the fetal heart rate signal for the identification of fetal distress," IEEE Trans Biomedical Engineering, 53: 119–125, 2006.

Chapter 17
Discussion and Future Work

Abstract Recently, the computational pulse diagnosis has attracted much attention. This book provides with several representative methods of computational pulse diagnosis. The ideas, algorithms, and experimental evaluation are also provided for the better understanding of these methods. In this chapter, we will give a further discussion about the book and present some remarks on the future development of computational pulse diagnosis.

17.1 Recapitulation

Wrist pulse conveys important information about the pathologic changes. As a traditional diagnosis technique, pulse diagnosis interprets health condition by analyzing the tactile radial arterial palpation. However, it is a subjective skill which needs years of training and practice to master [1–3]. Computational pulse diagnosis aims to use sensor technology to acquire pulse signal and interpret health condition by analyzing sampled pulse signal using machine learning technology. In general, it involves four major stages, i.e., acquisition, preprocessing, feature extraction, and classification.

Acquisition Pulse acquisition aims to obtain the pulse signal comprehensively and objectively. By far, a number of sensors and systems have been developed for acquiring pulse signal. Kaniusas et al. adopt the magnetoelastic skin curvature sensor to design a mechanical electrocardiography system for the non-disturbing measurement of blood pressure signal [4]. Humphreys et al. [5] present a system capable of capturing two photoplethysmography signals at two different wavelengths simultaneously to give a quick indication of the cardiac rhythm. Chen et al. present a liquid sensor system to measure the pulse signal [6]. Tyan et al. develop a pressure pulse monitoring system [7]. Lu et al. present a wrist pressure signal device with three channels of biosensors for telemedicine [8]. Wu et al. propose an air pressure pulse signal measurement system [9]. In view of the acquisition, position is an important factor, and multiple-channel and sensor fusion can provide comprehensive information; in Part II, we introduce two platforms: one is a compound

© Springer Nature Singapore Pte Ltd. 2018

D. Zhang et al., *Computational Pulse Signal Analysis*,

https://doi.org/10.1007/978-981-10-4044-3_17

multiple-channel pulse signal acquisition pressure system with positioning and sensor array design and the other is a fusion system which replaces the pressure sensor array to photoelectric sensor array to acquire more pulse information.

Compared with other pulse signal acquisition systems, our device can acquire comprehensive multiple-channel pulse signals, i.e., three-channel of main signals together with the sub-signals, and thus more diagnostic features, e.g., pulse width, could be extracted. We provide a systemic solution for the X-, Y-, and Z-axis sensor positioning. The fusion system can also acquire the photoelectric signal simultaneously. Related diagnosis experiment result shows that the proposed systems can acquire more information and achieve better diagnosis accuracy.

Preprocessing During the pulse signal acquisition, interference and other factors may introduce corruptions in pulse signals, e.g., high-frequency noise, baseline drift, saturation, and artifact are some common corruptions. High-frequency noise can be removed by denoising methods [10–15]. In Part III, we present some methods to handle other corruptions, e.g., the baseline drift, the saturation, and the artifact.

For baseline drift, we propose an ER-based method to detect the baseline drift level and a two-step wavelet-based cascaded adaptive filter to remove the baseline drift. Our strategy is that if the drift is not severe, we use cubic spline estimation to remove the baseline drift to avoid the distortion from wavelet filter. When the ER of a pulse signal is high, it must be filtered by a discrete Meyer wavelet filter before the cubic spline estimation.

For the detection of saturation, we develop two criteria from its definition and achieve 100% detection accuracy with the time resolution same as the sampling frequency. For the artifact detection considering that the similarity should be an effective feature, we transform the pulse signal into a complex network according to the similarity between pulse cycles, and then the artifact part of pulse signal will be transformed into isolated node in the network. The experimental result shows that the proposed method can achieve better performance than statistic-based method.

Finally, an optimal preprocessing framework was presented, where we also address the denoising, interval selection, segmentation, and other preprocessing details which enrich the pulse preprocessing. The experiments show that after the preprocessing, the quality of the pulse signal can be significantly improved.

Feature Extraction The property of the pulse signal is characterized by features. Good features are crucial to the diagnosis performance. In Part IV, we present several effective feature extraction methods to characterize the rhythms, spectrum, and inter-cycle variations.

First, we present a Lempel-Ziv-complexity-analysis-based feature VR and VC to characterize the rhythms of pulse. Second, we use Hilbert-Huang transform that extracted a series of spectrum features to characterize the spectrum of pulse signal; third, we present a 2-D description of pulse signal and decomposed pulse signal into periodic components and nonperiodic components. Finally, we present some methods to characterize the inter-cycle variations of pulse signal including the simple combination method, multiscale sample entropy, and complex network. The experimental results show the features proposed in this book are effective in pulse diagnosis.

Pulse Analysis Pulse analysis is to provide some reasonable interpretation based on pulse features. A lot of machine learning methods have been applied for pulse diagnosis such as neural network, support vector machine, k-nearest neighbor algorithm, dynamic time warping, etc. [16–21]. In Part V, we present some examples of effective classifiers. By incorporating the state-of-the-art time series matching method, we develop two pulse classifiers, i.e., EDKC and GEKC, to address the intra-class variation and the local time shifting problems in pulse patterns. Fuzzy C-means and auto-regressive model are also studied for pulse classification. Since we have extracted different type of pulse feature, we propose an MKL framework for integrating heterogeneous features. By designing appropriate kernel functions for different features, MKL provides a flexible way to combine information from different feature extraction and matching methods. Most of the present features can achieve higher than or comparable performance with those state-of-the-art pulse classification methods.

Comparison Since several kinds of pulse signals were discussed in this book, in the last part, we discussed the dependency and complementarity of these pulse signals to reveal their relationship. Since the ECG signal is also driven by cardiac contraction and relaxation and has been used for disease diagnosis, the comparison between pulse signal and ECG signal was also studied in Part VI.

In Part VI, the physical meanings, correlations, sensitivities to physiological and pathological factors, and the diagnosis performance of pulse signals acquired by different types of sensors were studied. Our analyses show that:

1. The changes in the elastic property and thickness of the vessel wall can be more readily detected using pressure signals.
2. The changes in the area of the cross section and blood composition can be more readily captured using photoelectric signals.
3. The changes in the blood viscosity and the blood flow state can be more effectively characterized using ultrasonic signals.

Thus, we conclude that each sensor is more appropriate for the diagnosis of some specific disease that the changes of physiological factors can be effectively reflected by the sensor, and different types of signals are complementary. Case studies verified the statements, and we find the combination of different signals may further improve the diagnosis performance. In the comparative study of ECG and pulse signals for the diagnosis of some specific non-cardiac diseases, we found, at least for the diagnosis of some specific diseases, pulse signal is valuable and can outperform ECG signal.

17.2   Future Work

In the future, we will continue our studies on computational pulse analysis. For pulse acquisition, we will reduce the weight and size of our acquisition system to make it more portable and use our system to construct a large-scale dataset of pulse signal. For pulse preprocessing, we will develop algorithms to further evaluate the quality of sampled pulse signal. For feature extraction and classification, we will develop more effective approaches to utilize the multichannel signals acquired under different pressures to improve the accuracy and degree of automation of computational pulse diagnosis. Moreover, we will extend the pulse diagnosis experiments to include more types of disease.

References

1. S. Walsh, and E. King, Pulse Diagnosis: A Clinical Guide, Sydney Australia: Elsevier, 2008.
2. R. Amber, and B. Brooke, Pulse Diagnosis Detailed Interpretations For Eastern & Western Holistic Treatments, Santa Fe, New Mexico: Aurora Press, 1993.
3. C. T. Lee and L. Y. Wei, "Spectrum analysis of human pulse," IEEE Trans. Biomed. Eng., vol. BME-30, no. 6, pp. 348–352, Jun. 1983.
4. E. Kaniusas, H. Pfutzner, L. Mehnen, J. Kosel, C. Tellez-Blanco, G. Varoneckas, A. Alonderis, T. Meydan, M. Vazquez, M. Rohn, A. M. Merlo, and B. Marquardt, "Method for continuous nondisturbing monitoring of blood pressure by magnetoelastic skin curvature sensor and ECG," IEEE Sensors Journal, vol. 6, no. 3, pp. 819–828, Jun, 2006.
5. K. Humphreys, T. Ward, and C. Markham, "Noncontact simultaneous dual wavelength photoplethysmography: A further step toward noncontact pulse oximetry," Rev. Sci. Instrum., vol. 78, no. 4, pp. 044304-1–044304-6, 2007.
6. L. Chen, H. Atsumi, M. Yagihashi, F. Mizuno, H. Narita, and H. Fujimoto, "A preliminary research on analysis of pulse diagnosis," in Proceedings of IEEE International Conference on Complex Medical Engineering, Beijing, China, 2007, pp. 1807–1812.
7. C. C. Tyan, S. H. Liu, J. Y. Chen, J. J. Chen, and W. M. Liang, "A novel noninvasive measurement technique for analyzing the pressure pulse waveform of the radial artery," IEEE Transactions on Biomedical Engineering, vol. 55, no. 1, pp. 288–297, Jan, 2008.
8. S. Lu, R. Wang, L. Cui, Z. Zhao, Y. Yu, and Z. Shan, "Wireless networked Chinese telemedicine system: method and apparatus for remote pulse information retrieval and diagnosis," in Proceedings of IEEE International Conference on Pervasive Computing and Communications, Hong Kong, China, 2008, pp. 698–703.
9. H.-T. Wu, C.-H. Lee, and A.-B. Liu, "Assessment of endothelial function using arterial pressure signals," Journal of Signal Processing Systems, vol. 64, no. 2, pp. 223–232, 2011.
10. L. Jing, S. Hao, G. Yinjing, and S. Hongyu, "Pulse Signal De-Noising Based on Integer Lifting Scheme Wavelet Transform," in International Conference on Bioinformatics and Biomedical Engineering, WuHan, China, 2007, pp. 936–939.
11. S. Su, Q. Yan-Yan, and Q. Jun-Fei, "Research on de-noising of pulse signal based on fuzzy threshold in wavelet packet domain," in International Conference on Wavelet Analysis and Pattern Recognition, Beijing, China, 2007, pp. 103–106.
12. G. Rui, W. Yiqin, Y. Jianjun, L. Fufeng, and Y. Haixia, "Wavelet based De-noising of pulse signal," in IEEE International Symposium on IT in Medicine and Education, Xiamen, China, 2008, pp. 617–620.

13. C. Fengxiang, H. Wenxue, Z. Tao, J. Jung, and L. Xulong, "Research on Wavelet Denoising for Pulse Signal Based on Improved Wavelet Thresholding," in International Conference on Pervasive Computing Signal Processing and Applications, Harbin, China, 2010, pp. 564–567.
14. D. Wang and D. Zhang, "Analysis of pulse waveforms preprocessing," in International Conference on Computerized Healthcare, Hong Kong, 2012, pp. 175–180.
15. H. Wang, X. Wang, J. R. Deller, and J. Fu, "A Shape-Preserving Preprocessing for Human Pulse Signals Based on Adaptive Parameter Determination," IEEE Transactions on Biomedical Circuits and Systems, vol. 8, pp. 594–604, 2013.
16. L. Xu, M. Q.-H. Meng, K. Wang, W. Lu, and N. Li, "Pulse images recognition using fuzzy neural network," Expert Systems with Applications, vol. 36, no. 2, pp. 3805–3811, 2009.
17. C. Chiu, B. Liau, S. Yeh, and C. Hsu, "Artificial neural networks classification of arterial pulse waveforms in cardiovascular diseases," in Proceedings of the 4th Kuala Lumpur International Conference on Biomedical Engineering, Springer, 2008.
18. W. Zuo, D. Zhang, and K. Wang, "On kernel difference weighted k-nearest neighbor classification," Pattern Analysis and Applications, vol. 11, no. 3–4, pp. 247–257, 2008.
19. Zhang D, Zhang L, Zhang D, Zheng Y. Wavelet based analysis of Doppler ultrasonic wrist-pulse signals. In: Proceedings of the ICBBE 2008 conference, vol. 2. 2008. p. 539–43.
20. Burges C. A tutorial on support vector machines for pattern recognition. Data Mining and Knowledge Discovery 1998;2:121–67.
21. L. Wang, K.-Q. Wang, and L.-S. Xu, "Recognizing wrist pulse waveforms with improved dynamic time warping algorithm," in Proceedings of the International Conference on Machine Learning and Cybernetics, pp. 3644–3649, August 2004.

Index

© Springer Nature Singapore Pte Ltd. 2018
D. Zhang et al., *Computational Pulse Signal Analysis*,
https://doi.org/10.1007/978-981-10-4044-3

Printed in the United States
By Bookmasters